Deaconesses in Nursing Care

T0139532

Medizin, Gesellschaft und Geschichte

Jahrbuch
des Instituts für Geschichte der Medizin
der Robert Bosch Stiftung

herausgegeben von
Robert Jütte

Beiheft 62

Deaconesses in Nursing Care

International Transfer of a Female Model
of Life and Work in the 19th and 20th Century

Edited by Susanne Kreutzer and Karen Nolte

Franz Steiner Verlag Stuttgart
2016

Gedruckt mit freundlicher Unterstützung der Robert Bosch Stiftung GmbH

Coverabbildung:
Diakonissen aus Niesky im Leprosenhaus in Jerusalem um 1876
Archiv der Fliedner Kulturstiftung

Bibliografische Information der Deutschen Nationalbibliothek:
Die Deutsche Nationalbibliothek verzeichnet diese Publikation in der Deutschen
Nationalbibliografie; detaillierte bibliografische Daten sind im Internet über
<http://dnb.d-nb.de> abrufbar.

© Franz Steiner Verlag, Stuttgart 2016
Druck: Laupp & Göbel GmbH, Nehren
Gedruckt auf säurefreiem, alterungsbeständigem Papier.
Printed in Germany
ISBN 978-3-515-11355-7 (Print)
ISBN 978-3-515-11358-8 (E-Book)

Contents

Deaconesses in nursing care. A transnational history

Susanne Kreutzer / Karen Nolte

Introduction

The academic discipline of history is currently focusing on transnational phenomena. Transnational history investigates the "different levels of interaction, connection, circulation, intersections, and interlacing" of a phenomenon that exceeds the framework of national boundaries.[1] Hence, it is not merely a comparative history but an approach that, in addition to the comparative perspective, focuses on analysing the transfer "of material objects, concepts, and cultural semiotic systems [...] among different and relatively clearly identifiable cultures that can be delimited against each other, resulting in a cultural mix and interaction".[2]

As well as unlocking new research questions, the transnational approach has led to the emergence of new historical research areas and topics. Using the concept of "transfer history",[3] there has been a growing interest in historical studies of religious communities because they were early "global players".[4] Internationally, sisters – just like missionaries – belonged to the best-connected professions of the nineteenth century. Originating usually in France, many Catholic sisterhoods settled in numerous other European and non-European countries. Likewise, Protestant deaconess motherhouses became a popular German export in the nineteenth century. More than half of the apostolic congregations in England during the 1880s came from France; others came from Belgium, Ireland, Italy, Germany, the Netherlands and Austria. Institutions and foundations of English origin constituted only a minority.[5]

Yet, what happened when nursing care organisations and the concepts of nursing that they embodied began their international journey? This anthology examines this question, focusing on the example of Protestant deaconesses who worked as nurses. At the centre we have a nursing organisation that was founded in the 1830s in Germany, but was subsequently exported to many European and even non-European countries. If the deaconess motherhouses wanted to stand a chance of survival in these countries, they had to adapt to the specific cultural and societal contexts. Because of these adaptation processes, the deaconess motherhouses are particularly suitable for an international comparative and transfer history. Simultaneously, only the transfer and subsequent contact with the other culture can illuminate the specificity of the

---

1 Patel (2005).
2 Middell (2000), p. 8.
3 Paulmann (1998), pp. 649–685; Espagne (1999).
4 Mettele (2006); Habermas (2008); Hauser (2011).
5 O'Brien (1997).

various traditions of nursing that had been shaped within their own nations and were now engaged in a transfer abroad.

The foundation of the model of deaconesses in Kaiserswerth, Germany

The community of deaconesses was conceptualised during the first half of the nineteenth century by the pastor Theodor Fliedner (1800–1864) in Kaiserswerth near Düsseldorf. From the outset it could be regarded as a "transnational space".[6] Young women from petit bourgeois and lower classes moved from all parts of Germany to Kaiserswerth to be trained in nursing care.[7] After a brief but thorough training period covering the care of body and soul, they were sent out to work in hospitals, clinics, community care, and private care in all parts of the German Reich, but also to other countries. Fliedner's concept of a community of deaconesses followed the model of the Catholic *Sisters of Mercy* and simultaneously recalled early Christian traditions of female work within the parish.

The Protestant motherhouse system regarded itself as a community of faith, service and life for unmarried women. It was based on the simple principle of exchange: the young women received thorough training and the security of lifelong provision for retirement, if they in return were willing to dedicate their lives completely to service in the community and to work with people who were unwell and in need.[8] In this way, the motherhouse assumed parental custody and control over the young women. The leaders of the motherhouse were the principals, i.e. a married couple. In Fliedner's model it was the theological principal and his wife (later the Mother Superior) who served the community as "parents". The sisters were regarded as the daughters of the motherhouse. In nineteenth-century Germany, belonging to such a surrogate family was a crucial prerequisite for guaranteeing the necessary amount of respectability for young unmarried women living and working away from their original families. In contrast to Catholic nuns, who bound themselves to their order with a vow, deaconesses could leave the community again. However, the leaders of the motherhouse were interested in binding the thoroughly trained deaconesses to the community for their entire lifetime.

The work of the deaconesses took place in the context of Protestant efforts to solve the *social question* that, as a result of industrialisation, was becoming more pressing in the nineteenth century. The work of the deaconesses was conceptualised as aid provided as part of the so-called *Inner Mission* to the impoverished population. Fliedner and other protagonists of the *Inner Mission* believed that poverty and disease could largely be attributed to a lack of faith. For that reason the deaconesses had to take care not only of the physical but also the spiritual well-being of their patients. Joint care of body and soul was

---

6   Soine (2013).
7   Schmidt (1998).
8   Köser (2006); Schmidt (2005), pp. 33–44.

the key to the deaconesses' understanding of nursing care. In addition to nursing care, the deaconesses were also engaged in numerous areas of welfare, education, and community work.[9]

In other countries, deaconesses were also used to remedy social shortcomings, to take care of Protestant parishes, and to lead the 'heathens' to the Christian faith. Thus, as early as the middle of the nineteenth century, the first deaconesses were sent to Palestine and to the Lebanon as part of the so-called *Outer Mission* or placement abroad.[10] The idea was to perform the same missionary work as the *Inner Mission*, but in another country or "outside". Not only in the German speaking regions but also in many other countries, institutions for deaconesses were founded, following the model in Kaiserswerth. Sometimes the initiative for these houses came from German motherhouses; sometimes local women used the Kaiserswerth concept to set up the institutions.

The evaluation of the deaconess model is highly controversial among scholars. The studies on the history of deaconesses in nursing care that were published in the 1990s emerged within the context of research on women and followed the parameters of emancipation and self-determination current at that time. Hence, these studies emphasise the normative constraints and repressive patriarchal character of the communities of deaconesses.[11] This thesis of suppression, however, adheres to a one-dimensional concept of power and does not explain why so many young women joined the community of deaconesses. In recent years there have been an increasing number of studies that have analysed the internal logic of the communities of deaconesses. For instance, the theologian Silke Köser follows Max Weber in her argument that a power relationship has to be borne by both parties: the rulers and the ruled. She shows how the principal couple at the deaconess motherhouse in Kaiserswerth managed to establish the hierarchical structure and subsequently the power of the principals in the deaconess motherhouse by creating a specific motherhouse culture and a collective deaconess identity. According to Köser, crucial factors in establishing this "collective identity" were the specific dress of the deaconesses, the initiation of the deaconesses through a confirmation ceremony, the celebration of the community through continuous correspondence with the nurses who worked elsewhere and, finally, the regular return of deaconesses to the motherhouse.[12]

In addition, the nursing care provided by the deaconesses has been more closely analysed in recent years. These studies reveal that in the Christian tradition, nurses enjoyed a high level of autonomy and appreciation.[13] In particular, this applied to the institutions belonging to the motherhouse, which had been set up by communities of sisters who thus also owned them. In these

9   Nolte (2013), pp. 167–82.
10   Kaminsky (2010); Habermas (2008).
11   Bischoff (1994); Schmidt (2005).
12   Köser (2006).
13   Kreutzer (2014); Nolte (2013); Weber-Reich (2003).

houses, the physicians did not manage to assert their claim to leadership until late into the second half of the twentieth century.[14] In addition, the Christian understanding of disease gave the carers a high status because, according to this concept, disease affected not only the body but also the soul of the patients. At the end of the nineteenth century, physicians increasingly focussed on the physical aspect of a disease, i. e. its symptoms, diagnosis, and treatment, while the nurses' task was to consider the personality of the patient as a whole. Due to the significance given to personal attention and the efforts to provide spiritual counsel, the nursing staff secured its own autonomous and highly respected area of duty. For this reason, the relationship between nurses and doctors was not regarded as hierarchical but as complementary, and the work of the nursing staff was situated between the tasks of the physicians and the pastors.

So far, there has been no systematic study of the extent to which this model was transferred to other countries and adapted to the new surroundings. There has been some research on the history of deaconesses in nursing care and the organisation of the motherhouses in several individual countries. There are also some initial comparative studies available that address the transfer of the communities of deaconesses, emphasising nursing care in the Scandinavian countries and the United States.[15] However, a systematic, comparative perspective on the transnational development of the communities is lacking. In which countries did deaconess motherhouses successfully establish themselves? Where were they doomed to fail and how can we explain the differences? To what extent was the German model adapted to the new national context during the transfer process and which social factors had an impact? Of particular interest are the different gender relationships, the frameworks provided by welfare states, and the dominant denomination in the various countries. Looking at these issues, we will link the history of deaconesses to overarching issues in the history of the respective societies.

Research on the history of deaconesses in nursing care is conducted in various disciplines: history, history of medicine, history of nursing care, and in diaconal institutions. The differences in research situations and research questions are reflected in the present publication. The goal of this book is to provide a single space for a dialogue between the multifaceted research projects. It is structured as follows:

---

14   Schmuhl (2003).
15   Andersson (2002); Christiansson (2006); Kreutzer (2010); Kreutzer (2012); Malchau-Dietz (2013); Markkola (2011); Markkola (2013); Martinsen (1984); Nelson (2001); Okkenhaug (2013); Soine (2013).

Germany – Foundation era of German deaconess motherhouses

Karen Nolte's article, in the first part of this volume, draws on Köser and discusses the self-understanding and everyday practice in nursing care experienced by the deaconesses in Kaiserswerth. In the German social and historical context, the life and working model of a deaconess was attractive not only because of the comparatively good training and "womb-to-tomb" social security it provided for women, but also because of the deaconesses' competencies, which allowed them to exceed professional boundaries in their everyday work. After all, these boundaries were regularly redefined in the regulations and instructions because of the practical experiences the deaconesses shared with their principals.

Deaconesses worked in all areas of nursing, as *Annett Büttner* illustrates in her article on the work of deaconesses in voluntary nursing care on the battlefield. She shows that denominational nurses played a pioneering role in the development and establishment of voluntary war nursing in the nineteenth century. Büttner describes the incredible challenges that the sisters and brothers had to face in the daily reality of war. By standing the test of the field, however, they increased acceptance of voluntary nursing on the battlefield. Furthermore, secular nursing care on the battlefield in Germany was organised following the denominational model.

Matthias Honold investigates the specific understanding of nursing care that emerged in the institution for deaconesses in Neuendettelsau, which had been founded in 1854 by the pastor Wilhelm Löhe (1808–1872). It was the first deaconess motherhouse to be founded in the countryside rather than in a town. Indeed, Löhe was inspired by the Kaiserswerth model when he founded his community of deaconesses. Yet, in contrast to Kaiserswerth, Neuendettelsau also welcomed and trained women who did not want to become deaconesses. In addition, the institution in Neuendettelsau focussed more on theoretical aspects in its curriculum.

Outer Mission – The transfer to Palestine

The second part of the book deals with the work of deaconesses in the Outer Mission in Jerusalem. *Uwe Kaminsky* introduces the deployment of Kaiserswerth deaconesses in Jerusalem as part of their *Orientarbeit (work in the Orient)*. The purpose of this work overseas was not to convert the heathens but to strengthen the Christian communities that were already there by building hospitals, orphanages and schools. While the efforts to win new deaconesses from the local population in Jerusalem were hardly successful, in Germany the *Orientarbeit* had a strong promotional effect. Kaiserswerth's work in the 'Holy Land' not only prompted people to donate money, it also boosted the attractiveness of the deaconess model, in particular for daughters from the higher social classes.

Ruth Wexler investigates the work of deaconesses in the *Leper Home* in Jerusalem and thus sheds light on a dual transfer: influenced by the model in Kaiserswerth, Hermann Plitt (1821–1900) established a deaconess institute within the context of the Moravian Church in 1866, which in 1883 moved from Gnadenfeld (Upper Silesia) to Niesky (Saxony). In 1874 the first deaconess from the motherhouse was sent to Jerusalem to care for lepers. Until 1950 there were approximately 50 deaconesses who worked in the *Leper Home* in Jerusalem. Wexler analyses the challenges that the sisters had to face in these completely different work and life conditions and how they tackled them.

Scandinavia – A successful transfer of the German model

The third part of the book focuses on the significance of Scandinavian deaconess motherhouses. *Susanne Malchau Dietz* illustrates that the model from Kaiserswerth was particularly successful in the Protestant countries in Scandinavia. This success story also influenced the structure of the motherhouses in the United States that had been established in the nineteenth and early twentieth centuries with the goal of taking care of the relevant immigrant communities. There were 11 deaconess motherhouses, four of which were of German and seven of Scandinavian origin. Using the example of the *Danish Deaconess Home* in Brush, Colorado, Dietz reveals the strategies that were used to recruit deaconesses from Denmark. She also shows how personal conflicts and power struggles could place a massive strain on everyday life in the communities.

Pirjo Markkola examines the significance of deaconesses for the history of caring for the poor and health care in Finland. The first Finnish deaconess motherhouses were established in the 1860s in the south of Finland, in Helsinki and Viborg. These still followed closely in the footsteps of the Fliedner model. They offered the first systematic training in nursing care in Finland. In contrast, the institutions for deaconesses that were founded in the 1890s in Sortaval and Oulu did not adopt the motherhouse model and only offered a significantly shortened training in community care. The reference motherhouse here was not Kaiserswerth but the *Lovisenberg Deaconess House* in Norway. Markkola reveals that community care that was subsidised by the state and Church became the main area of work for the deaconesses. She argues that the self-understanding of the deaconesses, which involved being responsible for both physical and spiritual matters, gave them the necessary flexibility to adapt to changing conditions in the twentieth century.

Limits of transfer – Great Britain and the United States

The fourth and final part illuminates the less successful history of transfer and investigates the reasons why the deaconess motherhouses gained only marginal significance in some countries. In the United Kingdom, institutions for deaconesses had been evolving from the beginning of the 1860s but they remained rather small and were of less significance by comparison. Using the examples of the *London Diocesan Deaconess Institution* and the *Evangelical Protestant Deaconess Institute and Training Hospital, Carmen M. Magnion* illustrates that these institutions could not succeed in the highly competitive medical marketplace in the United Kingdom and found themselves in dire straits in terms of funding. When, towards the end of the nineteenth century, the secular model of voluntary hospitals became fully established, there was hardly any demand for deaconesses as nurses in hospitals. The sisters could now work only in community care or in convalescent homes, where their pastoral care was still in demand.

Doris Riemann examines the foundation of the deaconess motherhouse in Baltimore in 1885, which specialised in community care, and she comments on the enormous difficulties of this transfer. While the deaconesses there initially looked to the German model and trained deaconesses in the care of body and soul, from the very beginning the motherhouse suffered from having too few new applicants. Furthermore, as early as the beginning of the twentieth century, the understanding of care that the deaconesses promoted came under massive pressure to become more academic and professional. Riemann shows how the deaconesses subsequently departed from their traditional understanding of care and transformed the female diaconate into a modern profession.

Finally, *Susanne Kreutzer* compares the development of the deaconess motherhouses in Germany, Sweden and the United States and uses one example from each country for her investigation: the *Henriettenstiftung* in Hanover, the *Ersta* institution for deaconesses in Stockholm and the *Philadelphia Deaconess Motherhouse* in Pennsylvania that specialised in hospital care. Kreutzer not only analyses the transfer of the German life and work model of the deaconess to those countries, but also the transformation from the formerly holistic understanding of caring for a unity of body and soul into an academic, professional and scientifically based concept of nursing. She analyses these developments within the specific context of each of the modern welfare states.

The present volume is based on an international workshop that took place in Kaiserswerth in 2013. We would like to thank Andrea Thiekötter for her generous support in organising the workshop at the *Fliedner University of Applied Sciences* and all the authors who contributed to this anthology. A special thank you goes to Robert Jütte and the *Robert Bosch Foundation* for accepting this volume for inclusion in the series. We would like to thank the *German Research Foundation (Deutsche Forschungsgemeinschaft)* for its financial support of this publication.

Bibliography

Andersson, Åsa: Ett högt och ädelt kall. Kalltankens betydelse för sjuksköterskeyrkets formering 1850–1930. Umeå 2002.

Bischoff, Claudia: Frauen in der Krankenpflege. Zur Entwicklung von Frauenrolle und Frauen-
berufstätigkeit im 19. und 20. Jahrhundert. Frankfurt/Main; New York 1994.

Budde, Gunilla; Conrad, Sebastian; Janz, Oliver (ed.): Transnationale Geschichte. Themen,
Tendenzen und Theorien. Göttingen 2006.

Christiansson, Elisabeth: Kyrklig och social reform. Motiveringar till diakoni 1845–1965.
Skellefteå 2006.

Fleischmann, Ellen; Grypma, Sonya; Marten, Michael; Okkenhaug, Inger Marie (ed.): Transnational and historical perspectives on global health, welfare and humanitarianism. Kristiansand 2013.

Espagne, Michel: Les transferts culturels franco-allemands. Paris 1999.

Habermas, Rebekka: Mission im 19. Jahrhundert. Globale Netze des Religiösen. In: Historische Zeitschrift 287 (2008), pp. 629–679.

Hauser, Julia: Waisen gewinnen. Mission zwischen Programmatik und Praxis in der Erzie-
hungsarbeit der Kaiserswerther Diakonissen in Beirut seit 1860. In: WerkstattGeschichte
57 (2011), pp. 9–30.

Hüwelmeier, Gertrud: Negotiating diversity. Catholic nuns as cosmopolitans. In: Schweize-
rische Zeitschrift für Religions- und Kulturgeschichte 102 (2008), pp. 105–107.

Kaminsky, Uwe: Innere Mission im Ausland. Der Aufbau religiöser und sozialer Infrastruktur
am Beispiel der Kaiserswerther Diakonie (1851–1975). Stuttgart 2010.

Köser, Silke: Denn eine Diakonisse darf kein Alltagsmensch sein. Kollektive Identitäten Kaiserswerther Diakonissen 1836–1914. Leipzig 2006.

Kreutzer, Susanne: Vom "Liebesdienst" zum modernen Frauenberuf. Die Reform der Krankenpflege nach 1945. Frankfurt/Main; New York 2005.

Kreutzer, Susanne: Nursing body and soul in the parish. Lutheran deaconess motherhouses
in Germany and the United States. In: Nursing History Review 18 (2010), pp. 134–150.

Kreutzer, Susanne: Rationalisierung evangelischer Krankenpflege. Westdeutsche und US-
amerikanische Diakonissenmutterhäuser im Vergleich, 1945–1970. In: Medizinhistorisches Journal 47 (2012), pp. 221–243.

Kreutzer, Susanne: Arbeits- und Lebensalltag evangelischer Krankenpflege. Organisation,
soziale Praxis und biographische Erfahrungen. Göttingen 2014.

Malchau-Dietz, Susanne: Køn, kald og kompetencer. Diakonissestiftelsens kvindefællesskab
og omsorgsuddannelser 1863–1955. København 2013.

Markkola, Pirjo: Women's spirituality, lived religion, and social reform in Finland, 1860–1920.
In: Perichoresis 9 (2011), pp. 143–182.

Markkola, Pirjo: Deaconesses go transnational. Knowledge transfer and deaconess education
in nineteenth-century Finland and Sweden. In: Fleischmann, Ellen; Grypma, Sonya; Marten, Michael; Okkenhaug, Inger Marie (ed.): Transnational and historical perspectives on
global health, welfare and humanitarianism. Kristiansand 2013, pp. 70–89.

Martinsen, Kari: Freidige og uforsagte diakonisser. Et omsorgsyrke vokser fram 1860–1905.
Aschehoug 1984.

Mettele, Gisela: Eine "Imagined Community" jenseits der Nation. Die Herrnhuter Brüder-
meine als transnationale Gemeinschaft. In: Geschichte und Gesellschaft 32 (2006), pp.
45–68.

Middell, Matthias: Kulturtransfer und Historische Komparatistik. Thesen zu ihrem Verhältnis. In: Comparativ. Zeitschrift für Globalgeschichte und vergleichende Gesellschafts-
forschung 10 (2000), pp. 7–41.

Nelson, Sioban: Say little, do much. Nursing, nuns, and hospitals in the nineteenth century.
Philadelphia 2001.

Nolte, Karen: Protestant nursing care in Germany in the 19th century. Concepts and social practice. In: D'Antonio, Patricia; Fairman, Judith A.; Whelan, Jean C. (ed): Routledge handbook on the global history of nursing. New York 2013, pp. 167–82.

O'Brien, Susan: French nuns in nineteenth-century England. In: Past and Present (1997), pp. 142–180.

Okkenhaug, Inger Marie: Norwegian nurses, relief and welfare in the United States and Middle East, ca. 1880–1915. In: Fleischmann, Ellen; Grypma, Sonya; Marten, Michael; Okkenhaug, Inger Marie (ed.): Transnational and historical perspectives on global health, welfare and humanitarianism. Kristiansand 2013, pp. 41–69.

Patel, Kiran Klaus: Transnationale Geschichte – Ein neues Paradigma?, H-Soz-u-Kult, 02/02/2005, <http://hsozkult.geschichte.hu-berlin.de/forum/id=573&type=artikel>.

Paulmann, Johannes: Internationaler Vergleich und interkultureller Transfer. Zwei Forschungsansätze zur europäischen Geschichte des 18. bis 20. Jahrhunderts. In: Historische Zeitschrift 267 (1998), pp. 649–685.

Schmidt, Jutta: Beruf: Schwester. Mutterhausdiakonie im 19. Jahrhundert. Frankfurt/Main; New York 1998.

Schmuhl, Hans-Walter: Ärzte in konfessionellen Kranken- und Pflegeanstalten 1908–1957. In: Kuhlemann, Frank-Michael; Schmuhl, Hans-Walter (ed.): Beruf und Religion im 19. und 20. Jahrhundert. Stuttgart 2003, pp. 176–194.

Soine, Aeleah: The motherhouse and its mission(s). Kaiserswerth and the convergence of transnational nursing knowledge, 1836–1865. In: Fleischmann, Ellen; Grypma, Sonya; Marten, Michael; Okkenhaug, Inger Marie (ed.): Transnational and historical perspectives on global health, welfare and humanitarianism. Kristiansand 2013, pp. 20–41.

Weber-Reich, Traudel: "Wir sind die Pionierinnen der Pflege…" Krankenschwestern und ihre Pflegestätten im 19. Jahrhundert am Beispiel Göttingen. Bern; Seattle 2003.

Germany – Foundation era of German
deaconess motherhouses

Deaconesses' self-understanding and everyday nursing practice in the first deaconess community in Kaiserswerth, Germany

Karen Nolte

Numerous scholars have researched the history, organisation, regulations and rules of the very first community of deaconesses. Pastor Theodor Fliedner founded it in 1836 in the small German town of Kaiserswerth near Düsseldorf.[1] However, the daily practice of the deaconesses in the area of nursing care has received little scholarly attention, even though the archive of the *Fliedner Kulturstiftung*, the cultural foundation named after Fliedner, keeps a large inventory of everyday sources.

The following article depicts the everyday practice in nursing care during the foundation of the first deaconess motherhouse in Kaiserswerth. The German social and medical developments during the first half of the nineteenth century form the context of my analysis. Crucial for this article is on the one hand the discourse on the *social question*, i.e. the reasons for the massive impoverishment within the urban proletariat. In this area I will uncover the specific Christian self-understanding of deaconesses in nursing care and their relationship to parish pastors and hospital chaplains. On the other hand, I will discuss the beginning of the systematic training of deaconesses in nursing care within the context of medical care for poor patients both in hospital and outside it. The self-understanding of the Protestant nurses from Kaiserswerth is at the centre of my investigation and I will uncover the relationship between doctors and nurses both as it was depicted in the rules of service and as it was experienced in everyday practice. While previous studies have tended to emphasise the patriarchal, hierarchical, and repressive character of the communities of deaconesses, this article reveals the deaconesses' opportunities and options as active agents in their everyday work. My research draws on social and religio-historical studies that previously examined the social structure, ideas, and organisation of the communities of deaconesses. In the following I will briefly summarise these studies.

Delineating the history of how the institution for deaconesses in Kaiserswerth was organised and structured, Anna Sticker was one of the first scholars who systematically collected, compiled, and commented on the normative texts. Subsequently, Ruth Felgentreff thoroughly reconstructed the history of the *diaconia* in Kaiserswerth. Since both researchers had themselves worked as deaconesses in Kaiserswerth, they also revealed an insider's insight into the first German community of deaconesses.[2] Utilising a gender historical perspective, Jutta Schmidt worked on the social structure of the deaconesses,

---

1   Nolte (2013), pp. 167–182.
2   Sticker (1960); Felgentreff (1998).

their motivations, and the ideals of the institution for deaconesses in Kaiserswerth. She found out that – against Fliedner's intentions – mainly women with
a rural or petty bourgeois background were attracted to the community of
deaconesses as a model of life and work.[3] Finally, Silke Köser has shown that
a "collective identity" was central to the constitution and stabilisation of a
community that was organised and shaped along strict hierarchical and patriarchal lines. Rites, symbols, and ritualised practices helped to found and to
strengthen the community of deaconesses. For example, the sisters were asked
to work through a catalogue of self-examining questions every day in order to
continuously renew their knowledge of the basic values of the community of
deaconesses and their tasks and duties. Thus, the active involvement of the
deaconesses was vital for the formation of a "collective identity".[4] Following
Köser's research, I will now establish how the deaconesses expressed their
self-understanding towards their patients, the doctors, and the pastors in their
everyday practice, and how they positioned themselves as members of the
community of deaconesses through their continuous contact with the motherhouse. I argue that this type of life was mainly attractive for women from the
petty bourgeois and lower classes because of the social security and the social
status it conferred on the women. Furthermore, it was enticing because of the
opportunities for autonomous action and independence that the deaconesses,
living and working far away from the motherhouse, gained.

The letters written by the deaconesses from Kaiserswerth are my main
source as they have been preserved in large quantities in the archive of the
Fliedner Kulturstiftung. The regular exchange of letters between the deaconesses who were working in various locations and the principals of the motherhouse was central to the creation and consolidation of their "collective identity". The nurses' letters are mainly characterised by the deaconesses' desire
to fulfil the expectations of their 'parents', as they called their principals. In
addition, the letters contain reports of the sisters' daily work and both their
personal and professional experiences. Some of the deaconesses were still
quite young and for them the 'parents' at the motherhouse were at times the
only familiar contact with whom they could share their thoughts and anxieties
when they were far away.

Thus, we find cracks in the self-portraits of the 'good' deaconess – and my
analysis focuses precisely on these cracks, which I use to discuss the daily
practice of the deaconesses working in nursing care. Furthermore, I am interested in the following questions: How were the deaconesses in Kaiserswerth
prepared as carers of patients and how did they themselves describe the nursing care? What was the relationship like between them and the patients? How
did the deaconesses describe their relationship with the doctors and pastors to
whom, according to the rules of service, they were subordinate?

3   Schmidt (1998).
4   Köser (2006).

The foundation of the Kaiserswerth Deaconess Institute and the *social question*

In 1836, the Protestant pastor Theodor Fliedner (1800–1864) founded the first institution for deaconesses in Kaiserswerth as an answer to pressing contemporary social problems and larger issues in society. With the industrialisation process that had begun in the nineteenth century in the rapidly growing metropolises, large parts of the petty bourgeois and lower classes became impoverished. Disease and poverty were closely linked, since wage workers had no social security in case of illness. By training his deaconesses as carers for poor people who were seriously ill, Fliedner was responding to the so-called *social question* that was the subject of intense debate among the bourgeoisie. Yet, he also saw an opportunity with his deaconesses to contribute to a re-Christianisation of society. The bourgeois concept of the *Inner Mission* was based on the assumption that spiritual and material impoverishment were causally linked. The leading figures of the *Inner Mission* observed with concern that the urban proletariat, influenced by social-democratic or socialist working class movements respectively, were moving further and further away from the Christian faith. Providing care for the poor and sick therefore did more than address the illnesses and material needs of the people in deprived urban areas. The goal was to draw these individuals away from the influence of the working class movement and guide them back to the Christian faith.

Theodor Fliedner used the Catholic female order of the *Sisters of Mercy* as a model for his community of deaconesses and combined the idea of a religious community of women with the early Christian concept of a deaconess. Referring to the early Christian *diaconia*, Fliedner was less interested in historic exactitude but rather in finding a basis on which to justify the professionalism of women as parish workers.[5] Fliedner sympathised with the *revival movement* that had been marking a religious awakening since the end of the eighteenth century, putting a practical Christian lifestyle for the individual at the centre of its Christian self-understanding. Due to the inter-denominational features of this religious *revival movement*, Fliedner had no fundamental reservations against Catholicism, which explains the mixture of Catholic and Protestant elements in the new community of deaconesses.[6]

At the institution for deaconesses in Kaiserswerth, women from the petty bourgeois classes were not only trained as educators and teachers but also as carers for poor patients and, as parish nurses, also as carers for people in need. Originally, Fliedner had intended women from the educated middle classes to become deaconesses. The only way for a bourgeois woman to earn a living in a manner befitting her social status was to work as a teacher. If the families of unmarried women from the bourgeoisie could not afford to feed their daughters, these penniless ladies secretly had to contribute to their keep with 'bashful wage labour', i.e. with sowing or other handiwork. To change

---

5   Schmidt (1998); Köser (2006).
6   Köser (2006), pp. 91–92.

this undignified living situation for unmarried bourgeois women, in 1865 the *Allgemeine Deutsche Frauenverein* (*General German Association of Women, ADF*) was founded, which led to the establishment of numerous other women's organisations and resulted finally the bourgeois women's movement.[7] In the nineteenth century, nursing care was still largely conducted by nursing attendants from the lower classes, who were paid but had received no formal training. As a result, this work was regarded as a servant's job. For that reason, women from the educated middle classes did not come to Kaiserswerth as Fliedner had intended to join the community of deaconesses and dedicate their life to the care of poor people and to nursing care. By contrast, for women from petty bourgeois circles and the lower classes, the institution for deaconesses was attractive,[8] as they received a sound education and vocational training here, which subsequently resulted in social advancement. Theodor Fliedner had designed a robe for the deaconesses that corresponded to the dresses of bourgeois married women and this uniform made the women's newly acquired social status visible to the public.[9]

As well as teaching the deaconesses to care for the sickly body, their training also comprised 'care for the soul': care for the spiritual well-being of the patients in a Christian sense. According to the Christian point of view, disease was either the result of a sinful lifestyle or, in pious Christians, it was a test of God, which they had to endure.[10] Since diseases often resulted in poverty, especially in the lower classes, the deaconesses from Kaiserswerth regarded the care they provided for body and soul as a crucial measure against the widespread impoverishment.[11] In the following, I will explain the details of how the deaconesses were trained.

Training for the care of body and soul

At the motherhouse in Kaiserswerth the principal instructed the nurses in how to care for the soul and the body. Theodor Fliedner had written an *Instruction für die erste Seelenpflege der Kranken* (*instructions for the initial care of the patient's soul*)[12] to be used during the lectures for his deaconesses on the care of the soul. Because illness and poverty were linked to a sinful lifestyle, care for the soul, i.e. religious instruction for predominantly poor patients, was central to Protestant nursing care. The importance of caring for the soul was expressed particularly clearly in dealings with severely ill or dying patients, as can be

7   Frevert (1986), pp. 63–145.
8   Schmidt (1998).
9   Nolte (2013).
10   Krankheit, TRE Vol. XIX, pp. 680–709.
11   Röper (1998).
12   Fliedner, Theodor: Instruction für die erste Seelenpflege der Kranken, Archive of the Fliedner Cultural Foundation in Kaiserswerth (AFCFK), Sign.: Rep. II: Fb.

seen in a passage from the handwritten *Medicinischer Cursus* (*medical course*) written by Fliedner:

> The beautiful holy duty of nursing care appears in its whole sincerity but also in its fullest meaning and importance at the bed of the mortally ill patient. Where the doctor's aid has met its limits, the love of the nurse continues to assist her patient with a caring hand and a mild disposition in the hour of struggle and fading, to bring him relief and comfort. Here, as it were, she doubles her eagerness and faithfulness [...].[13]

Care for the soul – as the deaconesses learned during their training – was the Lutheran nurses' area of competency that was independent from the doctors. The basis of providing good care for the soul was a thorough knowledge of the bible. In addition, the sisters received a repertoire of psalms, bible quotes and inspirational Christian writings so that they could give their patients religious lessons if necessary. Deaconesses were supposed to be able to interpret biblical texts and apply them to the specific situation of the patient. However, the pastors wished that they would do that only to a limited degree in order to differentiate clearly between their care for the soul and the spiritual guidance provided by the pastors.

Details of how the care for the soul was to be performed can also be found in Fliedner's *Instruction*: While the nurse was to start by paying attention to the patient's physical suffering, she was also supposed to carefully and 'silently' watch his or her behaviour. This had to happen right after taking on the patient so that the sister could gain insight into the condition of the patient's soul. Did he or she read from the *New Testament* that the deaconess had left in the patient's room? How did he or she behave during domestic prayers and devotions: in an "attentive, devotional, indifferent, or imprudent" manner?[14] Only then, a few days later, was the deaconess supposed to ask whether the patient had been confirmed and she had to check how well he or she knew the Ten Commandments and was ready to reflect on his or her contraventions of them. Subsequently, the sister had to report to the 'spiritual inspector' of the hospital on the 'religious condition' of the newcomer. She was to provide 'ignorant patients' with bible verses, inspirational excerpts and a hymnal. An important basis for caring for the soul was the following biblical quote: "Whoever does not accept the kingdom of God like a child will not enter it."[15] Accordingly, the following basic assumption applied to the care for the soul: the more the patient's knowledge could be compared to the knowledge of a child, the more promising were the efforts for the condition of the soul. This suggests that, according to contemporary ideas of the educated middle class, uneducated people were more open to religious ideas than educated people, young patients were more willing to take it in than older ones and women were more accessible to care for the soul than men.

Theodor Fliedner based his lessons in physical care on the manuals on health care produced by the physicians Carl Emil Gedike (1787–1867) and

---

13   Fliedner: Medicinischer Cursus.
14   Fliedner: Instruction.
15   New Testament, Mark 10:15; Luke 18:17.

Johann Friedrich Dieffenbach (1792–1847).[16] These handbooks followed the tradition of a number of instruction manuals on nursing care and had been written for the training of the nursing staff at the Berlin *Charité* hospital. With the development of both modern university hospitals and council hospitals from the end of the eighteenth century onwards, physicians started to write down their ideas on nursing care and to sketch out their idea of the ideal nurse. The Christian understanding of holistic care for body and soul contradicted the doctors' interests at times, since the sisters tended to follow the values and leading figures of their religious community, instead of submitting to the doctor's authority. The physicians' instructions on nursing care focussed on the care of the sick body and simultaneously defined the qualities of an ideally female nurse. The aim was the nurses' unconditional obedience to the doctors.[17] Theodor Fliedner used the physicians' instructions on physical care, which were in line with the latest medical findings of the time, and combined them with his ideas of Christian nursing care, which were based on an assumption of an inseparable link between body and soul.

A look at the manuscript entitled *Medicinischer Cursus* (*medical course*), shows that the nurses received a thorough overview of pathology and the common treatment methods that were used during the first half of the nineteenth century.[18] Scholars have often emphasised that the Protestant nurses focussed primarily on their missionary work at the patients' bedside and that physical care played a subordinate role. Yet, the manuscript of the *Medicinischer Cursus* reveals that the deaconesses learned far more than just a few nursing tricks. In addition to a basic grounding in anatomy and pathology, the nurses learned how the patient's room had to be furnished to adhere to the hygienic standards of the time. They were also trained in 'minor surgery' procedures, which had typically been the preserve of surgeons and non-academically trained medics (*Wundärzte*). While many of the practising medics claimed to be doctors, they were rather barber-surgeons. The nurses learnt the techniques of blood-letting, bleeding, leeching, and administering fontanels (that is creating an artificial wound containing pus to drain out the disease substances). They had to be able to perform these procedures upon the doctor's instruction in case a surgeon or other doctor was unavailable.[19] Surgeons without any academic training did not see themselves as pioneers who laid the groundwork for the academic physicians. Rather they assumed the title of a doctor and were in competition on the medical market with those physicians who had attended university. Learning to perform minor surgical procedures themselves enabled the deaconesses to work as healers and to cross into the territory of the doctor's expertise.[20]

---

16   Gedike (1854); Dieffenbach (1832).
17   Nolte (2013), pp. 167–182.
18   Fliedner, Theodor: Medicinischer Cursus, Vol. I–III, AFCFK, Sign.: Rep. II: Fd 1.3.
19   Fliedner: Medicinischer Cursus.
20   Stolberg (1998), pp. 69–85; Sander (1989).

In 1852, for instance, a Sister Dorothee wrote: "In the community we only had a few nursing cases but we were the busier with bleeding the patients and administering leeches."[21] In 1853 she wrote again: "Thus everything that occurs in the parish such as bleeding and leeching someone, as well as administrating enemas and being on night watch – as much as is in my power to do I will do."[22] Similarly, a Sister Lisette reported in 1846 that she went to a girl twice a day in order to make the bed, often to bleed her, and to administer 'blood suckers'.[23]

Other letters reveal that the deaconesses not only provided spiritual support to their severely ill patients but also monitored them very closely. Quite skilfully, they even provided pain therapies with opiates that the doctor had prescribed. For example, a Sister Mina reported in 1891 on a private care case:

> The past few weeks treated my dear patient quite badly. [...] On Wednesday, the 3rd of November, she was so weak that I could not but think that she would be called home in only a few days. However, the fever fell and she was able to eat a bit more and little by little she recovered somewhat.

> Her condition since then is that she has been suffering much more. After approximately seven days of getting worse, she experienced a painful cough that disappeared only momentarily with very few breaks in order to return with even more force. At times it is loose so that she can properly cough up, yet often it is so persistent and painful all day that her forehead is covered in sweat and she suffers from headaches. Also, she has often complained about back and chest pains since then. Thus, I have to pick up morphine more often than usual to ensure her night's' rest, but for her weak body, only a small dose is required. Yesterday she again had an exceptionally bad day where she was apathetic and lay there as if in a slumber. She did not want to take in anything either. Today she is a bit better again. Her life is hanging by a thread.[24]

Deaconesses working in the parish and deaconesses in private care in particular had to work at times quite independently and take their own autonomous decisions. This meant that they also performed tasks that touched on the doctors' area of expertise.[25]

The deaconesses acted with similar independence with regard to caring for the soul. The research of the past twenty years on female religiosity in the nineteenth century has emphasised the strong position of bourgeois women in the communication and practice of religion.[26] In Kaiserswerth, young women were trained to communicate the Christian faith to faithless people from the lower classes. Since the agents of the *Inner Mission* believed in a causal relationship between faithlessness and both disease and poverty, nursing care and care for the poor were always linked to providing religious instruction. Deacon-

---

21 Letter by Dorothee Haube 21/1/1852, AFCFK, Cleve 1845–1854, Sign.: 1337.
22 Letter by Dorothee Haube 11/2/1853, AFCFK, Cleve 1845–1854, Sign.: 1337.
23 Letter by Lisette Steiner 2/4/1850, AFCFK, Cleve 1845–1854, Sign.: 1337.
24 Letter by Mina Mätte 20/11/1891, AFCFK, Privatpflege [private care] 1888–1893, Sign.: DA 201.
25 Nolte (2010), pp. 87–108.
26 Habermas (1994); Götz von Olenhusen (1995), pp. 9–21; Gause (1998), pp. 309–327.

esses in Kaiserswerth learned to communicate the Word of God, and to explain and interpret biblical texts. The boundaries between the deaconesses' care for the soul and the spiritual guidance the pastors provided were not clearly defined. For this reason, Theodor Fliedner outlined what care for the soul entailed in the first edition of the *Haus- und Dienstordnung* (*house rules and service regulations*). He expanded on this set of regulations with additional papers that he published in the motherhouse journal *Der Armen- und Kranken-freund* (*the friend of the poor and the sick*). His intention was to clearly delineate the areas of caring for the soul and spiritual guidance. He believed that the deaconess should be a 'spiritual carer in private' while the pastor was supposed to be responsible for supervising the religious teachings of the patients and keeping an oversight of all things spiritual. The reality was different, however, since the deaconesses were present at the bedside at all times and they had to decide for themselves when to call for a pastor. In the section on the relationship between deaconesses and pastors I will further analyse the eager missionary work of the deaconesses at the bedside and the pastors' reactions to the, at times, quite broad interpretation of the deaconesses' area of competency relating to practical care for the soul.

Nursing care practice: Deaconesses and their patients

Deaconesses were well respected, particularly in the setting of domestic care, because they had received such a thorough education. Furthermore, the patients appreciated the religious support provided by the Protestant nurses, as one example from the end of the nineteenth century may illustrate. This story comes from a letter that a Sister Sophie wrote to the motherhouse: she not only describes how a pious woman who was suffering from uterine cancer was severely tested in her faith, but also how the husband and even the deaconess herself were doubting the love of God:

> Unfortunately, the condition of my dear patient is rather worrisome. During the last eight days the pain at the infected area is so severe that she does not know what to do. Both the local gynaecologist and the one from Remscheid said that it would be too dangerous to operate. They say the tumour would have to pass through on its own. Now, we are constantly giving her wraps for her body but we have been waiting in vain until now and we cannot see anything from the outside either.

> Her temperature is mostly 39 or 40 degrees. If the heavenly doctor does not send his aid soon, I fear that her little remaining strength will not last for much longer. It is a difficult test of faith, in particular for the severely ill lady, but also for her husband and myself who have to wait in vain for so long for the help of the Lord. And her faith is small, but she is quite willing to be reprimanded through the word of God and allows herself to be encouraged to have patience and hope. Today I read to her some passages from Job.[27]

---

27 Letter by Sophie Stock 1893, AFCFK, Privatpflege [private care] 1888–1893, Sign.:
    DA 201.

Sister Sophie went through her crisis of faith together with the patient's husband by reading to him the story of Job. This story is the ultimate example of the Christian understanding that disease is a test of God for righteous Christians.

However, the letters the deaconesses wrote also speak of the resistance shown by severely ill patients to care for the soul and how that clashed with the sisters' categorical desire to convert them. An example of such a confrontation comes from a letter the nurses Sister Louise and Sister Lisette wrote in 1847 when they worked as parish nurses:

> We also took care of a man who lives half an hour away from the town of Cleve. He was very ill with a chest infection and the doctor had no hope for him. We visited him once or twice daily because when we asked him to what extent his soul was prepared for the Lord when He would call for him, we saw that his soul was still very far away from the Lord. The patient answered, we are not there yet, I am not dying yet; and we told him that the Lord could come like a thief in the night and asked whether he could pass in front of Christ's judgement? He could not answer that.[28]

In fact the sisters managed with a – what we might call today – drastic intervention, where the dying man overcame his initial resistance and was willing to pray with them and to call for the pastor to receive communion. The continuation of the story reads like the narration of a miracle because the sisters reported how the man became pious and was healed completely. Yet, it was not this simple with all the patients. In 1853, a Sister Dorothee reported on a severely ill unmarried woman who had an illegitimate child and lived in great poverty. The deaconess described her first experiences with this patient:

> An unmarried person called for me because she was ill, as they told me. Beforehand she had wanted nothing to do with me because I had been forced to tell her the truth sometimes as if she had no more time left to live. Once she had told another woman that I could do nothing but talk. She said that the Good Lord that I spoke of was on holiday and that those who relied on Him would be cheated and other such chatter. I did not know what to do with her.[29]

The unmarried woman had long rejected care by a deaconess because she did not want to accept the attempts to convert her that went along with the nursing and care for the poor. When she was finally so ill that she could no longer manage on her own she allowed the sister to be called. The deaconess described the situation as follows:

> Boiling with fever, she was sitting erect in her bedstead. There was no bed, no sack of straw, indeed, not even straw. She did not wear a vest and had merely draped an old dress around her. On her back she had a huge abscess that the doctor called a plague-spot. I addressed her with the words: Oh Lehna, Lehna – to think of all the things that accompany sin. I procured for her first the necessary clothes, straw, linen, and a pillow, all of which I unfortunately had to beg for myself, and then I also provided her with food.[30]

---

28 Letter by Louise Türner and Lisette Steiner 24/9/1847, Cleve 1845–1854, Sign.: 1337.
29 Letter by Dorothee Haube 11/2/1853, Cleve 1845–1854, Sign.: 1337.
30 Letter by Dorothee Haube 11/2/1853, Cleve 1845–1854, Sign.: 1337.

The nurse saw the abscess literally as a sign of the woman's sinfulness and she continued – openly disgusted – to describe the lice and the dirt in the apartment, linking them to the condition of the woman's soul.[31]

> She also had a child who was ten years old and the lice were eating her alive. Unfortunately, here I could not do anything but provide food because I saw that the end would come quickly for the child's mother.[32]

In other letters, the deaconesses also link dirt with faithlessness, understanding the cleaning of the clothes and the houses as rituals of cleansing also in a metaphorical sense.[33] In contrast to the dying faithless man who was healed in a double sense, Sister Dorothee's mission was unsuccessful in the case of the sinful Lehna. Nonetheless she provided spiritual support when the woman was dying:

> Of course, I also called quickly for a clergyman who visited her faithfully and, I know this to be a fact, carried her in praying hands. Since she also had a friend around it was not necessary for me to be there the entire time and I visited her three times a day. I came and left again with the same heavy heart. Whether the spirit of the Lord was able to work at her heart in silence, I do not know: during the final night Sister Christine was also with her because I felt so eerie being alone with the dying woman.[34]

Sister Johanne in Elberfeld felt similarly when she failed in her care for the soul of a typesetter suffering from hydropsy. Even when the nurse reminded him of the Last Judgement she could not persuade him to change his ways. Although the man was facing his imminent death, even the pastor who had been called had to leave without having achieved anything:

> He said he could feel that his hours were numbered now and he asked me to send him a sensible man. He meant a pastor. Pastor Barner arrived, talked to him, but could not give him the Holy Communion that the man had demanded. Thus he lived for a few more days, cursing. Then the hour of his death arrived, he was unconscious, it was night, I was alone with him but I stood in the middle of the room, it was so eerie. I wonder what we would do if we did not have our Redeemer in such cases.[35]

These anecdotes of failed attempts at conversion in the deaconesses' letters allow insights into the everyday life of the deaconesses where it was not always 'uplifting' to step up to the bedside of a dying patient. These reports stand in contrast to the many reports published in the *Armen- und Krankenfreund*, which were ironed out for publication and tried to convince the reader otherwise. Thus, a Sister Henriette describes very vividly the fear she felt during the death struggle of a patient, in her letter to the motherhouse in Kaiserswerth:

> [...] a severely ill lady came who required all of my time. I did not have much to do with the children; I had to spend day and night with the patient. However, during the last

---

31 Nolte (2011), pp. 105–116.
32 Letter by Dorothee Haube 11/2/1853, Cleve 1845–1854, Sign.: 1337.
33 Nolte (2011), pp. 105–116.
34 Letter by Dorothee Haube 11/2/1853, Cleve 1845–1854, Sign.: 1337.
35 Letter by Johanne Niendecker 09/1/1862, AFCFK, Parish Elberfeld 1846–1862, Sign.: 1787.

eight days I was relieved every other night. Now she has died, but I will never forget that night. I have never seen anybody die so painfully, over and over again she opened her eyes wide and groaned horribly. O, it was gruesome. Sister Elisabeth was also there with me.[36]

The difficult battle with death in this description is an expression of the spiritual condition of the dying patient whose soul was burdened with sins that were unatoned. This might explain the nurse's fear that prompted her to take along a second sister for support, as had the other deaconesses in the previously described cases.

It is noteworthy that the deaconesses in the cases I have mentioned here were fearful of sinfully dying patients, as they express in their writings. At times the nurses even had to step away from the bedside, apparently so as not to endanger their own spiritual well-being. They seemed to fear that their faith would not be able to resist the refutation that those patients embodied because they had been unwilling to be converted.

The story of Sister Isabella illustrates that deaconesses sometimes also reached the limits of what they could achieve due to social differences: this nurse worked at the *Luisenhospital* in Aachen and was caring for a merchant suffering from a severe infection of typhus. When he recovered he asked for a newspaper. In response the nurse cautioned the seemingly prosperous patient as follows:

[…] whether he would not rather first read a psalm of thanksgiving and whether there was not a trace of gratefulness in his heart for the one who had helped him recover from his severe illness. The patient answered that only his good constitution, doctors, and nurses had helped him to recover; faith in a God had breathed in him when he was a young man but he had long given it up. [He said that] since he had grown out of God's tutelage and had begun standing on his own feet he was much happier; faith he would leave to weak and troubled people etc.[37]

The merchant did not want to listen to the deaconess's teachings. He possibly noticed that the nurse had a petty bourgeois background from her way of expressing herself and her *habitus*. At the end, however, the nurse was satisfied to learn that the now mortally ill wealthy man wanted to turn to faith after all: he was facing death and lost his battle. Now, she could assert her superiority over the materially wealthy but spiritually impoverished man and she finally noted without mercy: "The Lord had given him a long time to consider, he [the man] has no excuse."[38] Sister Isabella concluded that the rich merchant's turning to God had come too late for him to die blessedly and she triumphed in the end over the arrogant rich man. This way, in her eyes, the social hierarchy had justly been turned upside down.

36 Letter by Henriette Bücker 27/10/1878, AFCFK, Aachen Luisenhospital 1872–1881, Sign.: 1094.
37 Letter by Isabelle Kummer 24/1/1879, Aachen Luisenhospital 1872–1881, Sign.: 1094.
38 Letter by Isabelle Kummer 24/1/1879, Aachen Luisenhospital 1872–1881, Sign.: 1094.

Nursing practice: Deaconesses and physicians

Even newer scholarly articles on the history of nursing care hold onto the idea that it was in Christian nursing that the concept of an ideal nurse evolved and was nurtured. This perfect nurse was willing to make sacrifices, was "subservient to the doctor" and willing to subordinate herself.[39]

However, while the deaconesses granted the doctors their leading position in the realm of caring for the body, this area was not at all central to their own self-understanding as carers. As I illustrated at the beginning, while the deaconesses received a thorough training in physical care, it was care for the spiritual well-being of patients, caring for the soul, that formed the core of Protestant nursing care until well into the twentieth century. In this area of competency that was independent of the doctors, the nurses reported only to the leaders of the motherhouse. Yet at their workplaces, far away from the motherhouse, they acted at times quite independently of their spiritual 'parents'.

Considering the letters written by the deaconesses from Kaiserswerth, it becomes evident that the doctors played only a marginal role in the nurses' reports. They describe situations in which doctors gave orders regarding physical care, for instance in connection with pain management. Conflicts between doctors and nurses apparently arose only when the doctors interfered in the area of spiritual care. The Protestant sisters experienced an inner conflict when the doctors prohibited the nurses from discussing imminent death with mortally ill patients: on the one hand, the Protestant sisters were expected to confront the severely ill patients with their imminent end, to help them cleanse their soul so that they could finally die blessedly. On the other hand, according to the service regulations, they had to follow the doctors' orders obediently. In the nineteenth century, most doctors rejected the idea of enlightening dying patients about their hopeless prognosis because they feared that the patient's condition would worsen after such a shock to the system and the patient's life would be drastically shortened. In the pathology of the humours, which was central to medicine until far into the second half of the nineteenth century, the idea prevailed that an emotional upset, for example one caused by great fear, could result in a significant deterioration of the physical condition. While the deaconesses wanted to calm the soul by confronting the patients with their imminent death and causing them to repent of their sins, the doctors were convinced that such shocking facts should be withheld from the patients' sensitive souls for their benefit.[40] In 1852, a Sister Julie reported on such a conflict with a doctor on the question of informing a patient who received parish care in Cleve:

> My d[ear] patient is currently quite well, the pain has eased significantly during the past few weeks, but the body gradually begins to fade, her mood swings to being at times very cheerful; her memory is very sharp. The wound has been healing significantly for a quar-

---

39 Bischoff-Wanner (2011), pp. 13–36; Sieger (2005), pp. 196–216.
40 Nolte (2008), pp. 115–134.

ter of the year, but her whole condition appears to me as if she will soon dissolve. Yet her d[ear] parents faithfully hope that she is moving towards a recovery because the doctor interprets everything as a sign of recovery and claims that siblings and parents would otherwise not be able to bear the pain. I cannot talk to the doctor privately about this and I also think he would not honestly tell me about her condition.[41]

To be bound to silence contradicted the deaconess's duty to ensure that her mortally ill patients could have a blessed death. In other cases, the deaconesses sought help from the motherhouse when they could not reconcile with their conscience that they had to conceal a patient's imminent death from them. In case of doubt they could count on the support of the motherhouse when the doctors hindered their care for the soul.[42]

In the hospitals that were under the management of deaconesses, the doctors' interests were subordinate to the concepts of Christian nursing care. When hiring a physician in such a hospital, a certificate that the physician worked well with deaconesses was a very important document. The historian Fritz Dross has shown that no less a person than the famous surgeon Ferdinand Sauerbruch (1875–1951) failed to fulfil this requirement when, in 1900, he applied for the position of senior physician (Oberarzt) at the hospital in Fronberg. While he had worked as a doctor in residence (Assistenzarzt) at the deaconess hospital in Kassel, his application did not include a reference from a deaconess that asserted that he had worked well with a team of deaconesses. He did not qualify for the post.[43]

Nursing care practice: Deaconesses and pastors

The house rules and service regulations demanded that the deaconesses be subordinate to the pastor for their region. Yet, like the relationship between deaconesses and doctors, the reality was more complex. The deaconesses criticised the fact that the pastors did not visit poor and ill people often enough and the pastors regarded the eager missionary work of the deaconesses at the bedside with a critical eye. As mentioned above, Theodor Fliedner considered caring for the soul to be the centre of Christian nursing care, alongside the re-conversion of unfaithful Protestants, particularly those from the lower social stratum, and he believed that it had to accompany physical care. Nonetheless, he also used his first house rules and service regulations to warn against exaggerated eagerness.

During the 1870s, the deaconess institute itself for the first time publicly addressed criticisms aimed at the missionary work practised by the deaconesses at the patients' bedside. The second principal of the motherhouse in Kaiserswerth, Julius Disselhoff (1827–1896), lamented the fact that detractors

41   Letter by Julie Creuzinger 09/03/1852, AFCFK: Parish care in Cleve, 1845–1854, Sign.: 1337.
42   Nolte (2008), pp. 115–134.
43   Dross (2008), p. 177.

were accusing the people in charge at Kaiserswerth, telling them: 'It is not the Catholic Sisters who are campaigning; it is your sisters that are doing it.'[44] While Disselhoff fended off the criticism levelled against the care for the soul practised by his community of deaconesses, he seems to have felt compelled to address the accusations by recommending to 'his' sisters a gentler approach. Only when the deaconess had established a 'relationship of motherly friendship' with the patient, was she supposed to begin with the intensive care for the soul. He requested that the deaconess should have some life experience for this task, i.e. she was supposed to have known and experienced both sin and the mercy of the Lord.[45]

In 1893, the director of the deaconess institute in Altona, Theodor Schäfer (1846–1914), published a pamphlet on the work of the *female diaconia* (*Die weibliche Diakonie*). He was even more outspoken in criticising the rigorous missionary work that the deaconesses sometimes conducted at the patients' bedside. While he also emphasised the central role of caring for the soul in Protestant nursing care, he distinctly renounced the "spiritual bombardment" that he saw practised at times in the hospitals because he believed that it transformed care for the soul into a "Methodist torture treatment". One would not gain much, he believed, if the nurse converted the patient with "urges and pressure" to confess his faith. He noted that part of caring for the soul could also be "to leave a person alone as much as possible and to engage or bother him as little as possible". Instead, he suggested that the nurses should focus on the physical recovery of the patient.[46] Yet, the pastors' criticism of care for the soul in everyday practice must also be considered in the context of the competition which the deaconesses' care for the patients' souls presented for them, since the deaconesses had been practising this from the middle of the nineteenth century onwards. Principals and pastors made a great effort to delineate the deaconesses' care for the soul to maintain their own supervisory position in the spiritual guidance of the sick.[47] Thus, Theodor Schäfer quoted the founder of the motherhouse in Neuendettelsau, Wilhelm Löhe (1808–1872), in his writings on female diaconia as follows:

> Just as she [the nurse, K. N.] is not a doctor but follows the doctor's order with medication and care, so she does not assume the position of the shepherd either, but follows his orders in the choice of spiritual medication, which she must administer, and in the care for the soul, which she must conduct.[48]

This quote clearly illustrates that the deaconesses had to follow doctor's orders only with respect to physical care. The efforts to establish the pastor as a "spiritual doctor" in the care for the soul must be understood in the context that, in reality, the deaconesses' care for the soul could not be easily distinguished from the pastors' spiritual guidance of the patients. In fact, the dea-

---

44   Disselhoff (1872), p. 149.
45   Disselhoff (1872), pp. 150–152.
46   Schäfer (1893), pp. 160–161.
47   Kreutzer/Nolte (2010), pp. 45–56.
48   Schäfer (1893), p. 161.

conesses were present more often than the pastor when spiritual aid was needed. Thus, in 1899 Sister Sophie proudly described how she, instead of the pastor, had provided spiritual guidance for a dying woman.

> Mrs. Arns was a cheerful lady, aged 75, but was suffering in the chest and from hydropsy. Initially it looked as if we would have a long time of care. Last Saturday she was suddenly coughing blood. From that moment on her condition became critical and she completely lost her appetite which had been quite good before. She visibly lost her strength. The patient felt the end to be near and talked about it to her relatives who always reasoned her out of it. That was quite difficult for me. Her daughter, namely Doctor Füllrath's wife, and a daughter-in-law helped to care for her during the last days. Because she had to be lifted we always needed two people around her. Hence, I was never alone with the patient but I did not shy away from giving her the necessary words of comfort. They did not let a clergyman in to her. She was very restless and impatient but she recognised it as sin and on the last day, though still with a clear consciousness, she was as quiet and patient as a lamb which made me very happy as I had prayed for her and asked God for this. She recognised herself as a big sinner and I hope that our dear Lord received her with mercy.[49]

Since the pastor could not always be present, very often the deaconesses were in charge of providing the patients and the dying with spiritual support. Just as the deaconesses were able to replace surgeons and non-academically trained medics when these were not available, the sisters also provided care for the soul by themselves when the pastor could not be there. In other words, the boundary between the spiritual guidance the pastors provided and the deaconesses' care for the soul was not very distinct in everyday practice.

Conclusion

In this article I have provided some insights into the history of the everyday practice of the deaconesses from Kaiserswerth who worked in nursing care. The deaconesses were popular employees due to their training in physical care, which followed the latest curricula as developed by leading doctors of the time. Nonetheless, the collaboration between doctors and deaconesses included some conflicts, since the sisters' self-understanding as nurses was grounded essentially in those of their tasks that focused on care for the soul. Furthermore, missionary work at the bedside did not always correspond to the principles of the doctors. In the nineteenth century, a majority of doctors strictly rejected the idea of enlightening dying patients of their prognosis. The doctors feared that the message of death would cause a severe emotional upset and thus reduce the patient's life expectancy significantly. In rural communities the thorough training in physical care, including for minor surgical procedures, proved to be a blessing for the patients when surgeons and those doctors without any academic training were unavailable. In this case we can assume that the deaconesses' work could cross into the doctors' area of competency.

49 Letter by Sophie Stock 1893, AFCFK, Privatpflege [private care] 1888–1893, Sign.: DA 201.

Some of the patients displayed resistance to the sisters, which however only increased their eagerness to convert them. Yet, even within the diaconate, some felt that care for the soul as practised by the deaconesses was too forceful. Theodor Schäfer, the principal of the deaconess institute in Altona, called the intensive efforts of the deaconesses for the patients' spiritual well-being a "spiritual bombardment". Yet this criticism must also be read in the context of the competition that the deaconesses posed for the pastors in the area of spiritual guidance of patients. Principals and pastors were very eager to clearly delineate the care for the soul that the deaconesses provided in order to maintain their position as spiritual supervisors in the religious care provided to patients. With their dedicated care for the soul, the deaconesses also touched on the pastors' field of competence, since spiritual guidance of mortally ill and other patients played an important role in their self-understanding as parish pastors. Julius Disselhoff had emphasised that deaconesses were "spiritual carers in the private realm" while pastors were responsible for "broad perceptions"[50] within spiritual guidance. Yet the deaconesses' descriptions of their everyday practice reveal that they were the ones who were constantly present at the bedside of their patients and dying wards and, for that reason, they were the contact persons the patients spoke to when they felt their souls were suffering.

In the German social and historical context, the life and working model of a deaconess was attractive not only because of the comparatively good training and life-long social security it provided for women, but also because of the deaconesses' competencies, which allowed them to exceed the scope of their physical everyday work. After all, these boundaries were regularly redefined in their orders and instructions because of the practical experiences that the deaconesses so faithfully shared with their principals.

Bibliography

Literature

Bischoff-Wanner, Claudia: Pflege im historischen Vergleich. In: Schaeffer Doris; Wingenfeld, Klaus (ed.): Handbuch der Pflegewissenschaft. Weinheim 2011, pp. 13–36.
Dieffenbach, Johann Friedrich: Anleitung zur Krankenwartung. Berlin 1832.
Gause, Ute: Frauen und Frömmigkeit im 19. Jahrhundert. Der Aufbruch in die Öffentlichkeit. In: Pietismus und Neuzeit 24 (1998), pp. 309–327.
Disselhoff, Julius: Die geistliche Seite der Diakonissen-Thätigkeit. In: Der Armen- und Krankenfreund 24, September-Oktober (1872), pp. 149–162.
Dross, Fritz: "Der Kampfplatz der Liebe". Das Fronberg-Krankenhaus der Kaiserwerther Diakonie. In: Medizinhistorisches Journal 43 (2008), pp. 149–182.
Felgentreff, Ruth: Das Diakoniewerk Kaiserswerth 1836–1998. Von der Diakonissenanstalt zum Diakoniewerk – ein Überblick. Düsseldorf-Kaiserswerth 1998.
Frevert, Ute: Frauen-Geschichte. Zwischen bürgerlicher Verbesserung und neuer Weiblichkeit (edition suhrkamp, 284). Frankfurt/Main 1986.

50   Disselhoff (1872), p. 153.

Gedike, Carl Emil: Handbuch der Krankenwartung. Zum Gebrauch für die Kranken-
    wart-Schule der K. Berliner Charité-Heilanstalt sowie zum Selbstunterricht. Berlin 1854.
Götz von Olenhusen, Irmtraud: Die Feminisierung von Religion und Kirche im 19. und
    20. Jahrhundert. In: Götz von Olenhusen, Irmtraud (ed.): Frauen unter dem Patriarchat
    der Kirchen. Stuttgart 1995, pp. 9–21.
Köser, Silke: Denn eine Diakonisse darf kein Alltagsmensch sein. Kollektive Identitäten Kai-
    serswerther Diakonissen 1836–1914. Leipzig 2006.
Krankheit. In: Theologische Realenzyklopädie, Bd. XIX: Kirchenrechtsquellen – Kreuz. Ber-
    lin; New York 1990, pp. 680–709.
Kreutzer, Susanne; Nolte, Karen: Seelsorgerin "im Kleinen". Krankenseelsorge durch Dia-
    konissen im 19. und 20. Jahrhundert. In: Zeitschrift für medizinische Ethik 56 (2010),
    pp. 45–56.
Nolte, Karen: Protestant nursing care in Germany in the 19th century. Concepts and social
    practice. In: D'Antonio, Patricia; Fairman, Julie A.; Whelan, Jean C. (ed.): Routledge
    handbook on the global history of nursing. New York 2013, pp. 167–182.
Nolte, Karen: "Local missionaries". Community deaconesses in early 19th century health
    care. In: Dinges, Martin; Jütte, Robert (ed.): The transmission of health practices (c. 1500
    to 2000). Stuttgart 2011, pp. 105–116.
Nolte, Karen: Pflege von Sterbenden im 19. Jahrhundert. Eine ethikgeschichtliche Annähe-
    rung. In: Kreutzer, Susanne (ed.): Transformationen pflegerischen Handelns. Institutionelle
    Kontexte und soziale Praxis vom 19. bis 21. Jahrhundert. Göttingen 2010, pp. 87–108.
Nolte, Karen: Telling the painful truth. Nurses and physicians in the nineteenth century. In:
    Nursing History Review 16 (2008), pp. 115–134.
Röper, Ursula; Jüllig, Carola (ed.): Die Macht der Nächstenliebe. Einhundertfünfzig Jahre
    Innere Mission und Diakonie 1848–1998. Berlin 1998.
Sander, Sabine: Handwerkschirurgen. Sozialgeschichte einer verdrängten Berufsgruppe. Göt-
    tingen 1989.
Schäfer, Theodor: Die Arbeit der weiblichen Diakonie. Stuttgart 1893.
Schmidt, Jutta: Beruf: Schwester. Mutterhausdiakonie im 19. Jahrhundert. Frankfurt/Main;
    New York 1998.
Sieger, Margot: Kaiserswerther Kranken-Schwestern und die Veränderung der Pflege im
    20. Jahrhundert. In: Gause, Ute; Lissner, Cordula (ed.): Kosmos Diakonissenmutterhaus.
    Geschichte und Gedächtnis einer protestantischen Frauengemeinschaft. Leipzig 2005,
    pp. 196–216.
Sticker, Anna: Die Entstehung der neuzeitlichen Krankenpflege. Deutsche Quellenstücke aus
    der ersten Hälfte des 19. Jahrhunderts. Stuttgart 1960.
Stolberg, Michael: Heilkundige. Professionalisierung und Medikalisierung. In: Paul, Norbert;
    Schlich, Thomas (ed.): Medizingeschichte. Aufgaben, Probleme, Perspektiven. Frankfurt/
    Main; New York 1998, pp. 69–85.

Archives

Archives of the Fliedner Cultural Foundation (AFCFK)
Letters by the sisters:
    – Aachen Luisenhospital 1872–1881, Sign.: 1094
    – Cleve 1845–1854, Sign.: 1337
    – Parish Elberfeld 1846–1862, Sign.: 1787
    – Private Care 1888–1893, Sign.: DA 201.
Theodor Fliedner: Instruction für die erste Seelenpflege der Kranken, Archiv der Fliedner
    Kulturstiftung in Kaiserswerth, Sign.: Rep. II: Fb.
Theodor Fliedner: Medicinischer Cursus, Volume I–III, Sign.: Rep. II: Fd 1.3

Denominational sisters and brothers as pioneers of battlefield nursing care

Annett Büttner

In establishing the world's first Protestant deaconess motherhouse in 1836, pastor Theodor Fliedner (1800–1864) created a milestone in the history of nursing. For the first time in the history of the then 300-year-old Protestant Church, Protestant sisters were made available for nursing care. By contrast, the Catholic Church had founded sister- and brotherhoods that cared for patients as far back as the Middle Ages. After this pioneering start, there were many imitators who founded institutions for deaconesses all over Europe and in North America. Within only ten years, communities of deaconesses developed in Berlin, Paris, Strasbourg, Dresden, Utrecht and Bern, often with Fliedner's aid. In 1886 there were already 57 institutions with more than 6,300 nurses.[1] The international spread of the deaconess organisation can be likened to not-for-profit franchising.

While the Catholic associations trained their nurses only through hands-on nursing at the bedside, Fliedner had a new approach. He introduced a theoretical curriculum that was taught by a physician or an experienced nurse, and he used the textbooks that were available at the time.[2] Fliedner's work was also groundbreaking in other domains, such as care for prisoners and early years education for small children. In the middle of the nineteenth century a completely new area of work followed: nursing care on the battlefield. It is this domain that forms the topic of the present paper.

At the beginning of the nineteenth century, the military medical service in European armies was rudimentary. The military leaders generally did not pay much attention to it and hence it barely managed to fulfil its tasks. However, the massive battles that had become more typical required additional measures, and volunteer nursing care on the battlefield evolved. This process took a significant amount of time. Initially, during the anti-Napoleonic wars, there were German women's associations and the international initiatives of Florence Nightingale (1820–1910) and Henry Dunant (1828–1910). Eventually, denominational and secular volunteer male and female nurses served during the German wars from 1864 to 1870/71, which are also known as the Imperial Wars of Unification (German-Danish War 1864, Prussian-Austrian War 1866, German-French War 1870/71).[3] Since the structure of the *Red Cross* was not well developed during these wars, the denominational associations bore the main burden of volunteer nursing, and thus they can be rightfully regarded as its pioneers. In this article, I will discuss the largely unknown commitment that the *Kaiserswerth Deaconess Institute* and other deaconess mother-

1   Disselhoff (1886), p. 256.
2   Hummel (1986); Kruse (1995).
3   Grundhewer (1987), pp. 29–36; Riesenberger (1992), pp. 14–32.

houses demonstrated to nursing care on the battlefield. The nurses travelled on their own initiative to the base hospitals and gained model status for secular nurses because of the high quality of their work, their discipline, and their vocational ethos. I focus in particular on the pre-history of their services, their organisational structures and daily life at the base hospitals.[4] I was the first to analyse the archives of the motherhouses and deaconess institutions and the military records in the state archives of Saxony, Bavaria and Württemberg with a focus on volunteer nursing care on the battlefield. These sources are particularly significant, as the central archives of the Reich were almost completely destroyed during World War II and, as a result, the wartime deployment of deaconesses during the nineteenth century has remained largely unknown.[5]

The development of volunteer nursing care on the battlefield

It might be useful to begin this analysis with a brief explanation of the term "nursing care on the battlefield". In the publications at the time, this term was used more often than the alternative "care for the wounded". The reason for this is the simple fact that, until then in large wars, more soldiers had died in epidemics and from infections than in the battles themselves. During the German-French War this pattern was disrupted for the first time due to the improved care the volunteer nurses and the military medical service provided.

The issue of caring for sick and wounded soldiers has been troubling mankind for as long as wars have been in existence but it was only during the second half of the seventeenth century, after numerous interim steps, that an independent military medical service evolved.[6] The lack of funds and appreciation of the need by state and army leaders hindered its adequate development. The massive battles during the anti-Napoleonic wars of liberation clearly revealed the shortcomings of the existing medical service. More comprehensive aid measures were required. For the first time, volunteer female nurses temporarily emerged on the battlefield. These ladies came from women's associations that had been founded by members of the nobility and the upper bourgeoisie.[7]

In the following long period of peace, the military medical service in Europe continued to receive very little attention and still had a very low public profile. By contrast, civil nursing saw a renewed growth and increasing professionalisation during the heyday of Catholic orders and congregations and the development of Protestant deaconess motherhouses.

---

4   This paper draws on my doctoral dissertation on denominational nursing care on the battlefield during the nineteenth century. Cf. Büttner (2013).
5   Devantier (2008).
6   Ring (1962).
7   Frevert (1996).

Only after the disasters of the Crimean War[8] and the Sardinian War[9] at the beginning of the second half of the nineteenth century was there an international public debate about the need for reforming the military medical service. During this time, Florence Nightingale[10] and Henry Dunant[11], the first representatives of volunteer nursing care to be recognised all over Europe, proposed different methods of how to care for wounded soldiers. While Nightingale favoured expanding the military medical service, Dunant's suggestion of employing volunteers for a limited period of time was adopted because it was more cost-effective.[12] Military leaders, doctors, and politicians with a broader vision recognised the advantages of this system for the state, so that, after only a short period of preparation, the 1864 *Geneva Convention* could be signed. For the first time, the neutrality of medical services and their staff was incorporated into international law. In the following years, many regional and national *Red Cross* organisations were founded with numerous different names. This development was facilitated by members of the press who, for the first time, covered the wars and immediately informed the public about shortcomings at the base hospitals.[13] Now, base hospitals that did not meet the required standard were seen as a national disgrace. In addition, after the introduction of general conscription, soldiers were no longer mercenaries whose professional risk was to get killed or wounded, but members of all classes of society. If, for instance, the breadwinner of a family could no longer provide, in some circumstances the authorities would have had to step in and support the family.

In this setting, and with the international network of the motherhouse diaconia, it is plausible that the *Kaiserswerth Deaconess Institute* was actively involved in the development of volunteer nursing care on the battlefield.[14] As early as the end of the 1840s, its founder and leader, Theodor Fliedner, had offered to provide deaconesses and male nurses to care for Prussian soldiers. These came from troops that had fought in 1848 against the Danish independence and in 1849 had participated in the end of the revolt in the Grand Duchy of Baden. However, the Prussian military rejected these offers.[15] In hindsight, Julius Disselhoff (1827–1896), Fliedner's successor as principal of the institute, noted:

8   The Crimean War took place from 1853 to 1856 between Russia on the one side and the Ottoman Empire, France and England on the other side.
9   In the Second Italian War of Independence that is also known as the Sardinian War of 1859, the Austrian army fought against the troops of Piemont-Sardinia and France. On 24/6/1859 Dunant unintentionally became a witness to the battle at Solferino.
10   Goldie (1987). Nightingale had received major inspiration for her reforms of British nursing from Kaiserswerth. Kaiserswerther Diakonie (2001).
11   Dunant (1863).
12   Riesenberger (1992), pp. 16–17; Heudtlass (1977), p. 70.
13   Förster (1997), p. 5; Grundhewer (1987), p. 31.
14   Kaiserswerth, which was at the time still an independent town, was located in the Rhineland, which, as of 1815, belonged to Prussia. On the international network of deaconess motherhouses cf. Büttner (2006).
15   Gerhardt (1937), pp. 261, 475; AFCFK, Fliedner Estate Rep. IV a Vol. 2 Letters from Caroline Fliedner to Theodor Fliedner dated 10/7/1849 and 22/7/1849.

While King Friedrich Wilhelm IV was a friend and supporter of the issue of deaconesses in every respect, this institution – it was not yet even 13 years old – had not taken hold to such an extent that one could have comprehended the entirely new idea of sending deaconesses to war. It stayed that way until the beginning of the sixties.[16]

Initially, socially defined gender roles made the utilisation of women on the battlefield appear unthinkable.[17] As will be illustrated below, this attitude changed during the German-Danish War of 1864.

Working in base hospitals, the denominational associations not only followed the Christian-humanitarian impulse to help, but also pursued specific non-Christian objectives. Despite the unquestioned need for social organisations within the Protestant churches, the foundation of the cloister-like community of a deaconess motherhouse was regarded with suspicion, even within German Protestant circles. Due to this immense pressure from the outside and the strained financial situation, especially during the first decades of the deaconess movement, close connections to the bourgeoisie and aristocratic upper classes were crucial for its survival. The deaconess institute used the excellent relationship between Theodor Fliedner and the Prussian king, Friedrich Wilhelm IV (1795–1861), who was close to the Church, as a means of gaining acceptance in Protestant circles, which soon recognised the socially disciplining character of the deaconesses' work in hospitals, parishes and nurseries. For this reason, the Prussian ministry of the interior and the king supported the new institution with substantial funds, most of which were used for acquiring properties.[18] Relations with the Protestant Prussian state can thus be regarded as a key constituent for the successful foundation and development of the institution in Kaiserswerth. For its leaders and the nurses there was no question that in the event of war, the institute would help the state that had supported its development. Historians have coined the term *National Protestantism* for the ideas underlying the close connection between Protestant circles and the Prussian and later German state in the nineteenth century – the much-cited alliance of throne and altar.[19] These ideas implied a "systematic correlation" and a "true symbiosis of the religious and national element".[20] This close connection was facilitated by the structural conditions of German Protestantism. In the Protestant German states, the sovereign was simultaneously the head of the regional Churches, while in the Catholic world the Church looked towards Rome and the pope.

---

16   Disselhoff (1886), p. 207.
17   Frevert (1996); Hagemann (1998).
18   Friedrich Wilhelm IV had already visited Kaiserswerth multiple times as crown prince. In numerous personal conversations Fliedner explained his ideas and the king did not shy away from accepting theological advice from Fliedner. Fliedner helped him with the foundation of the Bethanien motherhouse in Berlin. Cf. the correspondence between the deaconess institute and the king and various government authorities in: Geheimes Staatsarchiv Preußischer Kulturbesitz Berlin, I.HA Rep. 89 Geh. Zivilkabinett No. 24390; Gerhardt (1937), pp. 44–45, 106–107, 224–226.
19   Cf. Lehmann/Gailus (2005); Hübinger (2000).
20   Krumeich (2000), p. 1.

The *Order of St. John*, which was close to the Prussian rulers, also played a crucial part in the development of volunteer nursing care in Prussia. This order provided financial support to the deaconess motherhouses, where later the majority of its sisters received their training.[21] Already at the beginning of 1857 – and thus a few years before Dunant – it had started its own initiative to provide material and personnel support for the military medical service in the event of a war.[22] In 1863, representatives from this order paved Dunant's way into the houses of the rulers and highest authorities of the various German states.

Nursing care on the battlefield, like the development of the world's first deaconess motherhouse in Kaiserswerth, also served the purpose of providing an alternative to the Catholic competition. Catholic sisters also worked as nurses during the Imperial Wars of Unification and at times there was fierce competition as to who would work in the base hospitals. The *Order of Malta*, the Catholic counterpart to the *Order of St. John*, had been revived only shortly before the German-Danish War and had not received state recognition within the German Federation.[23] Active involvement in caring for the wounded on the battlefield provided a good opportunity to demonstrate the order's usefulness. Simultaneously, the Catholic motherhouses hoped to gain secular recognition of their social work, which was not a given, and in particular not in Protestant Prussia.[24] Both denominations pursued missionary goals within the population.

As the following examples may show, the German-Danish War illustrations published by the two large denominations were quite similar in structure and message – at times they overlapped to an astonishing extent. The appearance of the deaconess from Kaiserswerth seems to have been adapted from an image of a Sister of Mercy. The latter had appeared on a collectible card that had presumably been made at the time of the war, while the illustration from Kaiserswerth only appeared in a publication from 1866.

21   Fliedner Cultural Foundation Kaiserswerth (2013).
22   Geheimes Staatsarchiv, I. HA Rep. 77, Ministerium des Innern Abt. I Generalabteilung Sect. 27 Tit. 530 No. 6: Tätigkeit des Johanniterordens im Falle eines Krieges 1857–1871, p. 10–15.
23   Twickel (1988).
24   Schweikardt (2008).

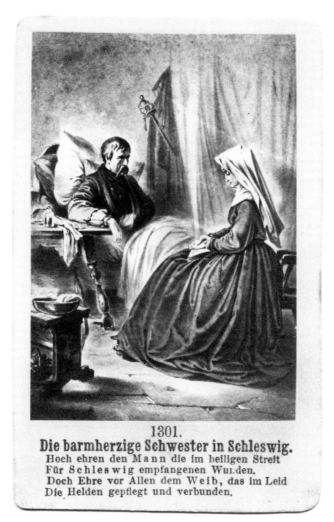

Figure 1: Sister of Mercy in the German-Danish War 1864 (Source: Photo collection in the archives of the Fliedner Cultural Foundation Kaiserswerth)

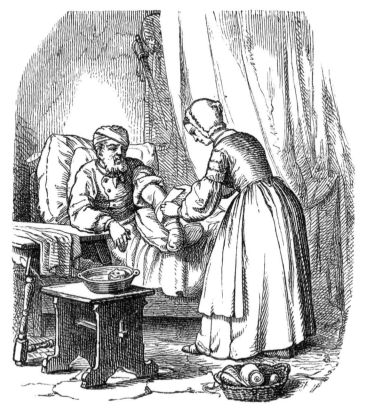

Im Kriegslazarett.

Figure 2: Deaconess in Schleswig 1864 (Source: Kaiserswerth Deaconess Institute (ed.):
Christlicher Volkskalender 1866, p. 115)

The first utilisation of denominational nurses in the German-Danish War

During the first of the three Imperial Wars of Unification, the international development of volunteer nursing care on the battlefield described previously played only an indirect role. In 1864, the secular organisations of volunteer nurses were still in the early phases of development. The committee from Geneva only sent two observers to the fighting armies. For the first time these wore the *Red Cross* brassard.[25] Apart from a few exceptions, such as the *Women's Association in Baden*, there were no non-denominational sisterhoods.[26] Secular women's associations had been founded during the time of the Imperial Wars of Unification, largely on the initiative of the wives of sovereign

25 Appia (1864).
26 Lutzer (2002); Riesenberger (2002), pp. 27–33.

princes. However, in the short intervening period they had been unable to set up qualified training programmes in nursing care. Thus the main occupation of the women in these associations was to organise wound-dressing materials and clothes for the wounded and ill soldiers. The female volunteers worked mainly behind the lines in the hospitals of the reserves. Often their amateurish work evoked criticism from the doctors, boards of motherhouses, and deaconesses.[27] Denominational nurses thus bore the main burden of volunteer care for the ill and wounded. Among them were Protestant deaconesses from Kaiserswerth and the Bethanien motherhouse in Berlin, Catholic sisters from the congregation of *St. Elizabeth* (Grey Sisters), representatives of various congregations of St. Francis, sisters from the *Order of St. Clemens* and sisters of *St. Vincent de Paul* but also deacons from *Rauhes Haus* Hamburg.

Their first deployment as nurses on the battlefield occurred entirely on the initiative of the boards of the motherhouses and deaconess institutes. After the beginning of the German-Danish War in February 1864, they had asked for assignments from the Prussian Ministry of War and other military offices, or they went directly to the battlefields of their own accord. The family ties and social contacts between the *Order of St. John* and leading employees in deaconess institutions facilitated the quick assignment of trained nurses to the base hospitals. For instance, the Mother Superior of the *Bethanien deaconess motherhouse* in Berlin, Anna zu Stolberg-Wernigerode (1819–1868), accompanied her brother, the chancellor of the *Order of St. John*, Eberhard zu Stolberg-Wernigerode (1810–1872), to Altona near Hamburg as early as 31 January 1864. Here she helped set up a base hospital and subsequently coordinated the assignment of deaconesses from her motherhouse. A contemporary reporter celebrated her as the "first deaconess who has ever been active on a battlefield".[28] Later she was dubbed the first 'war nurse'.[29]

In the light of the example set by the Berlin motherhouse, the motherhouse in Kaiserswerth also wanted to be involved as quickly as possible in caring for ill and wounded soldiers. In the month of January it had restricted itself to collecting winter clothes and dressing materials for the troops. Since no official orders came for the nurses, Fliedner's son-in-law and employee, Pastor Julius Disselhoff, travelled to Berlin on 8 February 1864 to offer the services of deaconesses and male attendants. The minister of war accepted the offer with the "most heartfelt thanks for the patriotism it revealed",[30] and he asked for ten female and two male nurses to be sent to the military hospitals in Kiel, where they would receive further instructions. Fliedner, who was already suffering severely from a lung disease, was still able to say good-bye to

27 CADN, Mutterhausregistratur B IX, Letter from Karoline Kienlein of Kissingen to principal Löhe 17/7/1866; B IXe, Letter from Löhe to Auguste Jakobi 27/8/1870. Due to their negative experiences in 1866, some deaconess motherhouses no longer worked with volunteer nurses during the German-French War. Büttner (2013), pp. 244–245, 408.

28 Wellmer (1868), p. 106.

29 Bruhn (1916), pp. 79–80.

30 AFKS, 2–1 DA 1195 Letter from Roons to the directors 11/2/1864.

his deaconesses in person. Pastor Disselhoff accompanied them to Schleswig Holstein, visiting the hospital in Altona along the way, which had been set up by the *Knights of St. John.* Here he received reliable information that the assigned hospitals had already been taken on by Sisters of Mercy and Protestant deaconesses from other houses, while there was still a high demand for aid at the Austrian hospital in Gottorf Castle in Schleswig. Changing plans, Disselhoff, the deaconesses, and male nurses reached Schleswig by train on 12 February. That same evening they received their briefing about the hospital, which did not yet have any equipment. There was chaos "comparable to an anthill that has suddenly been destroyed".[31] Approximately 500 patients – Austrians, Danes and some Prussians – were lying in their bloodstained clothes on straw mats on the floor, covered only by their coats and uncared for, so that the nurses found ample work to do.

This example illustrates the fact that while the nurses were welcomed verbally, the military did not ease their way into the hospitals and they were often forced to find their places of work themselves. Since there was no board that had an overview over all hospitals, the sisters were often also sent to places that no longer needed them. Initially the doctors looked at them with suspicion or sent them away because they were not convinced that the women could provide professional nursing care and insinuated a missionary zeal. The volunteer nurses were outside of the military structure and organisation. For that reason it was often chaotic and some nurses left because they did not find work.

Only once they had proven their usefulness in the course of the war were they purposefully called to the military hospitals. Their professional vocation in particular differed significantly from that of the military orderlies, many of whom were recruited among the invalid soldiers and had received very little training.[32] An independent observer attested to the orderlies' inactivity. Dr Klein, a chief staff surgeon from Württemberg, wrote:

> The orderlies are even more useless [than the hospital assistants]. In terms of nursing, most work was accomplished by the sisters and brothers which, in turn, had the effect of course, that the orderlies did absolutely nothing.[33]

The volunteer nurses followed two main strategies for their work during the next two wars: using individual initiative to get organised and improvising under extremely difficult circumstances. The following statement by a field deacon can be understood as a depiction of conditions that were typical: "I had to create my larger sphere of action by myself."[34]

The sisters and brothers had to master an everyday life as nurses in the base hospitals for which they had barely been prepared in their previous work. This applied even to the professional side of things, as they had very

---

31   Disselhoff (1886), p. 207.
32   As of 1832 in Prussia there was the profession of the military surgeon assistant and, as of 1852, the military orderly. Büttner (2013), pp. 36–40.
33   HSA Stuttgart, E 271 c Kriegsministerium Nr. 2153, Report by Dr Klein Aug. 1864, p. 12.
34   Fliegende Blätter 8 (1870), p. 262.

little knowledge about gunshot wounds and had not been trained as surgical assistants. Furthermore, psychologically they had to deal both with omnipresent death and their helplessness in the face of immeasurable numbers of patients. Simultaneously, they were lacking the most essential nursing accessories. The physical burden they endured during the three Imperial Wars of Unification is comparable to that of the soldiers: on the one hand there was the difficult journey to the front, involving open farm carts in the cold of winter and rain, on the other hand there was the danger of becoming ill or wounded themselves as they were very close to the front and because of the poor accommodation and food. The volunteers found comfort and support in their community and their Christian faith. They made an effort to organise church services in their denomination at their place of assignment. The male and female principals stayed in touch through letters and tried to locate and visit all members of their associations during their journeys through the war areas. Such visits were often brief, as evidenced by an example recounted by Pastor Disselhoff from Kaiserswerth. In 1866 he was able to stop only briefly in Dermbach near Salzungen (Thuringia):

> Of course, time did not allow me to rush to them during the day. I had to use the night even though I felt very sorry to have them woken up from their sleep which they needed so desperately. At midnight, from twelve until one, we enjoyed a quiet, beautiful hour in the presence of our Lord of Peace. Then I had to jump into the coach to rush on through the stormy, rainy night.[35]

The sources I studied contain very few specific details on the kind of injuries, symptoms and treatment methods. Only the worst wounds were briefly described and only very young probationary nurses directly expressed their horror about the appearance of the wounds.[36] Most nurses addressed the large suffering in general terms and hoped for a speedy end to the war. This behaviour undoubtedly served to reassure those who had stayed home and for whom the letters were intended as signs of life.[37] However, it also corresponded to a self-image, particularly among the sisters, that prevented them from showing off with detailed descriptions of their merits. Even following specific requests from the motherhouse to report on individual patients, one nurse merely wrote that she did not know what to tell.[38] For others the experience was apparently so depressing that they avoided mentioning it to protect themselves. A biography of a nurse from Niederbronn states: "Only rarely and with the utmost reluctance would she say a few words about her experiences there. The scenes re-emerged too violently in front of her soul."[39]

---

35 Armen- und Krankenfreund 7/8 (1866), p. 132.
36 AFCFK, 2–1 DA 1193, Letter from probationary nurse Cathinka Guldberg in Dresden 30/7/1866.
37 On the comparable practices in letters written by soldiers cf. Epkenhans (2006), p. XIII.
38 AFCFK, 2–1, 1199, Letter from Marie Krause 18/10/1870.
39 These thoughts refer to the operation in the Crimean War. Cf. Pfleger (1921), p. 124. In this vein, Friederike Leithold, a deaconess from Dresden, also only shared her traumatic war experiences in 1870/71 after a few years of distance. Cf. Leithold (1899), p. 273.

Most military hospitals were provisionally set up in churches, castles, schools, inns, barns, and even stables. In 1864, for the first time, tents and barracks were used as well. Their construction was modelled on images from the American civil war.

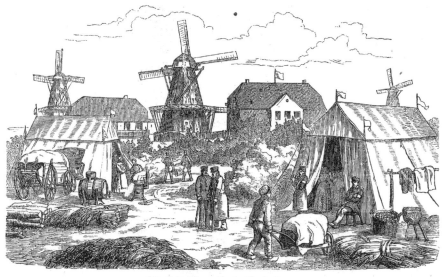

Die Kriegslazarethe in Sonderburg.

Figure 3: Tent hospital in Sonderburg/Denmark 1864 (Source: Kaiserswerth Deaconess Institute (ed.): Christlicher Volkskalender 1866, p. 118)

An innovation of the Imperial Wars of Unification was the provision of common care to all wounded, regardless of nationality. This cannot be attributed to the *Geneva Convention*, which had not yet been signed at the time of the German-Danish War. Rather, the international bias of the motherhouse diaconia facilitated this neutrality.[40] For example, in May 1864, two deaconesses from Kaiserswerth used a ceasefire to "fly from Kolding to Copenhagen like doves of peace to greet the Danish deaconesses and they were received in gracious audience by the Danish queen".[41] Such was the description – with the exaggerated heroic phrasings that were typical of the time. Danish deaconesses did not help during this war because their motherhouse had not been in existence for long enough. However, the Mother Superior had only recently returned to Denmark after her training in Kaiserswerth. Similarly, the first Mother Superiors of the deaconess institutes in Stockholm and Oslo had been trained in Kaiserswerth and subsequently transported the deaconess model to their home countries.[42] In 1864 the wounded from Denmark were

40 Büttner (2011).
41 Disselhoff (1886), p. 209. The Danish Queen Louise (1817–1898) was born Princess of Hesse-Kassel. Cf. also Büttner (2006).
42 Disselhoff (1886), pp. 330–335; Büttner (2006).

cared for by deaconesses from Stockholm, among others, some of whom had also received their training in Kaiserswerth and now greeted their sisters from Kaiserswerth in Copenhagen.[43]

Due to the work of the volunteers, the wounded and other patients often received aid faster than they would have from the Austrian military medical service, which was a very long way from the reinforcement units from home. The denominational nurses responded more flexibly to the needs of the wounded than the sluggish military medical service. Furthermore, the volunteer nurses pointed out shortcomings in the military administration and knew how to raise public awareness for these issues, such as the lack of equipment, winter clothes, and food supplies for the fighting troops at the front. Transport of the wounded was also significantly accelerated and professionalised through the involvement of the *Knights of St. John.*[44]

The denominational nurses were pioneers during the German-Danish War and the military quickly accepted them, recognising the usefulness of the women's 'invasion' of this space that had been conceptualised as an exclusively male sphere. The deaconesses had been exemplary in fulfilling the role assigned to their gender by society, which advised women to take on household and caring tasks. The acceptance of the denominational sisterhoods also resulted from the similarity of their codes of honour and conduct. With respect to their organisational structures and interior bias they shared a high affinity with the military. Thus, initially, they became the only accepted organisation in nursing care on the battlefield.[45] The different yet similar uniforms of the sisters and the military may serve as one example of this bond between the military and the denominational sisterhoods.

After this war, volunteer nursing care on the battlefield was generally accepted and could no longer be regarded as a humanitarian utopian dream.[46] During the early modern period, the main image of a woman on the battlefield had been that of a sutler travelling with the army. This picture was now superseded by the self-sacrificing 'nurse at the front'. A new myth was born.[47]

Work in the Prussian-Austrian and German-French War

The deployment of nurses in the Prussian-Austrian War of 1866 was managed for the first time by a central body, the *Royal Commissioner and the Military Inspector of Volunteer Nursing Care.* The commissioner served not only as a link to the Protestant deaconess motherhouses and deacon institutes but also to the

---

43 Gerhardt (1937), pp. 796–797 and AuKF, Jul–Aug. 1864, pp. 102 and 112–113. On the work of Swedish deaconesses and doctors cf. Gustafsson (2010), pp. 1249–1251.
44 Ressel (1866).
45 Büttner (2013), pp. 372–395.
46 Loeffler (1867), pp. IX–X.
47 The term of the nurse at the front was later largely coined through Elfriede von Pflugk-Harttung's nationalist publication about World War I, Pflugk-Harttung (1936). Cf. also Panke-Kochinke (2002), p. 28.

Catholic *Order of Malta* and the Sisters and Brothers of Mercy. At the time, this was seen as a way of immediately securing "a contained, strictly disciplined, ever ready and experienced base for practical nursing".[48] Yet since the commissioner had been appointed only shortly before the beginning of the war, he was not yet able to set up a thorough organisation of volunteer nursing care on the battlefield. Subsequently this role proved so successful that it was kept until World War II. During the first decades it was always the principal of the *Order of St. John* who was appointed to this position.

During the German-French War we can see attempts to integrate volunteer nursing care on the battlefield into the military medical service, for instance, when nurses were assigned to specific units of the army. However, since they often did not march out with them or followed only after the base hospitals had been dismantled, they were forced to reach their next destination at their own risk. In doing so, the nurses, who were used to the discipline of the motherhouse, exhibited a high level of improvisational talent and personal initiative. In 1870, for instance, a group of deaconesses from Neuendettelsau travelled independently through occupied France to get to their assigned destination, stopping in between at the houses of Catholic orders.[49] Similarly, sisters from other institutions for deaconesses moved independently through occupied terrain.[50]

In 1870/71, 220 Sisters from Kaiserswerth alone worked in base hospitals, 76 of whom were located near French battlefields. They were supported by five male attendants sent along by the principals of the institute. 144 worked in the hospitals of the reserves at home, many of which were set up in hospitals where deaconesses were already working.[51] The quota of nurses that were sent out in relation to their total number was nearly 40%, which had repercussions for their civilian areas of work, particularly in the Church parishes.[52] The sisters' deployment lasted at times for the entire duration of the war; one of them worked in base hospitals for 252 days.[53]

Nearly every association had to mourn victims of infectious diseases among their own members, since typhus, cholera and dysentery were constant companions of war. The funerals these sisters received were held with military honours, as the chronicles of the motherhouses and the sisters' letters describe with some pride.[54] These funerals wove their deaths into the secular symbolism of victims of war and epitomised society's high respect for their work. Through this ritual they were granted a female version of male heroism and the commemorative plaque in Kaiserswerth is an eloquent example of this.

---

48   Fontane (1979), Vol. 2, p. 312.
49   Correspondenzblatt Neuendettelsau 9 (1870), pp. 39–42.
50   Fröhlich (1880), pp. 35–37.
51   AFCFK, 2-1, 1201, 1200.
52   Disselhoff (1886), pp. 214, 221.
53   AFCFK, 2-1, 1201.
54   Cf. Büttner (2009), pp. 146–148.

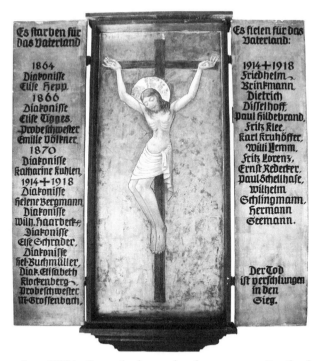

Figure 4: Plaque from 1933 in the motherhouse church commemorating the deaconesses from Kaiserswerth who passed away during their hospital service (Source: Photo collection from the archives of the Fliedner Cultural Foundation Kaiserswerth)

The male nurses had been recruited in 1864 from the brothers of *Rauhes Haus*[55] in Hamburg, who worked in the base hospitals of the *Order of St. John*[56] In 1866, volunteers and deacons from *Rauhes Haus*, the *Johannesstift Berlin*, and the institution for deacons in Duisburg worked in the base hospitals. They came under the Prussian field diaconia that had been founded in 1866 by Johann Hinrich Wichern (1808–1881). In Bavaria they were part of the *Field Diaconia of Erlangen*.[57] The volunteers were mainly students but also craftsmen and self-employed workers, and full-time deacons led their operations. The founder of the *Field Diaconia of Erlangen*, consistorial councillor August Ebrard (1818–1888), defined the new role as follows: "Field deacons are men who devote themselves in the strength of Christian faith and Christian love – voluntarily and without compensation – to the care, rescue and nursing of the wounded in the field, in other words the theatre of war."[58] The deployments were mostly very brief due to the fact that "the initial task of the field diaconia is not to provide city hospitals with caretakers who subsequently work for

55   Schmuhl (2005).
56   Büttner (2013), pp. 108–120.
57   Büttner (2013), pp. 108–121, 166–186 and 259–271.
58   Ebrard (1866), p. 3.

weeks on end as nurses, but rather to bring quick and massive aid to the places where a battle is being fought or has been fought and where the misery is immense at that very moment."[59]

Corresponding to the intentions of the *Inner Mission*, the field diaconia's role also involved providing spiritual care to support the military clergymen and distributing religious scripts to maintain and strengthen the Christian spirit in the army. Just as in 1864, additional areas of work included supporting the members of the *Order of St. John*, administering donations, and accompanying transports of the wounded back to the homeland. Fritz Fliedner coined the very appropriate term "kriegerisches Mädchen für alles" (military gofer) for the field deacons of the year 1866.[60]

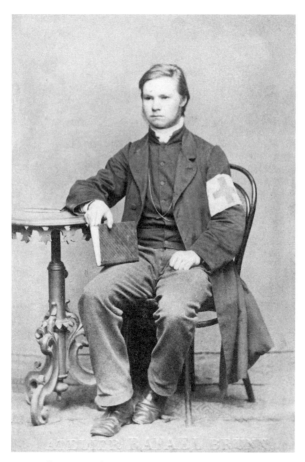

Figure 5: Fritz Fliedner (1845–1901), a son of Theodor Fliedner, as Prussian field deacon in Brünn (1866) (Source: Photo collection from the Fliedner Cultural Foundation Kaiserswerth)

59   Ebrard (1866), p. 36.
60   Fliedner (1901), p. 273.

While the letters written by the deacons from France provided descriptions of their deployment, with at times great attention to detail, they also focussed on the immense physical and psychological burden that could only be endured through their Christian motivation. The first report from the summer of 1870 already illustrates what the young men had to expect who – only a minute earlier – had been leading the life of a civilian:

> You will allow me to omit the description of the field covered in blood and the misery there. You will believe me though that at times I nearly collapsed and fainted because of all the pain and overexertion. As a companion of the surgeon generals W. and B., I have become used to the most horrible operations and amputations. Nonetheless, the feelings that you thought were dead, come to life again at the whimpering and moaning of the wounded and the sight of the dying [soldiers].[61]

Physicians and nurses often worked to the limits of their capacity. After the Battle of Wörth, in Reichshofen, approximately 11 field deacons were responsible for the care of 1,400 wounded. They barely had any sleep for eight days and even organised the transport of the patients with minor wounds back to Germany.[62]

The sisters and brothers of denominational associations working in the base hospitals during the Imperial Wars of Unification played a significant role in the establishment and further development of volunteer nursing care on the battlefield in general. As mentioned above, the work of the deaconesses and Catholic sisters convinced the initially sceptical leadership of the military medical service of the usefulness of deploying female nurses in a domain that had previously been dominated by men. In addition they became a model for new secular foundations such as the nursing organisations of the Red Cross that – at least in Germany – adopted the motherhouse system.[63]

Male field deacons distinguished themselves from non-denominational volunteers in their motivation, commitment and discipline, and facilitated thus the successful establishment of the Red Cross symbol. Because of untrained individuals with a low professional ethos who, in 1866, had travelled under the symbol of the Red Cross, all volunteers had been discredited.[64] It was an obvious fact

> that a large number of lowlifes marauded behind the frontline, wearing the brassard from Geneva, and Austrian officers reported that the emperor had explicitly given the order to shoot at all red crosses before he himself signed up to the Geneva Convention.[65]

Similarly, during the German-French War, numerous secular volunteers had flooded occupied France to satisfy their tourist curiosity and craving for sensation. They showed very little interest in nursing wounded and ill soldiers and

---

61   Letter from an unknown field deacon from the headquarters of the crown prince to Johann Hinrich Wichern 06/8/1870. Cited after: Fliegende Blätter 8 (1870), p. 259.
62   Report by Rathmann, a preacher, to the Central Committee for the Inner Mission on his journey to France in August 1870. Cited after: Fliegende Blätter 9 (1870), pp. 261, 280.
63   Riesenberger (2002), pp. 90–91; Büttner (2013), pp. 372–395.
64   Brassards with the symbol were offered for general sale. Erfahrungen (1867), p. 37.
65   Fliegende Blätter, Beiblatt 9 (1866), pp. 142–143.

the military had to use considerable efforts to remove them again.[66] The organisations of the *Red Cross* had not selected them carefully enough and many "visiting supporters" had undertaken the journey of their own accord. Since there was no strict organisation "there were some excesses that not only could not be excused but that were bad enough to discredit the white brassard".[67] Some even talked about a fiasco. The shortcomings caused the commander-in-chief of the Third Army, Crown Prince Friedrich Wilhelm (1831–1888) to issue an order on 22 August 1870 taking vigorous action against them. It determined that civilians who wore a *Red Cross* brassard but could not show an ID issued by an authorised body were to be immediately arrested and sent back home.[68] There was no longer a place for spontaneous auxiliary forces in occupied France.

Despite verbal expressions of friendliness for volunteer nursing, some military commanders had not yet realised the significance of a well-functioning medical service.[69] In particular they were unwilling to give up the monopoly of military strategy and tactics in favour of humanitarian needs. Equipment for the base hospitals was not transported at the same time the troops were moved, and in many battles it was not available. Often the more flexible denominational nurses and the doctors accompanying them reached the site before the military arrived and organised the initial care of the wounded, thus transforming what was intended to be a subsidiary activity into a primary task. At times it took days until the base hospitals were taken over by the military, at others they were left completely in the administration of the volunteer nursing staff.

In July 1866, for instance, two-thirds of the approximately 26,000 wounded after the battle of Sadowa had to be taken care of by volunteers. Pastor Disselhoff wrote about the deployment of deaconesses from Kaiserswerth:

> The main base hospital in the school was immediately taken on by four deaconesses. The wounded were lying not only in the rooms, but on carts in front of the building, on the street, against the walls of the building, downstairs in the corridor and upstairs in the halls. If one could get a fresh bundle of straw, one was happy. Furthermore, new transports with wounded soldiers arrived day and night, others were transported elsewhere. In between one could hear the loud screams and whimpering or the bleak moaning and the

---

66 In the German-French war alone, approximately 15,000 ID cards were issued to volunteers. Many had made the *Red Cross* brassards themselves. Cf. Sanitäts-Bericht (1884), p. 409.

67 Wichern (1886), p. 82; Seyferth (2007), pp. 424–425.

68 The bodies authorised to issue ID papers were: the *Royal Commissioner for volunteer nursing care in Prussia* (*Königliche Kommissar für die freiwillige Krankenpflege in Preußen*), the *Royal Military Commissioner in Bavaria* (*Königl. Militärkommissar in Bayern*) and the *Aid Association Württemberg* (*Württembergische Hilfsverein*). In November, the number of eligible groups was extended to span all delegates for the army and main frontlines of the *Royal Commissioner*. Sanitäts-Bericht (1884), Beilage 102, p. 275; Bericht über die Thätigkeit (1871), pp. 40–42; Grundhewer (1987), p. 38; Seyferth (2007), pp. 428–429.

69 During the German-French War only 18.8 % of the wounded returned to their units healed. In contrast, it was 88 % during World War I, a war that lasted significantly longer. Bleker (1987), p. 17.

sighs of the severely hit. There was not a single space in the building for the nurses to get a minute of rest. I occupied for them a tiny room that had one window. During the day it was the place for surgeries and amputations so that the blood was flowing on the floor boards. In the evening the nurses cleaned the floor, put down straw and straw bundles and lay down the way they were. In the morning, they moved everything away and the blood work began all over again.[70]

The sisters from Kaiserswerth who had travelled to Dresden in 1866 also worked to the limit of endurance. There they set up the base hospital in the cadet house. During the last days of June, hundreds of wounded soldiers arrived after the battles in Bohemia. There were also deaconesses from the *Elisabeth Hospital* in Berlin and Sisters of Mercy who cared for them.

The minute we had bedded, dressed and refreshed 150 wounded in the room of our deaconesses, the message came: Get them ready for transport! Because the arrival of new trains with injured soldiers had been scheduled. In 18 hours the whole room was filled, emptied, and refilled. During the first days of emergency, their [the deaconesses'] work nearly exceeded human strength. From 5 in the morning until nearly 11 at night they worked non-stop, went from one bedstead to the next, hastened from one horrible wound to an even more severe one. The doctors rotated but there was no relief for the nurses.[71]

Nonetheless, deployment in the base hospitals also had a tourist aspect for the nurses, who got to see countries and landscapes which they would never have seen otherwise. Their letters regularly contain descriptions of regional peculiarities, where possible with pictures in the letterhead.[72]

---

70   Der Armen- und Krankenfreund 7/8 (1866), p. 122.
71   Der Armen- und Krankenfreund 7/8 (1866), pp. 120–121.
72   During their return journey from their service in the base hospital, the Dresden deaconesses and their principal visited the Wartburg near Eisenach, which – because of Martin Luther's stay – is a particularly important place of remembrance for Protestants. Cf. Leithold (1899), p. 269.

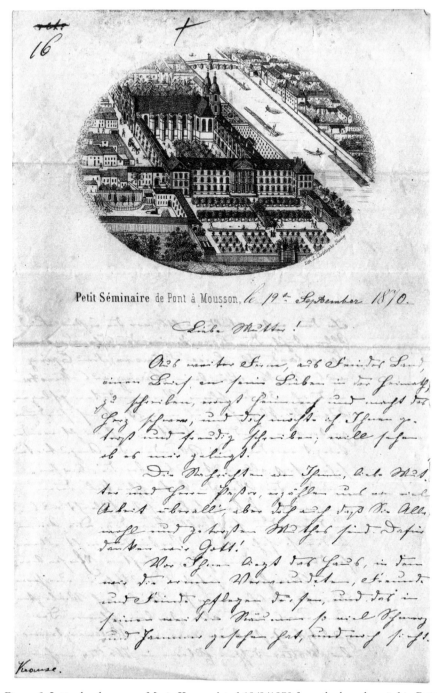

Figure 6: Letter by deaconess Marie Krause dated 19/9/1870 from the base hospital in Petit Séminaire de Pont à Mousson with a picture of a Premonstratensian abbey that hosted the base hospital. (Source: AFCFK 2–1, DA 1199)

For some deaconesses from Neuendettelsau, the highlight of their stay in the Palace of Versailles was attending the celebration for the proclamation of the German Reich in the Hall of Mirrors. They had managed to sneak into the hall through an antechamber without being noticed. Hidden behind standard bearers at the front they observed the scene in direct proximity without being seen themselves. Full of pride and self-confidence, the deaconess Sara Hahn wrote to Neuendettelsau: "Had we not gone inside, there would have been someone missing as we were the only ladies there anyway in that room full of important and less important uniforms of the German Reich."[73]

Even politically inactive deaconesses felt pride in the whole Reich rather than in an individual German nation, which was kindled by the knowledge of having been an eye-witness to a national event of historical importance and of having connected their own lives to the destiny of the country. Soon afterwards, Sara Hahn found the sheet music of Preludes by Bach and Phantasies by Mendelssohn and played them on the piano in the evening, an event that caused her to express her German-national convictions: "I was so happy to discover that music. France does not deserve to own those sheets."[74]

Despite their at times traumatic experiences in the base hospitals, the nursing staff did not question the war as such. The issue at hand was – in line with humanitarian progress – to minimise its negative outcome. As Niklas Luhmann has illustrated, it is one of the peculiarities of social institutions not to question the causes within society that necessitate their aid work in the first place. They merely work "on resolving issues that constantly re-appear as a result of implementing the existing structures and patterns of distribution. It is not their task, nor the task of aid, to come up with ideas for changing the structures that cause the concrete situations that require assistance."[75] Thus it does not come as a surprise that none of the sources I consulted contained a fundamental criticism of the war. Generic comments about the incredible misery that accompanied it were common, linked to the hope for a speedy end to the war and for peace.

Further development until World War I

The deployment of denominational and secular organisations during the Imperial Wars of Unification had revealed the opportunity for the development of volunteer nursing care as an addition to the military medical service. The latter was concerned primarily with practical rather than humanitarian issues. The goal was to maintain the combat strength of the army through quick recovery of the patients and wounded and to secure the workforce of fighting

---

73 Rößler (1982), p. 185. The original of the letter has not been preserved.
74 Correspondenzblatt Neuendettelsau 2 (1871), p. 5.
75 Luhmann (1975), p. 35.

civilians for the time after the war so as to minimise the funds needed for in-valid veterans.[76]

The development of volunteer nursing care after the Imperial Wars of Unification is a clear sign that the usefulness of the largely female volunteer denominational nurses was generally accepted. Yet there was no intention of actively involving them in the military organisation and leadership. Despite their achievements during the previous wars, the wartime medical regulations (*Kriegssanitätsordnung*) of 1878 allowed them only a subordinate role in the rear of the fighting troops and placed them under the para-military leadership of the *Imperial Commissioner* and the military courts.[77] In this way, the Ministry of War took into account the demands of the military and political authorities when incorporating and adapting volunteer nursing to military needs, and prevented the founding of parallel organisations.

Gustave Moynier (1826–1910), the president of the International Commit-tee of the *Red Cross* gained the impression that the high-ranking officers "ac-corded the patriotism of the Germans the privilege – like a favour – of laying their gifts at the feet of the military authority, which reserved the right to dis-pose of them as it saw fit [...]".[78] The sisters and brothers were merely per-ceived as cost-effective and efficient resources that were utilised with increas-ing effectiveness. The military administration exploited their self-sacrifice for the goals of the military medical service without granting them or the leader-ship of the motherhouses any say.

This becomes particularly evident when we consider the involvement of the sisters and deaconesses during the mobilisation plans from the end of the 1880s onwards. To obtain a precise overview over the numbers of available "trained [...] and morally reliable"[79] sisters in the event of war, the mother-house administrations reported the figures empire-wide from 1882 onwards to the regional organisations of the *Red Cross* or the *Order of St. John* once a year.[80] In return, these associations shared the costs of equipping the sisters. For each, a suitcase with items for personal use and wound dressing was purchased that was intended exclusively for deployment in war and was not allowed to be used in times of peace. The guiding principle was that each sister should take as much as she would need for four weeks and as much as she was able to

---

76   Riesenberger (2002), p. 59; Riesenberger (1992), pp. 46–47.
77   Kriegs-Sanitäts-Ordnung (1878), p. 179–181. In the Bavarian army, the subordination of private individuals to the military courts had occurred in 1870. Cf. Kriegsarchiv Mün-chen, Kriegsministerium B1212, Letter with illegible signature from St. Aubin 23/8/1870 to the delegate Prince of Thurn and Taxis.
78   Moynier (1883), p. 28.
79   Criegern-Thumitz (1890), p. 215.
80   Cf. among others Archive of the Stift Bethlehem Ludwigslust, 339. The number of sisters reported by this motherhouse increased from 16 in 1882 to 50 in 1908. For the Kaisers-werth motherhouse the number increased from 130 to 160 deaconesses. Cf. AFCFK 2–1, 517, 1205, 1209. For the Neuendettelsau motherhouse: CADN, Mutterhausregistratur B IX e Fasc. 8.

carry herself.[81] In March 1898, the *Imperial Commissioner* issued a secret order to the Central Committee of the regional organisation of the *Red Cross* to submit lists in the future that not only contained the total number of nursing staff but also the names of the available nurses. This measure was intended to ensure "that only truly useful and reliable staff are chosen for the special service, in short that only premium staff and material were assigned."[82]

Now the denominational sisters were an integral part of the national army logistics. The employment contracts that the deaconess motherhouses entered into on behalf of the serving deaconesses with the communities, nurseries, hospitals and other institutions that they staffed were amended to include an additional section that regulated the immediate recall of the sisters from the outposts to serve in base hospitals in times of war.[83] With this measure the number of nurses available for the military medical service could be significantly increased. Community deaconesses tended to be called up first, since they could be most easily spared. The hospitals were to serve as reserve hospitals and expected an increased number of patients in times of war. The deaconess motherhouses alone kept 54 reserve hospitals ready at the turn of the twentieth century. Together with the 42 hospitals of the *Order of St. John* and the 25 hospitals of the *Red Cross*, there were 40,000 beds available in the so-called associated hospitals of the reserve in the event of war.[84] Of the 5,482 deaconesses living in Germany in 1890, approximately 1,200 (21%) were prepared for the event of war.[85]

Apart from a few exceptions, the male field diaconia remained a unique feature of the Imperial Wars of Unification.[86] Their successor was the *Genossenschaft freiwilliger Krankenpfleger im Kriege* (*Association of Volunteer Workers in Medical Care*) that was initially set up by *Rauhes Haus* in Hamburg. From the very beginning it was a part of the *German Red Cross.*[87] The full-time deacons were drafted for regular military service or worked in base hospitals of the *Order of St. John.*

81   AFKCFK 2–1, 517, Protocol of the confidential conference of German deaconess houses of 9/3/1887 in Berlin. CADN Mutterhausarchiv, G II d 1.12, Letter from the foreman of the Order of St. John in Bavaria 6/5/1912.

82   Archive of the Stift Bethlehem Ludwigslust, 339, Letter from the Imperial Commissioner and military inspector of volunteer nursing care, Prince zu Solms-Baruth, 1/3/1898. The institutions for deacons also complied with the request to draw up such lists. Giese (1916), p. 3.

83   AFKCFK 2–1, 517, Protocol of the confidential conference of German deaconess houses of 9/3/1887 in Berlin, p. 2.; CADN Mutterhausarchiv, G II d 2.9 Draft of a letter regarding the service of the deaconesses during the war, n.d.; Archive of the Stift Bethlehem Ludwigslust, 339, Letter from the Stift Bethlehem Ludwigslust deaconess house 31/7/1897.

84   Cf. Cramer (1904), p. 27.

85   Criegern-Thumitz (1890), p. 217.

86   Cf. Giese (1916); Häusler (1995), p. 76.

87   Büttner (2013), pp. 412–417.

Thus the field diaconia became another example of the general phenomenon of how the state took over new types of tasks that the Inner Mission had previously performed and that were born of social affliction. Subsequently, the state ousted the volunteers from this area of work, which was by that point centrally organised.[88]

Conclusion

In the light of the achievements of denominational sisters and brothers on the battlefield, contemporaries regarded their first deployment as war nurses during the Imperial Wars of Unification both as useful and successful. Hence it became a model for future wars. The military also noted how the work of the *Order of St. John* and its subordinate deaconess motherhouses in particular raised public awareness of volunteer nursing, which led to its widespread recognition. It was during the German Imperial Wars of Unification that, for the first time, patients and wounded soldiers received care regardless of their nationality. The international network of the deaconess motherhouses made the sisters less prone to national pathos and facilitated contact with the wounded from the opposing side, allowing them to see them as patients in need and not as enemies. This was already the case during the German-Danish War of 1864, which took place before the *Geneva Convention* was signed. The first Mothers Superior of the Scandinavian motherhouses had been trained in Kaiserswerth and stayed in close contact with it until the end of their lives.

During the Imperial Wars of Unification, since there were hardly any secular associations of nurses such as the *Red Cross*, the denominational associations bore the main burden of the work. Their professional ethos and their organisational structures became the pattern in Germany for secular organisations in the area of volunteer nursing. Finally, while emphasising their supportive role for the state, we must not forget that numerous soldiers owed their lives to their work.

Bibliography

Literature

Appia, Louis: Les Blessés dans le Schleswig pendant la guerre de 1864. Rapport présenté au comité international de Genève. Geneva 1864.
Armen- und Krankenfreund. Eine Zeitschrift für die Diakonie der evangelischen Kirche [Friend of the poor and the sick. A publication of the diaconia of the Protestant Church]. Kaiserswerth, 1849–1939.
Bericht über die Thätigkeit der vom Militair-Inspecteur geleiteten Deutschen freiwilligen Krankenpflege während des Krieges 1870–1871. Berlin 1871.
Bleker, Johanna: Medizin im Dienst des Krieges. Krieg im Dienst der Medizin. In: Bleker, Johanna; Schmiedebach, Heinz-Peter (ed.): Medizin und Krieg. Vom Dilemma der Heilberufe 1865 bis 1985. Frankfurt/Main 1987, pp. 13–28.

88   Häusler (1995), p. 76.

Bruhn, E: Die erste Kriegsschwester. In: Der Reichsbote. Deutsche Wochenzeitung für Christentum und Volkstum, Sonntagsblatt 14/5/1916, pp. 79–80.

Büttner, Annett: Das internationale Netzwerk der evangelischen Mutterhausdiakonie. In: Women in Welfare. Soziale Arbeit in internationaler Perspektive. In: Ariadne. Forum für Frauen- und Geschlechtergeschichte 49 (2006), pp. 64–71.

Büttner, Annett: "Der Herr ist meines Lebens Kraft, vor wem sollte ich mich fürchten?" Die religiöse Deutung des vorzeitigen Todes durch evangelische Diakonissen im 19. Jahrhundert. In: Historical Social Research 34 (2009) 4, pp. 133–153.

Büttner, Annett: Pflege über Grenzen. Die Konfessionelle Krankenpflege in den Deutschen Reichseinigungskriegen. In: Kozon, Vlastimil (ed.): Geschichte der Pflege. Der Blick über die Grenzen. Vienna 2011, pp. 233–244.

Büttner, Annett: Die Konfessionelle Kriegskrankenpflege im 19. Jahrhundert. (Medizin, Gesellschaft und Geschichte 47) Stuttgart 2013.

Correspondenzblatt der Diaconissen von Neuendettelsau. Neuendettelsau, 1866–1871.

Cramer, Hermann: Militärische und freiwillige Krankenpflege in ihren gegenseitigen Beziehungen, unter besonderer Berücksichtigung des neuen Teils VI der Kriegssanitätsordnung vom 18.12.1902. Stuttgart 1904.

Criegern-Thumitz, Friedrich von: Lehrbuch der freiwilligen Kriegs-Krankenpflege beim Heere des Deutschen Reiches. Leipzig 1890.

Devantier, Sven Uwe: Das Heeresarchiv Potsdam. In: Archivar. Zeitschrift für Archivwesen 4 (2008), pp. 361–369.

Disselhoff, Julius: Die Kaiserswerther Diakonissen in den Kriegslazaretten. In: Der Armen- und Krankenfreund (1866), pp. 118–135.

Disselhoff, Julius: Die Arbeit unserer Diakonissen im Krieg. In: Jubilate! Denkschrift zur Jubelfeier der Erneuerung des apostolischen Diakonissen-Amtes und der fünfzigjährigen Wirksamkeit des Diakonissen-Mutterhauses zu Kaiserswerth am Rhein. Kaiserswerth 1886, pp. 207–221.

Dunant, Henry: Eine Erinnerung an Solferino. Basel 1863.

Ebrard, August: Die evangelische Felddiakonie in Baiern in dem deutschen Bundeskriege 1866. Erlangen 1866.

Epkenhans, Michael; Förster, Stig; Hagemann, Karen: Einführung. Biographien und Selbstzeugnisse in der Militärgeschichte – Möglichkeiten und Grenzen. In: Epkenhans, Michael; Förster, Stig; Hagemann, Karen (ed): Militärische Erinnerungskultur. Soldaten im Spiegel von Biographien, Memoiren und Selbstzeugnissen. Paderborn 2006, pp. IX–XVI.

Erfahrungen aus dem Krieg von 1866 über die Organisation der freiwilligen Hülfsthätigkeit und die Genfer Uebereinkunft von 1864 zur Verbesserung des Looses der im Felddienst verwundeten Militär-Personen. In: Mittheilungen der in den Feldhospitälern am Main thätig gewesenen Herren an den Hülfsverein im Grossh. Hessen für die Krankenpflege und Unterstützung der Soldaten im Felde. Darmstadt 1867.

Fliedner, Fritz: Aus meinem Leben. Erinnerungen und Erfahrungen. Berlin 1901.

Fliedner-Kulturstiftung Kaiserswerth: Der Johanniterorden und die Mutterhausdiakonie. Düsseldorf 2013.

Fliegende Blätter aus dem Rauhen Hause zu Horn bei Hamburg. Hamburg, 1864–1871.

Fontane, Theodor: Der deutsche Krieg von 1866, 2 vols., (1st edition Berlin 1870/71) 2nd edition Düsseldorf 1979.

Förster, Stig; Nagler, Jörg (ed.): On the road to total war. The American Civil War and the German Wars of Unification 1861–1871. Cambridge 1997.

Frevert, Ute: Nation, Krieg und Geschlecht im 19. Jahrhundert. In: Hettling, Manfred; Nolte, Paul (ed.): Nation und Gesellschaft in Deutschland. Munich 1996, pp. 151–170.

Fröhlich, Heinrich: Die Thätigkeit des Dresdner Diakonissenhauses in dem deutsch-französischen Kriege. Dresden n. d. [c. 1880].

Gerhardt, Martin: Theodor Fliedner. Ein Lebensbild, Vol. 2, Düsseldorf 1937.

Giese, Hermann: Evangelische männliche Felddiakonie 1914–16 der Duisburger Diakonen-Anstalt. Duisburg 1916.

Goldie, Sue M.: "I have done my duty". Florence Nightingale in the Crimean War 1854–56. Manchester 1987.

Grundhewer, Herbert: Von der freiwilligen Kriegskrankenpflege bis zur Einbindung des Roten Kreuzes in das Heeressanitätswesen. In: Bleker, Johanna; Schmiedebach, Heinz-Peter (ed.): Medizin und Krieg. Vom Dilemma der Heilberufe 1865 bis 1985. Frankfurt/Main 1987, pp. 29–44.

Gustafsson, Tomas: Svenska läkare vid fronten i dansk-tyska kriget 1864 [Swedish doctors at the front in the second Schleswig war in 1864]. In: Läkartidningen. Journal of the Swedish medical association, 18 (2010), pp. 1249–1251.

Hagemann, Karen: Venus und Mars. Reflexionen zu einer Geschlechtergeschichte von Militär und Krieg. In: Hagemann, Karen (ed.): Landsknechte, Soldatenfrauen, Nationalkrieger. Frankfurt/Main 1998, pp. 13–48.

Häusler, Michael: "Dienst an Kirche und Volk". Die Deutsche Diakonenschaft zwischen beruflicher Emanzipation und kirchlicher Formierung (1913–1947). Stuttgart 1995.

Heudtlass, Willy J.: Henry Dunant. Eine Biographie in Dokumenten und Bildern. Stuttgart 1977.

Hübinger, Gangolf: Kulturprotestantismus und Politik. Zum Verhältnis von Liberalismus und Protestantismus im wilhelminischen Deutschland. Tübingen 1994.

Hummel, Eva-Cornelia: Krankenpflege im Umbruch (1876–1914). Freiburg/Breisgau 1986.

Kaiserswerther Diakonie: Florence Nightingale. Kaiserswerth und die britische Legende. Düsseldorf 2001.

Kriegs-Sanitäts-Ordnung vom 10. Januar 1878 [wartime medical regulations]. Berlin 1878.

Krumeich, Gerd; Lehmann, Hartmut (ed.): Nation, Religion und Gewalt. Zur Einführung. In: Krumeich, Gerd; Lehmann, Hartmut (ed.): "Gott mit uns". Nation, Religion und Gewalt im 19. und frühen 20. Jahrhundert. Göttingen 2000, pp. 1–8.

Kruse, Anna-Paula: Krankenpflegeausbildung seit Mitte des 19. Jahrhunderts. 2nd edition Stuttgart 1995.

Lehmann, Hartmut; Gailus, Manfred (ed.): Nationalprotestantische Mentalitäten in Deutschland (1870–1970). Konturen, Entwicklungslinien und Umbrüche eines Weltbildes. (Veröffentlichungen des Max-Planck-Instituts für Geschichte 214) Göttingen 2005.

Leithold, Friederike: Erinnerungen aus meinem Diakonissenleben, ed. Luise von Ketelhodt. Leipzig 1899.

Loeffler, Friedrich: Generalbericht über den Gesundheitsdienst im Feldzuge gegen Dänemark. Berlin 1867.

Luhmann, Niklas: Formen des Helfens im Wandel gesellschaftlicher Bedingungen. In: Otto, Hans-Uwe; Schneider, Siegfried (ed.): Gesellschaftliche Perspektiven der Sozialarbeit, Vol. 1. 3rd edition Neuwied; Darmstadt 1975, pp. 35–51.

Lutzer, Kerstin: Der badische Frauenverein 1869–1918. Stuttgart 2002.

Moynier, Gustave: Das Rote Kreuz, seine Vergangenheit und seine Zukunft. Minden 1883.

Panke-Kochinke, Birgit; Schaidhammer-Placke, Monika: Frontschwestern und Friedensengel. Kriegskrankenpflege im Ersten und Zweiten Weltkrieg. Ein Quellen- und Fotoband. Frankfurt/Main 2002.

Pfleger, Luzian: Die Kongregation der Schwestern vom Allerheiligsten Heilande, genannt: "Niederbronner Schwestern". Freiburg/Breisgau 1921.

Pflugk-Harttung, Elfriede: Frontschwestern. Ein deutsches Ehrenbuch. Berlin 1936.

Ressel, Julius: Die Kriegs-Hospitäler des St. Johanniter-Ordens im dänischen Feldzuge von 1864. Breslau 1866.

Riesenberger, Dieter: Für Humanität in Krieg und Frieden. Das Internationale Rote Kreuz 1863–1977. Göttingen 1992.

Riesenberger, Dieter: Das Deutsche Rote Kreuz. Eine Geschichte 1864–1990. Paderborn 2002.

Ring, Friedrich: Zur Geschichte der Militärmedizin in Deutschland. Berlin 1962.

Rößler, Hans: "Heil Dir im Siegerkranz, Herrscher des Vaterlands!" Neuendettelsau und der Krieg 1870/71. In: Unter Stroh- und Ziegeldächern. Aus der Neuendettelsauer Geschichte, ed. Rößler. Neuendettelsau 1982, pp. 184–191.

Sanitäts-Bericht über die Deutschen Heere im Krieg gegen Frankreich 1870/71, report by Militär-Medizinal-Abtheilung des Königlich Preussischen Kriegsministeriums, Vol. 1. Berlin 1884.

Schmuhl, Hans-Walter: Senfkorn und Sauerteig. Die Geschichte des Rauhen Hauses zu Hamburg 1833–2008. Hamburg 2008.

Schweikardt, Christoph: Cholera and Kulturkampf. Government decision making and the impetus to establish nursing as a secular occupation in Prussia in the 1870s. In: Nursing History Review 16 (2008), pp. 99–114.

Seyferth, Alexander: Die Heimatfront 1870/71. Paderborn 2007.

Twickel, Maximilian von: Die nationalen Assoziationen des Malteserordens in Deutschland. Die rheinisch-westfälische Malteser-Genossenschaft. In: Wienand, Adam (ed.): Der Johanniterorden. Der Malteserorden. Cologne 1988, pp. 453–481.

Wellmer, Arnold: Anna Gräfin zu Stolberg-Wernigerode, Oberin von Bethanien. Bielefeld 1868.

Wichern, Johannes: Die freiwillige Pflege im Felde verwundeter und erkrankter Krieger durch die deutschen Vereine vom roten Kreuz. Hamburg 1886.

Archives

Archives of the Fliedner Cultural Foundation (AFCFK)

1–1 Nachlass Fliedner (Fliedner estate)

Rep. IV a Vol. 2: Letters from Caroline Fliedner 1849

2–1 Diakonissenanstalt (DA) (Deaconess Institute)

516 Zusammenarbeit mit dem Johanniterorden (Collaboration with the Order of St. John) 1852–1886

517 Zusammenarbeit mit dem Johanniterorden 1887–1909

1193 Diakonissen in den Kriegslazaretten (Deaconesses in the base hospitals) 1866–1867

1194 Schwesternbriefe aus den Lazaretten in Schleswig u. a. Orten (Letters from the nurses in the base hospitals in Schleswig and other locations) 1864

1195 Krankenpflege durch Diakonissen im Deutsch-Dänischen Krieg (Nursing by deaconesses in the German-Danish War) 1864

1199 Schwesternbriefe aus den französischen Kriegslazaretten (Letters from nurses in the French base hospitals) 1870–1871

1200 Schwesternbriefe aus den Kriegslazaretten in Deutschland (Letters from nurses in the base hospitals in Germany) 1870–1871

1201 Aussendung von Diakonissen auf den Kriegsschauplatz (Sending deaconesses to the front) 1870–1871

1205 Vorbereitung für den Einsatz von Diakonissen im Kriegsfall (Preparation for deploying deaconesses in the event of war) 1905–1914

1206 Bereitschaftserklärungen von Schwestern für den Lazaretteinsatz (Declarations of intent from nurses regarding deployment in base hospitals) 1887

Central archive of the Neuendettelsau diaconia (CADN)

Mutterhausregistratur (Motherhouse registry)

B IX Briefe der auswärtigen Schwestern (Letters from external deaconesses) 1866

B IXe Anmeldung von Freiwilligen zum Lazarettdienst (Registration of volunteers for service in base hospitals) 1866, 1870

B IX e Fasc. 8 Ausbildung von Krankenpflegerinnen für den Krieg (Training of female nurses for the war) 1899–1908

Mutterhausarchiv (Archive of the motherhouse)

G II d 2.9 Diakonissendienst im Krieg (Deaconess service during the war) 1889

G II d 1.12 Bayerischer Verein zur Pflege und Unterstützung im Felde verwundeter und erkrankter Krieger (Bavarian Association for the care and support of soldiers wounded or taken ill during the war) 1895–1914

Archive of the Stift Bethlehem Ludwigslust

339 Einsatz von Schwestern im Kriegsfall (Deployment of nurses in the event of war) 1882–1911

Prussian Privy State Archives (Geheimes Staatsarchiv Preußischer Kulturbesitz Berlin)

I.HA Rep. 89 Geheimes Zivilkabinett (Secret Civil Cabinet)

24390 Verein zu Düsseldorf für christliche Krankenpflege in der Rheinprovinz und in Westfalen (Dusseldorf Association for Christian nursing in the Rhein province and in Westfalia) 1836–1843

I. HA Rep. 77 Ministerium des Innern (Ministry of the Interior)

Abt. I Generalabteilung Sect. 27 Tit. 530 Nr. 6: Tätigkeit des Johanniterordens im Falle eines Krieges (Activities of the Order of St. John in the event of war) 1857–1871

State Archives (HSA, Hauptstaatsarchiv) Stuttgart

E 271 c Kriegsministerium (Ministery of War)

2153 Bedarf an Packpferden und Ausrüstungsgegenständen (Packhorse and equipment requirements) 1864–1866

Kriegsarchiv München (War archive Munich)

Kriegsministerium, Alter Bestand (Ministry of War, old records)

B1212 Freiwillige Krankenpflege im Deutsch-Französischer Krieg (Volunteer nursing care in the German-French War) 1870–1871

Wilhelm Löhe and the nursing education of the Neuendettelsau deaconesses[1]

Matthias Honold

The first deaconess institute in Bavaria was established in Neuendettelsau in 1854 by Wilhelm Löhe.[2] Theodor Fliedner had founded the first deaconess institute in Kaiserswerth 18 years earlier and Wilhelm Löhe had been following the progress of the various motherhouses and the *Inner Mission* in general for several years. He had been attempting to set up deaconess organisations ever since 1837, when he took up office as pastor in Neuendettelsau.[3] The developments that followed the Wittenberg *Church Conference (Kirchentag)* in 1848 – at which Johann Hinrich Wichern gave his famous impromptu speech that marked the start of the organised *Inner Mission* – intensified Löhe's views of the diaconate and *Inner Mission* and led to the establishment of a women's diaconal association in Bavaria and the opening of the first Bavarian deaconess institute in 1854.

Two aspects of the *Neuendettelsau Deaconess Institute* were remarkable at the time: firstly, it was the first time an institution of this type had been established outside a town. Neuendettelsau was a village in central Franconia with just 500 inhabitants. Secondly, the institute also offered training to young women who did not intend to become deaconesses. In this, Löhe's concept differed from that of Theodor Fliedner. One of his intentions was that, once they had finished their training, deaconesses would themselves become active in towns and villages, setting up new deaconess institutions or expanding existing ones. Löhe hoped to attract rural women – a social class that generally did not have access to further education – to train up as deaconesses for his work, as the following citation shows:

"When we pastors go out into our villages to visit the sick, we find everywhere women who minister more than others to the sick and suffering because they have a talent within them that prompts them to do so. They are following a natural impulse", writes Löhe at the start of his concept paper on the *female diaconate within the Protestant church of Bavaria and the establishment of*

---

1   See also: Riedel (2004), pp. 177–189.
2   Wilhelm Löhe (1808–1872). Wilhelm Löhe was born in 1808 in the provincial Franconian town of Fürth, which had come just into the Kingdom of Bavaria. He spent his childhood and a part of his school years there. It was clear from an early age that the only possible profession for Wilhelm was that of pastor. He studied theology in Erlangen and Berlin. After his examinations, he set out on a pilgrimage. He occupied more than ten posts as a vicar and parish administrator, before taking up his first and only posting as a pastor in 1837 in the small Franconian village of Neuendettelsau. It was from here that he organised his diaconal and missionary activities, which would make him known beyond his local village and even outside of Bavaria.
3   See: Stempel-de Fallois (2001).

deaconess institutes (*Bedenken über weibliche Diakonie innerhalb der protestantischen Kirche Bayerns, insbesonderheit über zu errichtende Diakonissenanstalten*), in which he set out his thoughts and those of his friends, so as to pave the way for the opening of the first deaconess institute in Bavaria.

Having found suitable women, Wilhelm Löhe started providing education for deaconesses and young women in Neuendettelsau on 9 May 1854. Women came together here to receive an education; the motherhouse idea was not the main focus.

The deaconess institute got off to a very good start. As early as 1875, it ranks fourth in a list of motherhouses according to the number of deaconesses in service. Only the deaconess institutes in Kaiserswerth, Berlin-Bethanien and Dresden were able to report higher numbers of deaconesses. The deaconess institute in Stuttgart had the same number as the Neuendettelsau institute.[4] The *Neuendettelsau Institute* was unusual at the time because all the other deaconess institutes established in the mid-nineteenth century were located in urban areas. The *Neuendettelsau Institute* remained an anomaly throughout the middle and second half of the nineteenth century.

What then were the theoretical considerations underpinning Löhe's work?

Diaconal work in concentric circles: Benevolent societies for female diaconate and Löhe's concept of diaconal work

"What they call Inner Mission these days has its levels and limits. It is like concentric circles, like the ripples formed when a stone falls into a lake. There is the outer, human circle; then a second, narrower, Christian circle; and the third, narrowest, Church circle." This is how Wilhelm Löhe explained his views of diaconal work in 1851.[5] Once the deaconess institute was established, Löhe's practical implementation of diaconal work followed a similar structure. The assistance provided by the deaconesses was to comprise all three areas, with the inner circle – diaconal work rooted in the Church – being the most important. Later, Löhe was to say: "All diaconal work starts from the altar."[6] Here Löhe was already defining the focus of his concept of nursing within the *Inner Mission*. Outward deeds, the (physical) care of those in need, were to influence inner well-being and win back this group of people for the Church – the aim of the *Inner Mission*.

Originally, Löhe's intention was to train young women and deaconesses in Neuendettelsau who would then go back to their parishes, to their own families or to other families, to carry out diaconal work. To this end, he set up a *Lutheran women's diaconal association* (*Lutherischer Verein für weibliche Diakonie*) on 27 February 1854. The idea was that it would lead to the formation of branch associations to support deaconess institutions. Initially, branch associa-

---

4   See Jenner (2004), pp. 87–88.
5   Götz (1933) pp. 73–74 (Bericht der Gesellschaft für innere Mission 1851).
6   See: Correspondenzblatt der Diaconissen von Neuendettelsau No. 12 (1868), p. 46.

tions were set up in Nuremberg, Fürth, Altdorf, Gunzenhausen, Hersbruck and Wendelstein and took on a range of different fields of activity. However, they did not prosper. The fields of activity were not expanded and no further associations were set up. The idea failed to catch on, so Löhe decided to pursue the motherhouse model of diaconate. In addition, the deaconesses started demanding social security, which was initially to be provided through local work.

Löhe's deaconess concept

As we have seen in the passage from Löhe's *Bedenken über die weibliche Diakonie* quoted at the start, the pastor believed women represented the ideal nursing staff for his project. In a number of key texts, Löhe dealt with the image of women and his views on the deaconess role.

As early as 1852, i.e. before the deaconess institute was established, Löhe was preparing a paper on female virtue entitled *Von der weiblichen Einfalt*, which was printed a year later.[7] This paper can be seen as a key text presenting Löhe's ideas about the female diaconate. Two other fundamental papers by Löhe discuss the image of women and of deaconesses. The papers were published between 1858 and 1860 in *Correspondenzblatt* under the headings *Von den Diakonissen (On deaconesses)*[8] and *Von der Barmherzigkeit (On charity)*[9]. They were part of the teaching given to deaconesses and pupils and reveal a key focus of the teaching. For Löhe, the concept of charity was a vital element: "A deaconess is a servant of charity, how could she be otherwise than charitable," he writes.[10] For Löhe it was extremely important that trainee deaconesses thought about the concept of charity. "Servants of charity and those who are to become such should [...] receive teaching on charity itself."[11] The 74th article of Löhe's paper deals with the comprehensive education of deaconesses that he believed was necessary. "Knowledge and study, however, are not enough for the education that a deaconess should receive; her training requires suitable education and sanctification of the soul."[12] The 75th article deals with Löhe's views of the concepts of practice and talent. Löhe was fully aware that not every deaconess was well suited to every occupation, and that

---

7   See Köser (2008), p. 405.
8   See Ganzert (1962), pp. 447–453. Ganzert writes in his notes that the essay on the office and career of deaconesses according to the Word of God and history came first and foremost in deaconess teaching. Ganzert (1962), p. 704. The essay was first printed in Correspondenzblatt der Diaconissen von Neuendettelsau (1858), volumes 1 and 2.
9   See Löhe (1927). First printed in: Correspondenzblatt der Diaconissen von Neuendettelsau (1859), volumes 3 and 4 to 6 (1860) (with interruptions). Löhe had already published a similar essay under the title *Von der seligen Übung der Barmherzigkeit (On the holy practice of charity)* in Correspondenzblatt (1858), volumes 3 and 4.
10   Ganzert (1962), p. 463.
11   Ganzert (1962), p. 466.
12   Ganzert (1962), pp. 520–521.

deaconesses should be trained and put to work in areas that matched their abilities and inclinations. When it came to taking such decisions, their leaders were to assist them in making the right career choice.

In the article *Von den Diakonissen* Löhe also presents his views on the deaconess career path:

> If you want a ladder for the profession of deaconess, I give you the following:
>
> First become a maidservant and learn all household chores thoroughly, from the lowliest to the best. Shame on the young woman who does not achieve the first level.
>
> Go for a time into a nursery and learn how to look after children. Shame on the deaconess who is put to shame by the nursery nurse.
>
> Receive instruction as a teacher of young children and do not rest until you know and can do what she is expected to know and do: the task is not very great.
>
> If you have the talent for it, receive instruction as a school teacher; do not rest until you have done what you can for the girls' school, not to bring it out of the hand of the pastor, for God has set him there as a shepherd, but to hand the school over from the male school teacher into female hands.
>
> Receive instruction in how to manage the refuge house within a parish, namely the female refuge house; avoid the male refuge house and the large refuges that are unnatural and seldom last long.
>
> Receive instruction as a nurse for the sick in body and do not forget that your spiritual vocation is of greater significance than your physical role.
>
> Receive instruction in caring for those with emotional disorders: not in a rationalistic hospital or madhouse, but somewhere where people know how to use the simple remedy of God's Word for every emotional disorder.
>
> After all this, if you are able, become a parish deaconess.[13]

These objectives were implemented at the deaconess institute, which later became the motherhouse.

Would-be deaconesses were offered the appropriate teaching at the deaconess institute to enable them to climb this career ladder.

Wilhelm Löhe and nursing education

It was the first time that a German deaconess institute had been set up not in a city but in a rural area and Löhe made the most of this situation when it came to training nurses. Without any contact with the large hospitals in the cities, and therefore without the influence of hospital doctors, he was able to develop a comprehensive nursing course and implement it at the new deaconess institute.[14]

---

13   Correspondenzblatt der Diaconissen von Neuendettelsau, 2 (1858), p. 7. See also Schoenauer (2013), pp. 408–419.

14   See also Riedel (2012), pp. 39–47.

In the institute's first annual report, Löhe sets out his principles of nursing, although it should be noted here that Löhe was not only thinking of nursing, but also of training women to work in girls' schools and in childcare. This training was open to all women, including those who did not intend to become deaconesses. Löhe's concept differed from the other deaconess institutes at the time. Löhe intentionally built his *Neuendettelsau Institute* as an educational institution for women. Young women who did not plan to become deaconesses were trained alongside deaconess students. This meant that a high value was placed on the subjects covered by a general education. It also meant that additional vocational subjects were taught. The training in Neuendettelsau was therefore designed not only to provide a nursing education, but also to provide training in the areas of childcare and teaching.

The comprehensive training model developed by Löhe focused primarily on the professional arenas in which women of the mid-nineteenth century were allowed to work. Many occupations were not yet available to women. According to Löhe, the trained deaconess was to be a "light bearer in the darkness".[15] Linked to this ideal was a comprehensive education in general subjects, vocational training in nursing and teaching, and a theological preparation.

In the field of nursing education, Wilhelm Löhe's curriculum in Neuendettelsau covered three main aspects: physical care, spiritual care and general knowledge. This was an unusual approach in the mid-nineteenth century. Löhe saw humans as creatures of God, composed of body and soul, in which body and soul are in constant interaction, so that a person's mental condition has a great influence on the body. For Löhe, it was essential that the healing process be accompanied by spiritual care. In addition to faith, he repeatedly emphasised cheerfulness of spirit, focusing on "spiritual nursing". Löhe presented his views in a paper entitled *Vom Einfluß der leiblichen Krankheiten auf das psychische Befinden des Kranken, sowie die Anwendung geistlicher Mittel zur Hebung der daraus hervorgehenden Gefahr der Seele* (*On the influence of bodily diseases on the mental condition of the patient, and the use of spiritual means to avert the associated risk to the soul*). This text, which was originally dictated by Löhe to the deaconess students in class, was first published in *Der evangelische Geistliche*. In 1858, this dictated section was published as a separate document by publisher Samuel Gottlieb Liesching in Stuttgart.

In this manuscript, Löhe explores his concept of comprehensive care for both body and soul. He begins the lesson with the following words: "Man consists of body and soul. But the human soul also comprehends the spirit, so this paper talks about body, soul, and spirit".[16] In today's language, Löhe's approach would be described as 'holistic', and the concept of spirit is used from a theological perspective. Humans are connected to the triune Godhead by the Holy Spirit, which is higher than the soul. Löhe's text also addresses clinical conditions:

15 Löhe (1927), p. 124.
16 Löhe (1858), p. 5.

We are not talking here about the condition of people affected by disease, we are simply talking about the action of the body and its diseases upon the lower region of the soul, which is the seat of the emotions; we are talking, simply put, about the so-called psychological effects of physical diseases.[17]

Löhe describes the link between body and soul/spirit as follows: "The body and soul of people are in constant interaction; not that the spirit acts directly on the body, nor the body on the spirit, but the spirit affects the soul, which affects the body directly, just as, ultimately, the body acts upon the soul, and by this means also indirectly upon the spirit."[18]

It was important to Löhe that the deaconesses should internalise this relationship in their training and take it into account later on when caring for the sick. He was well aware that this was a tall order for the deaconesses: "The ability to recognise the effects of each disease on a patient's mental state is an art that we should wish every deaconess to possess."[19] In the classroom, this aspect was taught under "Pastoral care of the physically ill: those suffering from acute and chronic diseases, the infirm, the convalescent, the ailing, and the dying – the blind, the deaf, the dumb – the first visit to a patient."[20]

The dictated manuscript about the influence of physical diseases on a patient's mental state was intended by Löhe specifically for the students who had chosen nursing as their professional field of work:

Here now, my worthy students, is the introduction to the subject in the title of this dictation; and I hope that at least now you will recognise that answering this question and dealing with this subject are of major importance for those who have chosen nursing as their favourite occupation in the deaconess house.[21]

Here Löhe once again clearly indicates that training at the deaconess institute was highly differentiated and that the students were given intensive training to match their professional aspirations. This approach meant that there was no rigid lesson plan at the deaconess institute. Instead, teaching was adjusted according to the available teachers and upcoming subjects.

In a second publication from 1856, Löhe goes into his concept of spiritual nursing. In the preface to the publication entitled *Dr. Gottfried Olearius Anweisung zur Krankenseelsorge* (*Dr Gottfried Olearius's guide to pastoral care of the sick*), Löhe describes the difficulties of providing such instruction:

In the deaconess house in Neuendettelsau, instruction is given in spiritual nursing. The author has undertaken this task for two semesters and admits to having encountered many difficulties. The lack of precedent meant that he not only had to find teaching material himself, but also had to determine the scope and limits of the teaching.[22]

---

17 Löhe (1858), pp. 5–6.
18 Löhe (1858), p. 6.
19 Löhe (1858), p. 7.
20 Erster Bericht über den Fortgang und Bestand der Diakonissenanstalt zu Neuendettelsau 1854/1855, Nördlingen (1855), p. 33.
21 Löhe (1858), pp. 7–8.
22 Löhe (1871), p. III.

In the preface, Löhe writes about the teaching situation at the *Neuendettelsau Deaconess Institute* to explain the reason behind the publication. There was a lack of suitable teaching materials that students could use to revise classes and deepen their knowledge.

> The poor students either had to learn from the mouth of the teacher – and then they worried that they would not remember – or they had to take notes, for which some of them were not skilled enough, and the teacher feared his lecture would be distorted, or the teacher had to give dictation, but that takes so much time and is also a boring occupation, especially for those with little writing experience.[23]

This description also offers a glimpse into the teaching situation at the deaconess institute. While most of the girls and young women came from middle-class families, the level of education varied widely. The age range was also very large. Women up to the age of 35 years were accepted for training alongside girls as young as 16. The teaching therefore had to be adapted accordingly. In addition to the nursing education, there was general education in subjects such as reading, penmanship, German language, arithmetic, and basic theology.[24]

The importance Löhe attached to a comprehensive deaconess education, and the advantages he believed it offered over general nursing training can be seen in the following statement:

> It raises the value of the Christian deaconess service. Ultimately, anyone can learn the physical skills of nursing provided they have the right disposition for it; by contrast, psychological nursing is a high grace of God, and the pinnacle of this is pastoral love, which derives its truth from the Word of God.[25]

The second annual report from 1855 reveals that these beliefs were put into practice at the institute:

> The hospital of the institute has also done more than just accomplish its main purpose, that of giving students the opportunity to practise nursing. Some of the sick have found healing or relief and some have found something even better: an awakening to eternal life and salvation of the soul.[26]

Setting up a hospital ward within the deaconess institute must also be seen in the context of Löhe's training concept. The idea was that students would apply their theoretical knowledge from the classroom in practical nursing tasks. It was a dual-track education system, which Löhe also applied in other fields, such as in the training of kindergarten and school teachers.

---

23   Löhe (1871), p. IV.
24   See: Erster Bericht über den Fortgang und Bestand der Diakonissenanstalt zu Neuendettelsau 1854/1855, Nördlingen (1855), pp. 31–32.
25   Löhe (1858), p. 67.
26   Zweiter Bericht über Bestand und Fortgang der Diakonissenanstalt zu Neuendettelsau, Nördlingen (1855), p. 20.

Practical nursing training at the *Neuendettelsau Deaconess Institute*

As a theologian, of course, Wilhelm Löhe had no medical or nursing training. Nursing was taught by a doctor, Dr Schilffarth, a friend from the neighbouring town. The deaconesses and students had classes in nursing three times a week. The teaching was divided into three main areas: preparatory, theoretical and practical classes. In the first annual report, Dr Schilffarth provides a comprehensive overview of the teaching content:

"The preparatory part deals with knowledge in the fields of anatomy and physiology that is essential for proper nursing practice, and these subjects were taught in the following order." This preparatory part was further subdivided into three areas. The first part dealt with the parts of the human body, the second with the structure of bones, cartilage, ligaments, muscles, glands, hair, nails, fat and bone marrow, skin, and blood and other bodily fluids. The third part covered the nervous system, blood circulation, respiration, digestion and sensory organs. In this way, the deaconesses learned the basics of the structure of the human body. They were then expected to apply this knowledge to nursing.

The nursing part of the course was divided into theoretical and practical teaching. Theoretical classes were based on *Anleitung zur Krankenwartung*, an introductory nursing book by Dr Gedike, and *Lehr- und Handbuch für Bader*, a textbook and handbook for surgeons by Dr Haus. The lessons covered the following subjects:

> 1. On patient care in general; 2. On the qualities necessary for nursing; 3. On the sick room; 4. On cleaning and improving the air: a) by ventilation; b) by fumigation; 5. On warming the sick room; 6. On lights and lighting; 7. On storing equipment [...] 8. On cleanliness [...] 9. On the clothes and linen of the patient; 10. On food and drink for the patient; 11. On administering internal medicines [...] 12. On injections [...] 13. On baths [...] 14. On the use of Priesnitz's cold water therapy; 15. On compresses [...] 16. On plasters [...] 17. On rubs and ointments; 18. On various nursing implements; 19. On bedsores; 20. On assistance during blood-letting; 21. On leeches; 22. On assistance during surgical operations and autopsies; 23. On caring for the dying and the dead; 24. On precautions to be taken with infectious diseases; 25. On medical records; 26. On the treatment of simple and superficial wounds; 27. On emergency treatment in general; 28. On emergency treatment for the seemingly dead; 29. On emergency treatment for external injuries; 30. On emergency treatment for sudden internal disorders and diseases; 31. On dressings; 32. On caring for the feeble-minded and mentally sick; 33. On caring for new-born infants; 34. On caring for women in childbed.[27]

The theoretical part of the training was very comprehensive. It is interesting to note the wide range of topics covered, including medical records (see point 25) and hygiene, which included both the cleanliness of the sick room and washing the patient. The teaching covered both intensive treatment and the various nursing activities. A particular focus of the training provided in Neuendettelsau was point 32: caring for the feeble-minded and mentally sick. When

---

27   Erster Bericht über den Bestand der Diakonissenanstalt zu Neuendettelsau 1854/1855, Nördlingen (1855), pp. 35–37.

he set up the deaconess institute in Neuendettelsau, Wilhelm Löhe had set himself the task of devoting himself to the so-called lunatics and cretins, who at that time were completely marginalised.

The priority Wilhelm Löhe gave to nursing training for deaconesses is reflected in the fact that the doctor started giving lessons in nursing just three days after the deaconess institute opened.

Nursing training lasted two semesters. The theoretical part came first and took the form of lectures. Where necessary, notes were produced so that lessons could be repeated. Practical training is described by the doctor: "Finally, application of the instruction, at the sick bed in the institute and in private homes, forms the practical part of the deaconess training."[28]

Lessons given by the doctor in the first month following the opening of the *Neuendettelsau Deaconess Institute* on 9 May 1854 covered bones, ligaments, muscles, glands, fat and bone marrow, skin, hair and the nervous system and external sensory organs. Lessons were summarised in dictations and then revised in separate repetition classes supervised by the female director of the deaconess institute. The following report demonstrates the practical focus of the teaching: "At last the group of pupils was delighted when a cow's eye was dissected: it was with deep emotion that they beheld the obvious wisdom of the Lord."[29]

To summarise, we can say that Löhe developed the following principles for nursing care:
– The training concept is based on three pillars: bodily care, spiritual care and training.
– The approach is generalist and comprehensive.
– The patient is the 'object' of charity.
– Body and soul are connected. A patient's mental state affects the illness.
– Health stems from a holistic approach.
– Mental health care derives its wisdom from the Word of God.
– Spiritual health care derives its wisdom from the Word of God.
– A treatment plan is drawn up as a basis for treating the sick.
– Nursing care is based on daily prayer and intercession.
– Empathetic counselling is a component of nursing care.[30]

The practical application of knowledge after graduation

After their training in Neuendettelsau, most of the deaconesses served in hospitals, children's facilities and in parish nursing.

28   Erster Bericht über den Bestand der Diakonissenanstalt zu Neuendettelsau 1854/1855, Nördlingen (1855), p. 38.
29   Der erste Monat der Diakonissenanstalt zu Neuendettelsau, in: Correspondenzblatt der Gesellschaft für innere Mission nach dem Sinne der lutherischen Kirche, July 1854, p. 27.
30   See Riedel (2008), pp. 16–17.

Neuendettelsau deaconesses were working at the hospital in Fürth, for instance, from as early as 1856. However, their biggest operational arena, the *Nuremberg hospital*, was not taken over until 1875, after Löhe's death.

The following assessment by Hermann Beck in his monograph *Die innere Mission in Bayern diesseits des Rheins*, which was published in 1880, shows how highly the work of the Neuendettelsau deaconesses was valued:

> The work of the deaconess house enjoys recognition throughout Protestant Bavaria, even in circles that have no real connection with the Church. Evidence may be seen in the fact that the City of Nuremberg placed nursing services at the city's hospital in the hands of the Neuendettelsau deaconesses in October 1875 and has transferred to them the management of the entire inventory and kitchen. The hospitals in Fürth, Hof, Lindau, Ansbach, Kulmbach, Memmingen, Regensburg and Oettingen are also run either partially or exclusively by deaconesses.[31]

Work in the parishes, which was still being developed in the middle of the nineteenth century, was also carried out by the Neuendettelsau deaconesses in the early years: "After all this, if you are able, become a parish deaconess." This was the highest level of care, in Löhe's view. In parish nursing, deaconesses had to apply all their skills, from housekeeping to childcare and nursing. The deaconess had to prove her ability in all areas, as can be seen in the following passages detailing the work of a parish deaconess.

In 1878, a Neuendettelsau deaconess started working at the newly founded diaconal station in Ansbach, a small town in Franconia, and kept a record of her work. The report covers the first few weeks following the opening of the diaconal station and the long excerpt that follows describes her day-to-day nursing tasks:

> Monday, 4 March
> Made 16 introductory visits. Visited old Sophie Wutzer. Went to old Mrs Dorndörfer in Wolfsschlucht who has severe paralysis dorsalis agitas, prayed with her and promised to come often.
>
> Tuesday, 5 March
> Visited Mrs Dorndörfer, who was a little better, brought her wine and eggs, combed her hair and bathed her and prayed with her.
>
> Went to see Mrs Kleinod, who is sick following childbirth and whose husband is bankrupt. The new-born twins died but three living children make a lot of disturbance. Started clearing up, combed the children's hair and put them to bed in the evening.
>
> 6 March
> Spent the entire day with Mrs Kleinod, washed and dressed the children, tidied the rooms, soaked the linen for the washerwoman, instructed the maid how to clean the kitchen. Brought Mrs Dorndörfer soup at midday, on the way back visited Mrs Pfaffenberger and brought her some eggs and read to her from the Passion story, then to Mrs Stutzer, who was delighted with a picture of Christ, read to her. Later I went to Mrs Holbein, who is suffering from caries of the hip, promised to come and see to her dressings.
>
> 7 March
> Went to Mrs Kleinod in the morning, prepared the children for kindergarten, tidied the cupboards and dressers, mended some clothes for the children. At midday brought soup

31 Beck (1880), pp. 30–31.

and eggs to Mrs Holbein. Visited Mrs Pfaffenberger and read to her, brought eggs to Mrs Wellhöfer. Then back to Mrs Kleinod and in the evening changed Mrs Hohlbein's dressings.

8 March
To Mrs Kleinod early in the morning, changed Mrs Hohlbein's dressings at midday, made the bed and found her an air cushion. Visited Mrs Dorndörfer, found her very unsettled again, prayed with her. Then to Mrs Kleinod until the evening, put the children to bed and prayed with them. Then home.

23 March
Early Saturday morning at home, then took coffee to old Mr Gusten, then to Mrs Kleinod, who is very weak again, but the children are well. Later I paid two visits to a seamstress named Huber on Theresienstrasse, who has her legs in plaster, and to a consumptive young sculptor named Derzdörfer, in whom the disease is already advanced, but he appears patient and resigned. Both patients live in the same house. At midday I went to visit Mrs Hommel, found her very agitated, then home to sleep a little. Back to Mrs Hommel in the afternoon, who was calmer, then to Mrs Kleinod and old Mr Gusten and in the evening back to the Hommels for the night watch.

Tuesday 16 July
Old Mr Kögler died today. I visited him every day in the last few days. He was often not completely lucid, but he asked for prayers. I have again advised Mrs Schauffler that she should take steps to remarry her husband, from whom she is divorced, since she is living with him. I visited a really nice family, very pious, worthy people, the old ones are called Popp, the young ones are called Reichelshöfer. They live and work together. The young man has had very severe pneumonia, now he would like to be read to from time to time, and the old woman in particular is asking to be read to because she is blind in one eye and can no longer read. She says we are wretchedly poor when we can no longer read God's Word. Hearing a few words does us good but we soon hunger for more.[32]

These records illustrate clearly how varied the tasks of a parish deaconess were at the time.

Conclusion

A report in the journal *Die Diakonisse* in 1926 shows how pioneering Wilhelm Löhe's training concept had been in the middle of the nineteenth century. In an article entitled *Von der Ausbildung der Diakonissen* (*On the training of deaconesses*), Pastor Hickel from Darmstadt writes:

> The most modern of the fathers of the diaconate, Wilhelm Löhe in Neuendettelsau, went one step further. He had originally dismissed the Fliednerian view of a professional diaconate from the not unjustified concern that one should not turn Christian assistance and love into a profession for the few. So his intention was not to found a motherhouse, which would, in his view, also have been a working community in the sense of Christian love, but rather to train teachers of Christian love who, from their base in small hospitals, would then – according to his plan – get hold of local young women and train them in the service of Christian love.

---

32 Zentralarchiv Diakonie Neuendettelsau: Bestand Mutterhausarchiv Handschriften, GIIc 4.5.

However, this concept did not catch on, so Löhe followed the motherhouse approach, but without neglecting the training aspect.

> But he held fast to one point: the importance of training the nurses. It is astonishing how much he achieved here and how much he attempted to include in the purview of the deaconess. In doing so, he did the deaconess movement a great service: he showed that there is nothing superfluous for the service of Christian love in training all of an individual's abilities; rather that it is only in doing so that individuals are properly equipped to serve fully.[33]

Bibliography

Beck, Hermann: Die innere Mission in Bayern diesseits des Rheins. Hamburg 1880.

Ganzert, Klaus (ed.): Wilhelm Löhe. Gesammelte Werke vol. 4. Aus dem Kalender der Diakonissenanstalt. Neuendettelsau 1864.

Götz, Justus (ed.): Im Dienst der Kirche. Quellen und Urkunden zum Verständnis Neuendettelsauer Art und Geschichte. 2nd Edition Neuendettelsau 1933. Bericht der Gesellschaft für inneren Mission 1851, p. 73.

Hickel, Theodor: Von der Ausbildung der Diakonissen. In: Die Diakonisse, Januar 1926, pp. 14–19.

Jenner, Harald: Von Neuendettelsau in alle Welt. Entwicklung und Bedeutung der Diakonissenanstalt Neuendettelsau / Diakonie Neuendettelsau 1854–1891/1900. Neuendettelsau [2004].

Köser, Silke: "Weibliche Einfalt" und "innere Herrlichkeit eines männlich vollendeten Charakters". Geschlechterrollen und Frauenbild bei Wilhelm Löhe. In: Schoenauer, Hermann (ed.): Wilhelm Löhe 1808–1872. Seine Bedeutung für Kirche und Diakonie. Stuttgart 2008, pp. 391–409.

Löhe, Wilhelm (ed.): Dr. Gottfried Olearius Anweisung zur Krankenseelsorge. Mit einigen einleitenden Sätzen und zwei Anhängen versehen. Für junge Geistliche, Krankenpfleger und Krankenpflegerinnen. 2nd Edition Nürnberg 1871.

Löhe, Wilhelm: Von dem Einfluß der leiblichen Krankheiten auf das psychische Befinden des Kranken, sowie von der Anwendung geistlicher Mittel zur Hebung der daraus hervorgehenden Gefahr für die Seele. Stuttgart 1858.

Löhe, Wilhelm: Von der Barmherzigkeit. Sechs Kapitel für jedermann, zuletzt ein siebentes für Dienerinnen der Barmherzigkeit. 4th Edition Neuendettelsau 1927.

Riedel, Manfred: Innovation für die Pflege aus der Tradition. Pflegeleitbild – Gestern – Heute – Morgen, in: Schoenauer, Hermann et al. (ed.): Tradition und Innovation. Diakonische Entwicklungen am Beispiel der Diakonie Neuendettelsau. Stuttgart 2004, pp. 177–189.

Riedel, Manfred: Die Reform der Krankenpflege durch Löhe. In: Diakonie Neuendettelsau (ed.): Löhe-Journal. 200 Jahre Wilhelm Löhe. Neuendettelsau 2008, pp. 16–17.

Riedel, Manfred: Wilhelm Löhe und die Pflege. In: "Du sollst ein Segen sein!" Der christliche Auftrag im Pflegealltag. Tagungsband zum 3. Christlichen Pflegekongress vom 29. bis 31.10.2009 in Neuendettelsau. Jena 2012, pp. 39–47.

Schoenauer, Hermann: Evangelische Schwestern im Dienst des Nächsten. Die Diakonissen von Neuendettelsau in Geschichte und Gegenwart. In: Henkel, Jürgen / Wyrwoll, Nikolaus (ed.): Askese versus Konsumgesellschaft. Aktualität und Spiritualität von Mönchtum und Ordensleben im 21. Jahrhundert. Hermannstadt/Sibiu; Bonn 2013, pp. 408–419.

Stempel de Fallois, Anne: Das diakonische Wirken Wilhelm Löhes. Von den Anfängen bis zur Gründung des Mutterhauses Neuendettelsau (1926–1854). Stuttgart; Berlin; Köln 2001.

---

33 Hickel (1926), p. 15.

Archive

Zentralarchiv Diakonie Neuendettelsau, Bestand Mutterhausarchiv
Handschriften, GII 4,5 [Diarium der Gemeindeschwester in Ansbach 1878].

Outer Mission – the transfer to Palestine

The establishment of nursing care in the parish. Kaiserswerth deaconesses in Jerusalem

Uwe Kaminsky

> The work of the sisters in Jerusalem is one of the strongest pillars of all our work in the 'Holy Land'. And I cannot imagine what would happen if we had to do without them.[1]

This comment was made by the head of the *Syrian Orphanage*, Theodor Schneller, at a promotional event held in Düsseldorf in 1902. Schneller was not the only one to highlight the important role played by the Kaiserswerth sisters in missionary affairs in Palestine. In general, the deaconesses' involvement in *Orientarbeit* (*work in the Orient*) in Palestine represented the backbone of German missionary activity.

This article presents a short history of the concept of *Orientarbeit*, shows the functions played by the Kaiserswerth deaconesses in Jerusalem, outlines their importance to the overall fabric of German Protestant work, and provides an interpretation concerning the end of their effectiveness. The aim in doing so is to help refine the explanations given for the 'entanglement' of the missionary and caring aspects of deaconess work.[2] The reason Kaiserswerth deaconesses were sent to Jerusalem was not to carry out missionary work among 'heathens', but to set up nursing care in existing Christian parishes in the Middle East.

Early history and concept of *Orientarbeit*

The *Kaiserswerth Deaconess Institute* founded by Theodor Fliedner in 1836 must be considered the cradle of female social welfare work. In Kaiserswerth, Theodor Fliedner (1800–1864) and his wives, Friederike (1800–1842) and Caroline (1811–1892), trained women for nursing, teaching and social welfare work in the community.[3] The *Kaiserswerth Deaconess Institute* served as a model for many other deaconess motherhouses that were founded later, both in Germany and elsewhere. The "motherhouse-based social work" model developed here played a key role in recruiting young women to a Protestant order that undertook social work and the activities of a people's church.[4]

As early as the 1840s, Fliedner was sending the deaconesses to England and the USA to work in hospitals and communities. In 1851, with the support of Prussia's Frederick William IV, he added *Orientarbeit* – work in the Levant.

---

1   Ludwig Schneller (1902), quoted in: Kaminsky (2010), p. 48.
2   For the German debate see Habermas (2008); for details about the difference between mission societies and deaconess institutes see Kaminsky (2013).
3   Köser (2006); Felgentreff (1998); Sticker (1961).
4   Friedrich (2005); Kaminsky (2010).

Shortly before 1849, Fliedner gave up his position as pastor in Kaiserswerth, and henceforth devoted himself solely to the further expansion of the institution and deaconess work overseas.

The Kaiserswerth *Orientarbeit* is one of a multitude of German colonial and missionary activities in Palestine.[5] For classification purposes, we need to outline a few of the basic conditions and concepts of the Kaiserswerth social work. On 7 December 1841, Baron Christian Carl Josias Bunsen and the Archbishop of Canterbury, acting for the Prussian and English monarchs respectively, signed a document establishing the joint *Bishopric of the United Church of England and Ireland* in Jerusalem. This arrangement was to last until 1886.[6] Palestine, as Christ's country of origin, from which the commission to spread the Gospel emanated, exercised a great spiritual and religious attraction. This "Christian yearning for Jerusalem" was particularly popular among Protestant Christians around the mid-nineteenth century, whose goal was to regain the 'Holy Land' for the message of the Gospel by exerting religious, cultural, and philanthropic influence.[7] This was to be a "peaceful crusade" in the 'Holy Land'[8] – a metaphor that both associated it with and disassociated it from the classic crusades. In Fliedner's report about his travels in the Orient in 1858 he provides an example of 'geopiety': the longing for the 'Holy Land', its biblical topography and geography, and the efforts to spread the Gospel.[9]

He saw Palestine as the Levant, "where the life-giving sun first cast its rays", and where people now "sit in darkness and shade of death, and Mohammed's deceptive moonlight casts only a dim twilight into the night, and where the female sex in particular languishes in the profoundest degradation and abasement [...]". Fliedner underscored "the diverse Protestant efforts to spread the Gospel for the salvation of these countries and peoples, including our sending out our deaconesses (even if our efforts amount only to the size of a mustard seed)".[10] His report is full of similar comments. In this setting, Fliedner was one of a series of forces vying with each other for religious influence and missionary superiority in Palestine.

In 1857, Fliedner distributed his *Proposal for Establishing a German-Evangelical Missionary Society for the Orient.*[11] In its summary form, it can be seen as a key that sheds light on Fliedner's own missionary efforts, as well as on the role of the *Orientarbeit* undertaken by the Kaiserswerth deaconesses as

---

5   Goren/Eisler (2011); Friedrich/Kaminsky/Löffler (2010); Murre-van den Berg (2006);
     Trimbur (2004); Eisler/Haag/Holtz (2003); Hanselmann (1971); Davis (1991); Ben-Arieh
     (1997); Roth (1973).
6   Lückhoff (1998); Hänsel (2003).
7   Foerster (1991); Kirchhoff (2003); Kirchhoff (2005).
8   Goren (2003a); Goren (2003c).
9   Murre-van den Berg (2010); Hammer (1986).
10   Fliedner (1858).
11   Fliedners Gedanken über eine Deutsch-Evangelische Missionsgesellschaft für das Mor-
     genland. In: Der Armen- und Krankenfreund, March-April 1901, pp. 59–62; Fliedner, G.
     (1910), pp. 655–660.

a 'home mission' abroad. Fliedner stated that he had tried in vain to interest the *Rhine* and *Basel Mission Societies* in the Levant. Under their rules, these mission societies could only operate among 'heathens' or non-Christians. However, in Fliedner's view, the German Church had a specific vocation to evangelise the Oriental churches. Besides sending missionary preachers to the area, Fliedner believed this should entail the establishment of hospitals, orphanages, and schools and other educational institutions. One of his intentions was to stop the 'brain drain' to Paris of the education-hungry youth of the Levant, which was already an issue in those days, as well as countering the ostensible moral dangers of 'European pseudoculture'.

The idea was that training local people would create a pool of personnel to undertake subsequent missionary activities. For Fliedner, this basically involved an 'internal reformation' of the local Christian churches, not the proselytisation of Muslims. Here he was making a romantic overestimation of Greek culture, assuming that the Greek population of the Ottoman Empire would eventually overcome its Muslim counterpart. In the case of Greeks, Copts, and Armenians, Fliedner laid great emphasis on systematic educational work among the female sex "on evangelical Christian bases", since he saw in the future mothers "the most reliable foundation for the education of the people".[12]

Ultimately, it was only at the Kaiserswerth stations overseas that efforts were made to put these missionary plans into practice. Elsewhere, they remained unfulfilled, together with plans to establish a seminary for travelling preachers and an evangelical association of teachers for the Levant. The idea of evangelising through a home mission that is reflected in these plans had already been tried out in Germany by this time and, with the encouragement of Johann Hinrich Wichern (1808–1881), had led in 1849 to the founding of the *Central Committee for Inner Mission*, a coordinating committee for efforts that combined social work with a requirement to undertake missionary work among the people. It involved bringing about a change in religious, social and, indirectly, political circumstances – by setting a good example, through a life of hands-on compassion, and by providing social welfare. As in Germany, there was a void in local communities that had to be filled to achieve this. The only solution was to focus on building sustainable communities abroad. Fliedner's requests to the Prussian king to send pastors to those communities where the deaconesses were active shed light on these efforts. The Protestant Church sent pastors not only to Jerusalem, but also to Smyrna, Alexandria, Cairo and Beirut.[13]

---

12 Ibid.; In a draft of the statutes of a *German-Protestant missionary society for the Orient*, Fliedner's stated aims were the "evangelisation of the people of the Orient, preferably in European, Asian and African Turkey and at its borders", quoted by Fliedner G. (1910), p. 313; Neubert-Preine (2001), pp. 31–43.

13 Fliedner, G. (1910), p. 297.

The *Kaiserswerth Deaconess Institute* as a provider of social infrastructure for Protestant outreach in the Orient

The Kaiserswerth *Orientarbeit* involved exporting a social welfare model and included exerting cultural influence through religion. In this sense, Kaiserswerth's involvement was not only one of the earliest in this region, but also one of the most enduring, since its offshoot, the *Talitha Kumi Evangelical Lutheran School* in Beit Jala (run since 1975 by the Berlin Mission), continues to exist to this day. The Kaiserswerth projects can be compared to other German missionary projects, like the establishment of a missionary colony in Jerusalem in 1846 by the *Pilgermissionsanstalt St. Chrischona* (*St. Chrischona Pilgrim Mission*) and Christian Friedrich Spittler, and to the *Syrian Orphanage*.[14] The *Orientarbeit* in Jerusalem began in 1851. For the Bishop of the Anglo-Prussian Bishopric, Samuel Gobat (1799–1879), Fliedner's 1850 offer to dispatch deaconesses as nurses was very opportune, since there were many cases of illness among the Germans and English at the *Jerusalem Mission* at that time.[15] Fliedner wanted to set up a training school of Christian nurses and teachers for the Levant. Consequently, his involvement in Palestine envisaged establishing a new *Deaconess Institute* as the starting point for more extensive work in the Levant. This coincided with the king's plans, since he was interested in expanding independent Prussian work in Palestine. The ethnically exclusive welfare programme, to be limited to missionary Europeans only, was broadened very soon after its inception to include independent educational activities, which took place in the context of a home mission abroad.

In the spring of 1851, Fliedner arrived in Jerusalem with four deaconesses, rather than the two requested, and occupied a house. They started providing nursing and education services. From the initial educational work, conducted on the roof of the deaconess house in Jerusalem, there very soon developed an independent institution in 1868, which still exists to this day and is known as *Talitha Kumi*.[16]

On his first trip to the Orient, Fliedner made preparations for dispatching deaconesses to Constantinople (1852) and Smyrna (1853) to work in nursing or education.[17] Apart from requests from local merchants, the Prussian government's interests also played a role in this situation.[18] As early as 1847 or 1849, the king had asked Fliedner to provide the *German Hospital* in Constantinople with deaconesses. In this context, Fliedner's close ties to the royal palace itself, which not only encouraged the dispatching of deaconesses, but also provided real estate and later donated funds to acquire property or build

---

14 Sinno (1982), pp. 45–80; Lückhoff (1998), pp. 165–190; Loeffler (2006).
15 The story of the foundation, often repeated, was reported first in "Erster Bericht über das Diakonissenhaus zu Jerusalem von Mitte April bis 10. September 1851", pp. 1–8; details in Kaminsky (2010), pp. 21–24.
16 Kaminsky (2010), pp. 27–29.
17 Pschichholz (2010); Pschichholz (2011).
18 Fuhrmann (2006).

houses, played an important role. Fliedner also managed to use the political interest in the deaconesses' work to expand it along the lines of his home mission concept.

The activities became increasingly institutionalised and specialised. One of the best examples of this is *Talitha Kumi*. This project started with the construction of a school building in 1868, from which there grew a large-scale educational institution for girls and, around the turn of the century, an elementary school, a nursery school, a domestic science school, a training institution for nursery school teachers, and a training institution for school teachers. When Fliedner died in 1864, only 12 of the 51 deaconesses working in the Orient were working as nurses in hospitals, whereas 39 were employed as teachers or educational personnel.[19]

In Palestine, more institutions of German social Protestantism came into existence. *The Syrian Orphanage* founded in 1860, which expanded under the name of Johann Ludwig Schneller to the biggest missionary institution in Palestine, can also be seen as social infrastructure for Prussian policy, although for Schneller, this had not been its most important purpose.[20]

Another institution was the private *Jesus Hilfe asylum*, which was built to care for the lepers near the Jaffa Gate. However, this charitable project only survived by being overtaken by the *Bruedergemeine Herrnhut* (*Moravian Church*) in 1881, who arranged for the lepers to be cared for by sisters from the deaconess house in Niesky.[21] The founding of the *Marienstift children's hospital* by the Duke of Mecklenburg-Schwerin in 1872 was a similar case of diversification into medical care by a private charity. The main function of the hospital was the treatment of severely ill children. There was even a kind of rooming-in for the mothers. But the institution was only sustainable with money from Germany, which dwindled towards the end of the century. Doctor Sandreczky, the head of the institution, committed suicide in 1899, allegedly because of illness and because of the debts he was responsible for.[22] In 1901 Kaiserswerth took over the house as an associated institution of the deaconess hospital.

The contribution of *Orientarbeit* to the formation of parishes

Wherever the deaconesses were, nursing was initially thought of as a service for the members of their own community, but it also became attractive to local residents: Christians and non-Christians alike. For example, whereas in the first year (1851/52) the 78 patients cared for at the *Jerusalem Hospital* included just five Muslims, by 1863 the figure had shot up to 312 Muslims out of a total of 473.[23]

19   Fliedner, G. (1910), p. 312.
20   Loeffler (2004).
21   Loeffler (2007). Compare also the article by Ruth Wexler in this volume.
22   Sinno (1982), pp. 158–162; Nissan/Martin-Fiedler (2011).
23   Fliedner, G. (1910), p. 293.

Things were different at *Talitha Kumi*, where the number of Muslim girls remained low, largely as a result of the threat of social isolation facing anyone who converted. The only girls for whom this was a more or less empty threat were orphans without any family to press claims to their labour. The direct proselytising of Muslims was prohibited in the Ottoman Empire. The few well-known cases led to some violent conflicts with the Muslim society of origin and the Ottoman authorities.[24]

Work overseas was mainly financed by donations – particularly from the Prussian State, as described above, and from the committees and associations set up by it. In addition to its primary home mission purpose, overseas work also had a major effect in terms of promoting the *Kaiserswerth Deaconess Institute* in the homeland.[25]

As well as boosting people's willingness to donate, the involvement abroad increased the attractiveness of the deaconesses' activities within Germany, as well as within the institution itself. The importance of the overseas facilities for the sisterhood should not be underestimated. These were places where sisters could learn and spend their novitiate period – places where they could grow into their duties and where the deaconesses, most of whom were not linguistically gifted, could be tried out in an alien setting. It was here that the 'heroines' of female deaconry emerged: women who were not only trained as nurses or educators, but were also able to collect donations, lead people, and administer real estate. The perfect example of such a woman was the "veteran of German evangelization work in the Orient", Charlotte Pilz (1819–1913), who lived in Jerusalem from the age of 34 onwards, initially as principal of the deaconess house there, then, from 1868, as principal of *Talitha Kumi*, where she remained until her death in 1903.[26]

The possibility of working abroad, particularly in Palestine, attracted so-called *Höhere Töchter*, women of higher social standing. By the end of the nineteenth century it had become very difficult to find new deaconesses, since there were now other alternatives for women who wanted to work. In particular, educated women from the higher classes were less willing to become deaconesses because of the self-denial and subordination that was asked of them.[27]

One example of a lady from a highly respected family becoming a Kaiserswerth deaconess in the later years was Theodore Barkhausen (1869–1959). She and her father, President of the *High Consistory* of the *German Protestant Church*, travelled with the German Emperor to Palestine in 1898. After the death of her father in 1905, she joined the Kaiserswerth motherhouse and

---

24   Sinno (1982), pp. 94–98.
25   Kaminsky (2010), pp. 46–51.
26   Eisler (2001), (2006).
27   Schmidt (1995): In 1898, 23 out of 49 deaconess houses were headed by Mother Superiors of noble birth. Schmidt (1998), p. 190.

became a successful and well-respected manager of the Kaiserswerth *Orientarbeit* in Jerusalem.[28]

The work of deaconesses serving in diaspora parishes was a successful model and attracted missionary organisations. They wanted to involve deaconesses in the missionary field, especially during the period of German imperialism. The *Kaiserswerth Deaconess Institute* and the deaconess institutes of the *Kaiserswerth General Conference* (1861) opposed the use of deaconesses for 'heathen' missions.

The *Kaiserswerth Deaconess Institute* saw such a "pioneering service" in the "still underdeveloped regions" as the duty of missionary societies, not of deaconess institutes. Another reason for this was the fact that the missionary societies wanted the deaconesses to spend their working lives in the field, but expected the deaconess institutes to train them and provide for their old age. There was also the question of who the deaconesses should report to: the mission organisation or the motherhouse.[29]

Fliedner did not want to convert non-Christians, but to support the process of building Christian parishes in the Orient. In most of the German deaconess institutes, the number of deaconesses involved in missions to 'heathens' was small until World War I. Much later, in 1931, the *Kaiserswerth Institute* took part in the missionary work of the *Rhenish Missionary Society* by sending three deaconesses to Sumatra. But such work never became an integral part of the Kaiserswerth project.

The visit by German Emperor Wilhelm II to Palestine in 1898 once again boosted German public interest in Palestine, as well as consolidating mutual trust between the royal palace and the *Deaconess Institute*.[30] The head of the *Kaiserswerth Deaconess Institute*, Zöllner, proclaimed a "crusade of love" against the Muslims to get more donations.[31] The author of a publication which covered the trip and the circumstances surrounding it extolled the work of the deaconesses as the "birthplace of a new, more noble life". He reported that more than fifty of the former pupils were working as teachers, 23 subsequently became deaconesses, others became Biblewomen, and a large number worked as domestics, "most of whom as Christian housekeepers convey the blessing that has been received".

> When it comes to dealing with the tasks facing Protestant Christianity in the Mohammedan world, hardly anyone is more suited than the German deaconesses, who in the silent service of love and through change without words help the cross to vanquish the crescent.[32]

---

28 Felgentreff (2002), pp. 51–56; Wilhelm Martens: Theodore Barkhausen in Jerusalem 1909–1950. Archiv der Fliedner Kulturstiftung, Gr Fl IVp 19/4.

29 Kaminsky (2013).

30 Krüger (2011); Petschulat (2009); Benner (2001); Ronnecker/Nieper/Neubert-Preine (1998); Das deutsche Kaiserpaar (1899).

31 Fuhrmann (2006), pp. 187–188.

32 Die deutsche Kaiserfahrt (1898), p. 174.

Between 1902 and 1904, the Kaiserswerth deaconesses opened schools and undertook community nursing in Jerusalem, Bethlehem and Haifa. In 1901, a new hospital building was opened outside the Old City of Jerusalem.[33]

As religiously motivated, trustworthy and particularly inexpensive personnel for the home mission abroad, deaconesses were unbeatable in their day – outstanding in the quality of their work, their motivation, and even their low cost. They received no salaries, only pocket money and home leave at regular intervals.

In addition to their social welfare work, the task of the Kaiserswerth deaconesses was to proclaim the Gospel and win over patients or pupils. This required a form of follow-up care, and often led to the deaconesses carrying out community nursing in the newly emerging Arab Protestant communities. Thus in 1911, for example, a sister in Bethlehem provided support to 39 families, assisted at the outpatients' clinic operated by the Swedish Jerusalem Society, and ran a sewing school.

In addition, the *Kaiserswerth Deaconess Institute* founded a Levantine teacher training college in Jerusalem, as well as a Levantine deaconesses school for "the young novitiates from the number of former pupils of our orphanages in the Levant who wish to take up the vocation of deaconess". As a result, Fliedner's desire for a training school or "cultivating ground" to train local sisters was fulfilled in 1911. Even if the prospect of establishing an independent sisterhood seemed unlikely, nevertheless it was necessary to maintain contact with the children who had received the appropriate education and with the young women after their time at the Protestant German institutions. An alumnae association called the *Zoar Association* was set up in Beirut. In Smyrna, its counterpart was known as the *Forget Me Not Association*, and its aim was "to promote the feeling of togetherness among its members and to keep the ties with the sisters alive". The situation in Jerusalem was similar: in 1911, the *Talitha Association* admitted around 60 former pupils.[34]

Cultivating grounds without plants – The problems of recruiting the next generation in the Levant

As indicated above, Theodor Fliedner's original idea was to sow the "mustard seed" in Jerusalem for subsequent independent work by deaconesses. The Kaiserswerth orphanages in Beirut, Smyrna, and Jerusalem acted as the "cultivating grounds" for this future development. In particular, the children of Eastern Christians from Armenia, Syria, and Palestine were educated here, some of them from a very young age. From the turn of the century they also had the possibility of continuing their training at a deaconess school in Jerusa-

---

33   Kaminsky (2010), p. 39; Eisler (2003).
34   Übersicht über den Stand der Arbeit der Kaiserswerther Diakonissen im Morgenland (D.[isselhoff]). In: Der Armen- und Krankenfreund, Jul-Aug 1903, p. 125; Stursberg (1911), p. 134.

lem. The first two Arab novitiates from the Beirut orphanage were confirmed as deaconesses in Jerusalem in February 1873.[35] The first formerly Muslim novitiates entered the diaconate in 1881 in Beirut.[36] However, it was rare for Arab Muslims to be recruited. Fliedner's approach was slanted far more towards strengthening existing Christian communities – an approach that was particularly evident in Jerusalem.

By 1886, 12 girls from *Talitha Kumi* are reported to have entered the sisterhood, and a further 14 by 1901. The 1911 special publication marking the institute's 75th anniversary listed a total of 43 novitiates and deaconesses who had joined in the Levant, of whom 18 were still active. In 1911 a total of 131 German and non-German sisters were involved in the Kaiserswerth *Orientarbeit* (in Cairo, Alexandria, Istanbul, Smyrna, Beirut, Haifa, Jerusalem and Bethlehem) in 28 fields of activity. For Palestine the corresponding figures were 27 – in just ten fields of activity. These figures may be viewed as very high, or – if perceived as the result of a good sixty years of activities – as low, depending on one's expectations. No independent sisterhood emerged from the local situation.

In the following, I summarise the biographies of two non-German sisters.[37] Rufka Schible (1859–1922) was born in Bhamdun, Lebanon. When she was four, her parents brought her to the deaconess school in Beirut, where she was raised by the deaconesses. She was confirmed in 1874, and in 1879 entered the sisterhood. She worked at the deaconess hospital in Alexandria for 26 years, and in 1905 came to Jerusalem as a community nurse. Here she became involved among other things in looking after the former pupils from *Talitha Kumi*.

Afife Samaan (1883–1959) was the daughter of a merchant in Nazareth. After her mother died in 1891, she had to help her grandmother look after the household as well as her three sisters and brothers. Two of her siblings were brought up in the English orphanage in Nazareth. When she was ten, she came to *Talitha Kumi* together with her three-year-old sister. In 1899, she was confirmed at the *Church of the Redeemer*, and then worked as an infant teacher and educator at *Talitha Kumi*. In 1918, she followed the German sisters into internment at Helouan, Egypt, and then to Germany. Here she worked as a teacher in a community home. In 1926, she was allowed to leave for *Talitha Kumi*, where she served until 1940. During World War II she again followed the German sisters into internment at the *Waldheim Colony*, which lasted until 1948. From 1950 she worked at the school called *Talitha Kumi* that opened in Beit Jala.

These two life histories show clearly how the *Kaiserswerth Deaconess Institute* was able to 'stock' the deaconess stations, or cultivating grounds, with 'plants' from their own educational work. In all instances, a German deaconess, who

---

35 Marschie Sab, die erste arabische Diakonissin. In: Der Armen- und Krankenfreund Nov–Dec 1880, pp. 161–166; Lückhoff (1998), p. 205.
36 In detail: Hauser (2008); Hauser (2011).
37 For more examples see Kaminsky (2009), pp. 92–95.

is referred to specifically in the biographies and who acted as a kind of foster mother or mentor, played a special role as a model for the young Arab and Armenian girls from Christian families. The special deaconess mentality, which demanded a high degree of self-denial and assimilation, was initially conveyed to the Arab or Armenian candidates by providing a living example, which they were then required to emulate. This also included limiting their contact with family and friends, and with the opposite sex in general. They also had to give up any ambition to become mothers themselves.

At the end of World War I, many of the Arab and Armenian deaconesses had to leave their familiar surroundings and their life stories are dominated by the disruption resulting from the loss of many of the fields in which they had previously worked. The *Victoria Hospital* in Cairo was one option for them. Ultimately, eight non-German deaconesses were able to remain there as nursing staff and helped to maintain the Kaiserswerth claim to ownership. The situation at the end of World War I was more difficult for those sisters who, together with the German deaconesses, had to leave their cultural milieu and go to Germany. This was the case, for example, of Afife Samaan (mentioned above), but presented an even greater problem for another Arab deaconess called Fumija Arbid.

Fumija Arbid (born 1881) worked from 1903 to 1909 "as a teaching sister in the school in Jerusalem connected with the *Talitha Kumi* boarding school",[38] according to a 1909 document. After World War I, the convalescent home for the deaconesses in Areya was given up and in 1920 she followed her German colleagues to Germany. Here she worked as a teacher at a school in Hilden, near Dusseldorf, until 1924. Her suffering in the alien setting in Germany has been recorded in several letters: "I cannot learn to be at home here. It is like living under pressure all the time."[39] She was sent back to Jerusalem in 1924, and from 1930 onwards she was also allowed, as a "community sister of the Arab community", to follow up former Talitha pupils. Nevertheless, it would appear that inwardly she felt distanced from the motherhouse, and in September 1932 she left the diaconate. The fact that Fumija Arbid, a deaconess who left the order in 1932, had been working in Jerusalem's Evangelical-Arab community since the end of 1930 and, after leaving the sisterhood, continued to be involved there, underscores the national and Church emancipation that had taken place in the interim. This situation also led to a rift among the former Talitha pupils. The alumnae communities in Jerusalem and Beirut, where Kaiserswerth had previously run schools, not only provided living examples of their own success through their educational work and the implementation of an intercultural network, they also generated reservoirs of new boys and girls for the school.

After World War I, only one local woman joined the Kaiserswerth diaconate on a permanent basis: Najla Moussa Sayegh (1902–1986), who from 1950 to 1975 headed the *Talitha Kumi* school (which was located in Beit Jala

---

38   Kaminsky (2010), p. 84.
39   Kaminsky (2010), p. 86.

from 1950 onwards).[40] For the *Deaconess Institute*, this absence of native "plants" for the cultivating grounds in the Levant meant they had to live off their capital. The local deaconesses were aging, and among the staff too the flowers cultivated in the Levant were starting to fade.

Conclusion

The Kaiserswerth deaconesses were important representatives of German culture and the Protestant religion, as well as promoting education and social welfare in what was then Palestine. They supported the development of German Protestant parishes in Jerusalem, Istanbul, Beirut, Alexandria and Cairo. The involvement of deaconesses in missionary work was not the aim of Fliedner's project. He wanted to strengthen existing Christian parishes, not convert 'heathens'. Furthermore, there were differences of opinion about the question of who would be in charge of any missionary work carried out by the deaconesses, so the number of deaconesses in the mission fields was low.

According to Theodor Fliedner's original approach, the aim of the work was to help establish a cultivating ground to produce local deaconesses. They did manage to make deaconesses out of a few of the Armenian and Arab girls educated at the schools, but the outcome was not a self-sustaining, local sisterhood. The involvement of the deaconesses also had an impact back in Germany, where working in the 'Holy Land' was considered very special. This helped with fundraising, as well as with demonstrating the reverent nature of the work of the *Kaiserswerth Deaconess Institute*.

Given the absence of women willing to be trained as deaconesses and to follow the path of Christian humility, subordination, and self-denial, in the long run the work of the deaconesses inevitably had to come to an end – not only in Germany, but in Palestine too. The end to local recruitment that came about with World War I was exacerbated by the cessation of German educational work in Palestine during and following both world wars. Consequently, the *Kaiserswerth Deaconess Institute* was forced to live off its capital, specifically when it came to local deaconesses.

Until the early 1930s, the deaconess model remained extremely attractive to women in Germany against the background of the economic crisis. Subsequently, and particularly from the 1950s onwards, it was affected by a permanent crisis, leading to the present-day dying out of deaconesses in Germany. As early as the inter-war period, it became impossible to deal adequately with the changes taking place in society in Palestine. Until Najla Moussa joined the diaconate, there had been no local growth in the sisterhood. Her retirement as head of the *Talitha Kumi School* in 1975 brought to an end the history of the Kaiserswerth deaconesses in Palestine.

---

40   Felgentreff (2001); Kaminsky (2010), pp. 87–91.

Bibliography

Barth, Boris; Osterhammel, Jürgen (ed.): Zivilisierungsmissionen. Imperiale Weltverbesserung seit dem 18. Jahrhundert. Konstanz 2005.

Ben-Arieh, Yehoshua; Davies, Moshe (ed.): Jerusalem in the mind of the Western world, 1800–1948 [With eyes toward Zion, V]. Westport; London 1997.

Benner, Thomas Hartmut: Die Strahlen der Krone. Die religiöse Dimension des Kaisertums unter Wilhelm II. vor dem Hintergrund der Orientreise 1898. Marburg 2001.

Das deutsche Kaiserpaar im Heiligen Lande im Herbst 1898. Mit Allerhöchster Ermächtigung Seiner Majestät des Kaisers und Königs bearbeitet nach authentischen Berichten und Akten. Berlin 1899.

Die Kaiserfahrt nach dem heiligen Lande. Berlin 1898.

Eisler, Jakob; Haag, Norbert; Holtz, Sabine: Kultureller Wandel in Palästina im frühen 20. Jahrhundert. Eine Bilddokumentation. Zugleich ein Nachschlagewerk der deutschen Missionseinrichtungen und Siedlungen von ihrer Gründung bis zum Zweiten Weltkrieg (edited by Verein für württembergische Kirchengeschichte in Verbindung mit dem Verein der Freunde der Hebräischen Universität Jerusalem in Baden-Württemberg e. V.). Epfendorf 2003.

Eisler, E. Jakob: Charlotte Pilz und die Anfänge Kaiserswerther Orientarbeit. In: Nothnagle, Almut; Abromeit, Hans-Jürgen; Foerster, Frank (ed.): Seht, wir gehen hinauf nach Jerusalem. Festschrift zum 150jährigen Jubiläum von Talitha Kumi und des Jerusalemsvereins. Leipzig 2001, pp. 78–95.

Eisler, E. Jakob: Frauen im Dienste des Jerusalemsvereins im Heiligen Land. In: Feldtkeller, Andreas; Nothnagle, Almut (ed.): Mission im Konfliktfeld von Islam, Judentum und Christentum. Eine Bestandsaufnahme zum 150-jährigen Jubiläum des Jerusalemsvereins. Frankfurt/Main 2003, pp. 45–56.

Eisler, E. Jakob: Charlotte Pilz (1819–1903). In: Hauff, Adelheid M. von (ed.): Frauen gestalten Diakonie. Vol. 2: Vom 18. bis zum 20. Jahrhundert. Stuttgart 2006, pp. 251–263.

Feldtkeller, Andreas; Nothnagle, Almut (ed.): Mission im Konfliktfeld von Islam, Judentum und Christentum. Eine Bestandsaufnahme zum 150-jährigen Jubiläum des Jerusalemsvereins. Frankfurt/Main 2003.

Felgentreff, Ruth: Bertha Harz und Najla Moussa Sayegh. Zwei Diakonissen – eine Aufgabe, ein Dienst. In: Nothnagle, Almut; Abromeit, Hans-Jürgen; Foerster, Frank (ed.): Seht, wir gehen hinauf nach Jerusalem. Festschrift zum 150jährigen Jubiläum von Talitha Kumi und des Jerusalemsvereins. Leipzig 2001, pp. 96–121.

Felgentreff, Ruth: Das Diakoniewerk Kaiserswerth 1836–1998. Von der Diakonissenanstalt zum Diakoniewerk – ein Überblick. Düsseldorf 1998.

Felgentreff, Ruth: Diakonisse Theodore Barkhausen. In: Mitteilungen aus Ökumene und Auslandsarbeit (2002), pp. 51–56.

Fliedner, Georg: Theodor Fliedner. Durch Gottes Gnade Erneuer des apostolischen Diakonissenamtes in der evangelischen Kirche. Sein Leben und Wirken. 3 Vol. Kaiserswerth 1908, 1910, 1912.

Fliedner, Theodor: Reisen in das heilige Land, nach Smyrna, Beirut, Constantinopel ... 1851, 1856 und 1857. Kaiserswerth [1858] [GrFl. II a 15].

Fliedner, Theodor: Vorschlag zur Gründung einer deutsch-evangelischen Missions-Gesellschaft für das Morgenland. Düsseldorf 1857 [GrFl. II a 14].

Foerster, Frank: Mission im Heiligen Land. Der Jerusalems-Verein zu Berlin 1852–1945. Gütersloh 1991.

Friedrich, Norbert: Mutterhaus- und Anstaltsdiakonie. Zu einer spezifischen Form der protestantischen Vereinsbildung im 19. und 20. Jahrhundert. In: Zeitschrift für Bayerische Kirchengeschichte 74 (2005), pp. 3–13.

Friedrich, Norbert; Jähnichen, Traugott (ed.): Sozialer Protestantismus im Kaiserreich. Problemkonstellationen – Lösungsperspektiven – Handlungsprofile. Münster 2005.

Friedrich, Norbert; Kaminsky, Uwe; Löffler, Roland (ed.): The social dimension of Christian missions in the Middle East. Historical studies of the 19th and 20th centuries. (Missionsgeschichtliches Archiv 16) Stuttgart 2010.

Fuhrmann, Malte: Der Traum vom deutschen Orient. Zwei deutsche Kolonien im Osmanischen Reich 1851–1918. Frankfurt/Main 2006.

Goren, Haim: Debating the Jews of Palestine. German discourses of colonization, 1840–1883. In: Leipziger Beiträge zur jüdischen Geschichte und Kultur 1 (2003), pp. 217–238. [2003a]

Goren, Haim (ed.): Germany and the Middle East. Past, present, and future. Jerusalem 2003. [2003b]

Goren, Haim: "Zieht hin und erforscht das Land". Die deutsche Palästinaforschung im 19. Jahrhundert. Göttingen 2003. [2003c]

Goren, Haim; Eisler, Jakob (ed.): Deutschland und Deutsche in Jerusalem. Jerusalem 2011.

Habermas, Rebekka: Mission im 19. Jahrhundert. Globale Netze des Religiösen. In: Historische Zeitschrift 287 (2008), pp. 629–679.

Hammer, Karl: Die christliche Jerusalemssehnsucht im 19. Jahrhundert. Der geistige und geschichtliche Hintergrund der Gründung Johann Ludwig Schnellers. In: Theologische Zeitschrift 42 (1986), pp. 255–266.

Hanselmann, Siegfried: Deutsche Evangelische Palästinamission. Handbuch ihrer Motive, Geschichte und Ergebnisse. Erlangen 1971.

Hänsel, Lars: Friedrich Wilhelm IV and Prussian Interests in the Middle East. In: Goren, Haim (ed.): Germany and the Middle East. Past, Present, and Future. Jerusalem 2003, pp. 15–25.

Hauff, Adelheid M. von (ed.): Frauen gestalten Diakonie. Vol. 2: Vom 18. bis zum 20. Jahrhundert. Stuttgart 2006.

Hauser, Julia: "… das hier so furchtbar verwahrloste weibliche Geschlecht aus dem Stande heben zu helfen." Der emanzipatorische Auftrag Kaiserswerther Diakonissen im Osmanischen Reich (1851–1918) und seine Ambivalenzen. In: Gippert, Wolfgang; Götte, Petra; Kleinau, Elke (ed.): Transkulturalität. Gender- und bildungshistorische Perspektiven. Bielefeld 2008, pp. 219–236.

Hauser, Julia: Waisen gewinnen. Mission zwischen Programmatik und Praxis in der Erziehungsanstalt der Kaiserswerther Diakonissen in Beirut seit 1860. In: WerkstattGeschichte 57 (2011), pp. 9–30.

Kaminsky, Uwe: Die innere Mission Kaiserswerths im Ausland. Von der Evangelisation zum Bemühen um die Dritte Welt. In: Friedrich, Norbert; Jähnichen, Traugott (ed.): Sozialer Protestantismus im Kaiserreich. Problemkonstellationen – Lösungsperspektiven – Handlungsprofile. Münster 2005, pp. 355–385.

Kaminsky, Uwe: German "Home Mission" abroad. The "Orientarbeit" of the Deaconess Institution Kaiserswerth in the Ottoman Empire. In: Murre-van den Berg, Heleen (ed.): New faith in Ancient Lands. Western mission in the Middle East in the nineteenth and early twentieth centuries. Leiden 2006, pp. 191–209.

Kaminsky, Uwe: Die Kaiserswerther Orientarbeit als soziale Infrastruktur zwischen Staat und Kirche. In: Tamcke, Martin; Manukyan, Arthur (ed.): Protestanten im Orient. Würzburg 2009, pp. 81–95.

Kaminsky, Uwe: Innere Mission im Ausland. Der Aufbau religiöser und sozialer Infrastruktur am Beispiel der Kaiserswerther Diakonie (1851–1975). (Missionsgeschichtliches Archiv 15) Stuttgart 2010.

Kaminsky, Uwe: Mutter, Tochter oder Zwillingsschwester? Unklare Familienverhältnisse zwischen Äußerer und Innerer Mission. In: Sarx, Tobias; Scheepers, Rajah; Stahl, Michael (ed.): Protestantismus und Gesellschaft. Beiträge zur Geschichte von Kirche und Diakonie im 19. und 20. Jahrhundert. Jochen-Christoph Kaiser zum 65. Geburtstag, (Reihe Konfession und Gesellschaft 47) Stuttgart 2013, pp. 93–104.

Kirchhoff, Markus: Konvergierende Topographien. Protestantische Palästinakunde, Wissenschaft des Judentums und Zionismus um 1900. In: Leipziger Beiträge zur jüdischen Geschichte und Kultur 1 (2003), pp. 239–262.
Kirchhoff, Markus: Text zu Land. Palästina im wissenschaftlichen Diskurs 1865–1920. Göttin-
   gen 2005.
Köser, Silke: Denn eine Diakonisse darf kein Alltagsmensch sein. Kollektive Identitäten Kai-
   serswerther Diakonissen 1836–1914. Leipzig 2006.
Krüger, Jürgen: Die Reise Kaiser Wilhelms II. nach Jerusalem. Geschichte und Bedeutung.
   In: Goren, Haim; Eisler, Jakob (ed.): Deutschland und Deutsche in Jerusalem. Jerusalem
   2011, pp. 19–31.
Laak, Dirk van: Über alles in der Welt. Deutscher Imperialismus im 19. und 20. Jahrhundert.
   München 2005.
Löffler, Roland: Das Aussätzigenasyl Jesushilfe. Zur Geschichte einer Herrnhuter Wohltätig-
   keitseinrichtung in Jerusalem. In: Unitas Fratrum 59/60 (2007), pp. 37–89.
Löffler, Roland: Die Gemeinden des Jerusalemsvereins in Palästina im Kontext des kirch-
   lichen und politischen Zeitgeschehens in der Mandatszeit. In: Nothnagle, Almut; Abromeit, Hans-Jürgen; Foerster, Frank (ed.): Seht, wir gehen hinauf nach Jerusalem. Festschrift zum 150jährigen Jubiläum von Talitha Kumi und des Jerusalemsvereins. Leipzig
   2001, pp. 185–212.
Löffler, Roland: Nationale und konfessionelle Identitätsbildungsprozesse in den arabisch-
   lutherischen und arabisch-anglikanischen Gemeinden Palästinas während der Mandatszeit. In: Feldtkeller, Andreas; Nothnagle, Almut (ed.): Mission im Konfliktfeld von Islam,
   Judentum und Christentum. Eine Bestandsaufnahme zum 150-jährigen Jubiläum des Jerusalemsvereins. Frankfurt/Main 2003, pp. 71–104.
Löffler, Roland: Protestanten in Palästina. Religionspolitik, Sozialer Protestantismus und Mission in den deutschen evangelischen und anglikanischen Institutionen des Heiligen Lan-
   des 1917–1939. Stuttgart 2008.
Löffler, Roland: Die langsame Metamorphose einer Missions- und Bildungseinrichtung zu
   einem sozialen Dienstleistungsbetrieb. Zur Geschichte des Syrischen Waisenhauses der
   Familie Schneller in Jerusalem 1860–1945. In: Trimbur, Dominique (ed.): Die Europäer in
   der Levante. Zwischen Politik, Wissenschaft und Religion (19.–20. Jahrhundert). Des Européens au Levant. Entre politique, science et religion (19.–20. siècle). München 2004,
   pp. 77–106.
Löffler, Roland: Sozialer Protestantismus in Übersee. Ein Plädoyer für die Integration der
   Äußeren in die Historiographie der Inneren Mission. In: Friedrich, Norbert; Jähnichen,
   Traugott (ed.): Sozialer Protestantismus im Kaiserreich: Problemkonstellationen – Lö-
   sungsperspektiven – Handlungsprofile. Münster 2005, pp. 321–353.
Löffler, Roland: The metamorphosis of a pietistic missionary and educational institution into
   a social services enterprise. The case of the Syrian Orphanage. In: Murre-van den Berg,
   Heleen (ed.): New faith in Ancient Lands. Western mission in the Middle East in the nine-
   teenth and early twentieth centuries. Leiden 2006, pp. 151–174.
Lückhoff, Martin: Anglikaner und Protestanten im Heiligen Land. Das gemeinsame Bistum
   Jerusalem (1841–1886). Wiesbaden 1998.
Murre-van den Berg, Heleen (ed.): New faith in Ancient Lands. Western mission in the
   Middle East in the nineteenth and early twentieth centuries. Leiden 2006.
Murre-van den Berg, Heleen: The study of western missions in the Middle East (1820–1920):
   An annotated bibliography. In: Friedrich, Norbert; Kaminsky, Uwe; Löffler, Roland (ed.).
   The social dimension of Christian missions in the Middle East. Historical studies of the
   19th and 20th centuries. (Missionsgeschichtliches Archiv 16) Stuttgart 2010, pp. 35–53.
Neubert-Preine, Thorsten: Diakonie für das Heilige Land. Die Gründung der Kaiserswerther
   Orientarbeit durch Theodor Fliedner. In: Nothnagle, Almut; Abromeit, Hans-Jürgen;
   Foerster, Frank (ed.): Seht, wir gehen hinauf nach Jerusalem. Festschrift zum 150jährigen
   Jubiläum von Talitha Kumi und des Jerusalemsvereins. Leipzig 2001, pp. 31–43.

Nothnagle, Almut; Abromeit, Hans-Jürgen; Foerster, Frank (ed.): Seht, wir gehen hinauf nach Jerusalem. Festschrift zum 150jährigen Jubiläum von Talitha Kumi und des Jerusalemsvereins. Leipzig 2001.

Petschulat, Tim O.: Wahrnehmungen zu den orientalischen Christen im Kontext der Kaiserreise Wilhelms II. (1898). In: Tamke, Martin; Manukyan, Arthur (ed.): Protestanten im Orient. Würzburg 2009, pp. 109–148.

Pschichholz, Christin: Considerations of the correlations between social welfare, missionary activities and foreign policy. German Protestant communities in Istanbul and Izmir and the Diaspora care. In: Friedrich, Norbert; Kaminsky, Uwe; Löffler, Roland (ed.): The social dimension of Christian mission in the Middle East. Historical studies of the 19th and 20th centuries. Stuttgart 2010, pp. 191–203.

Pschichholz, Christin: Zwischen Diaspora, Diakonie und deutscher Orientpolitik. Deutsch evangelische Gemeinden in Istanbul und Kleinasien in osmanischer Zeit. Stuttgart 2011.

Raheb, Mitri: Das reformatorische Erbe unter den Palästinensern. Zur Entstehung der Evangelisch-Lutherischen Kirche in Jordanien. Gütersloh 1990.

Ronecker, Karl-Heinz; Nieper, Jens; Neubert-Preine, Thorsten (ed.): Dem Erlöser der Welt zur Ehre. Festschrift zum hundertjährigen Jubiläum der Einweihung der evangelischen Erlöserkirche in Jerusalem. Leipzig 1998.

Roth, Erwin: Preußens Gloria im Heiligen Land. Die Deutschen und Jerusalem. München 1973.

Schmidt, Jutta: Beruf Schwester. Mutterhausdiakonie im 19. Jahrhundert. Frankfurt/Main; New York 1998.

Sinno, Abdel-Raouf: Deutsche Interessen in Syrien und Palästina 1841–1898. Aktivitäten religiöser Institutionen, wirtschaftliche und politische Einflüsse. Berlin 1982.

Sticker, Anna: Friederike Fliedner und die Anfänge der Frauendiakonie. Ein Quellenbuch. Neukirchen 1961.

Stursberg, Johannes (ed.): Jubilate! Denkschrift zur Jubelfeier der Erneuerung des apostolischen Diakonissen-Amtes (von Julius Disselhoff). Aus Anlaß der fünfundsiebzigjährigen Wirksamkeit des Diakonissen-Mutterhauses zu Kaiserswerth a. Rhein, durchgesehen und nach dem Stande vom 1911 neu herausgegeben. [Kaiserswerth] 1911.

Tamke, Martin; Manukyan, Arthur (ed.): Protestanten im Orient. Würzburg 2009.

Trimbur, Dominique (ed.): Die Europäer in der Levante. Zwischen Politik, Wissenschaft und Religion (19.–20. Jahrhundert). Des Européens au Levant. Entre politique, science et religion (19.–20. siècle). München 2004.

Deaconesses at the *Leper Home* in Jerusalem 1874–1950

Ruth Wexler

Around fifty deaconesses served at the *Leper Home* in Jerusalem during the years 1874–1950. These young women, who spent up to 38 years in Jerusalem, grew up in *Moravian Church* communities in Europe, and most of them trained at the *Emmaus Deaconess Institution* in Niesky, Germany, an institute of the *Moravian Church.*

The *Leper Home* in Jerusalem was a Protestant initiative to care for people suffering from leprosy. This disease, mistakenly identified with the leprosy mentioned in the Old Testament (zara'at in Hebrew), was regarded as a fearful, contagious and incurable disease.[1] In the mid-nineteenth century, several dozen lepers were living in dilapidated huts outside Jerusalem's Zion Gate in their own separate community, dependant for their livelihood on begging and the generosity of pilgrims.[2] The Anglican-German Bishopric in Jerusalem established the first *Leper Home* in 1867, offering the beggars free shelter, food and care. The *Moravian Church* was asked to assume responsibility for its management and sent staff from Europe to run the home and care for the patients. The deaconesses sent to care for the patients played a significant role in this unique institution. The circumstances during this eventful period in the history of Jerusalem and the nature of the *Leper Home* made their mission remarkably challenging, highlighting their striking self-devotion throughout the history of the home.

The main source used for studying the deaconesses' experiences are the 79 annual reports of the *Leper Home* in Jerusalem for the years 1867–1950. Some were "compiled from German" and some were written originally in English, differing in style and length over the years. They were sent out by the *Moravian Church's* Board of Directors to members of the Church throughout the world "to give an account of the Home and to win new friends". Readers are asked to pray for the success of the enterprise and to continue to provide financial support.[3]

The first report was written and signed by Bishop Latrobe, the Secretary of the *Moravian Church.* Later, both the Treasurer and Secretary of the *Moravian Church* signed the annual reports, in which they included edited accounts they

---

1   Leprosy is an ancient chronic infectious disease caused by Mycobacterium Leprae, transmitted by droplet infection, and affecting mainly the skin and the peripheral nerves. It is manifested by anaesthesia and paralysis of hands, feet, and eyes, which, left untreated, may result in severe disabilities. Anti-bacterial medication to eliminate the infection has been available since 1941, and a number of measures are used to prevent disabilities. Nowadays it is named Hansen disease after Armuer Hansen, who discovered the causative agent in 1873. See Yawalkar (2002).

2   Tobler (2005), pp. 47–49, 54–55.

3   1st annual report (hereafter AR) of the Leper Home in Jerusalem for the year 1867, p. 5. 14th AR 1885, p. 19.

received from the House-Father and the deaconesses stationed in Jerusalem, as well as their comments on the work, a list of contributions, and a financial statement. Periodically, unedited notes from the staff were included, as well as a medical report written by the doctor. From 1922 onwards, the Matron's detailed accounts became the main part of the annual reports. The Matron sent an account of the different activities within the home, accounts of special events in Jerusalem affecting the home, a detailed report on the health and spiritual state of the patients, and a report concerning the staff. As a result, even though the annual reports were written for specific purposes that may affect their content and style, they are a rich source of material for studying the deaconesses' experiences.

This article is divided into three sections: a) The *Deaconess Institution* within the *Moravian Church*; b) The *Leper Home* in Jerusalem; c) The deaconesses' experiences at the *Leper Home* in Jerusalem. These experiences, as reflected in the annual reports, are described through the following aspects: harsh physical conditions, the language challenge, the patients as people of the East, the spiritual work, caring for patients with an incurable disease, unrest and isolation in Jerusalem, and conflicts between Arabs and Jews. All these challenges serve to illustrate the deaconesses' remarkable devotion.

The *Deaconess Institution* within the *Moravian Church*

The *Moravian Church*, considered to be the first Protestant Church, desired to revive the practices of the early Church, and consecrated women as deaconesses in the years 1745–1790.[4] Besides assisting in ceremonial acts as in the early Church, they cared for the sick and trained the young girls of the com-

---

4   The *Moravian Church*'s religious heritage dates back to Jan Hus, a Catholic priest who led a reaction against the *Roman Catholic Church* in Bohemia and Moravia in the early fifteenth century and was sentenced to death for heresy in Constance, Germany, in 1415. Within fifty years of his death, a small group of his followers in Bohemia formed their own independent church known as the *Unitas Fratrum* or the *Unity of the Brethren*. The influence of German-speaking immigrants who joined the Brethren enabled close contact with the developing Reformation in Germany. The Brethren often found themselves caught in bitter wars between Catholics and Protestants, which forced them to flee. They persevered in small groups, holding on to their faith and tradition secretly until, in 1722, Count Nicolas Ludwig von Zinzendorf placed an estate he owned at the disposal of a group of refugees. They laid the foundations for the renewed *Church of the Brethren* and named it the *Moravian Church* after their country of origin. The new settlement, named Herrnhut, developed a strict social and religious system, in which the members were divided into groups by gender and marital status and the elected council of elders wielded great influence. This settlement was followed by many others that sprang up in Europe, South and North America, South and East Africa, and Asia during the nineteenth century. The *Moravian Church* was the first to undertake foreign missions as an organised Protestant Church. A mission to slaves in St. Thomas in the West Indies began in 1732; see Hutton (1909), pp. 35–36, 52, 141, 157, 163, 312, 314, 317; Schattschneider/Frank (2009), pp. 25–30, 39–48; Fries (2003), p. 18.

munity. This office of women had ceased by the time Hermann Plitt (1821–1900) arrived on the scene. He was the director of the *Theological Seminary* of the *Moravian Church* in Gnadenfeld in Upper Silesia[5] and was inspired by Theodor Fliedner's initiative in Kaiserswerth to renew the office of deaconess for the purpose of caring for the sick and the needy. Young unmarried women were offered education in theology, education and nursing, enabling them to earn their living respectably. Following this idea, in 1842 Plitt set up a deaconess institute within the *Moravian Church*. This innovative idea initially met with opposition from within the Church because it required the women to remain single and devote themselves entirely to their work.[6]

Plitt finally opened the *Deaconess Institute* in 1866 and named it *Heinrichsstift*. In a small house near Gnadenfeld, with modest rooms and means, two sisters[7] – one of whom had trained in the *Kaiserswerth Deaconess Home* in Frankfurt-am-Main – took care of the sick and the elderly.[8] With the help of a third sister, who joined in 1876, they performed home visits and took care of the children in the vicinity. As they slowly gained trust and recognition within the local Catholic environment, they needed a larger facility to be able to respond to the increasing demand. In 1870 the *Heinrichsstift Hospital*, the first in the area, was inaugurated. The sisters received their first motherhouse with a training centre for additional sisters, most of them members of *Moravian Church* communities. They adopted new areas of activity: community health care, setting up an infirmary at the Pedagogium in Niesky,[9] and overseas missionary work. In 1883, following years of steady growth, the motherhouse was relocated to Niesky and was named *Emmaus* to commemorate a significant event in early Christianity. Plitt, concerned about losing the uniqueness of the institution, was against joining Fliedner's organisation, but in 1898, following a change in management, the *Emmaus Deaconess Institute* (EDI) joined the *Kaiserswerth General Conference*.[10]

A total of 92 sisters were working in hospitals, doing community work, and teaching children in various facilities belonging to the *Moravian Church* when Pastor Theodor Schmidt was appointed head of the EDI in 1913. One of his first innovations was the introduction of a council, involving the sisters in the management of their own institution. Schmidt served as head of the EDI from 1913 to 1947, working hand in hand with Matron Padel as equal

---

5   Gnadenfeld (renamed Pawłowiczki) is a village founded by the Moravians in 1743 in Silesia, a region located along the Oder River, part of Poland since 1945; see http://en.wikipedia.org/wiki/Upper_Silesia (accessed 30/01/2015).

6   Heinke (2008), pp. 11–12.

7   The term sister is used for convenience. The terms deaconess, sister, and nurse are used interchangeably in the data that served as the basis for this article.

8   Goldner (1890), pp. 108–110.

9   Niesky is a town founded by Moravians in 1742 in East Saxony, a region located in the eastern part of Germany on the border with Poland and the Czech Republic, and was part of the German Democratic Republic until 1990; see http://en.wikipedia.org/wiki/Niesky accessed 15/01/2015.

10 Heinke (2008), p. 13.

partners, sharing responsibility for the work of the sisters wherever they
served. Many changes took place during this significant period. The number
of sisters increased to over 140, and a new building was bought for the motherhouse, separating it from the hospital for the first time. As well as training
their own sisters, they operated a housekeeping school and a school for infants. The work in the leprosy asylums in Jerusalem (since 1876) and in Surinam (since 1892) was highly appreciated and regarded as a means of expanding the horizons and strengthening the character of the few who were sent
there.[11]

World War II was a turbulent time for EDI, which was forced to flee from
Niesky. With the return to Niesky in the summer of 1945 a new era began for
EDI under the direction of Pastor Paul Fabricius, who put the emphasis on
developing, expanding, and modernising the hospital. Retirement homes
were created for the elderly in the surrounding community, where the sisters
continued to care for their retired colleagues. The work abroad in the *Bethesda
leprosy asylum* in Surinam in South America was suspended in 1947, as was the
work in the *Jesus Hilfe Leper Home* in Jerusalem in 1951.[12]

The *Leper Home* in Jerusalem

At the turn of the nineteenth century, Jerusalem was a forsaken, small city in
the Ottoman Empire. This began to change when Europeans, driven by religious awakening or economic and political motives, began arriving in the
Holy Land.[13] Within this eventful period, in the years 1862–1925, 15 different
hospitals were established outside the Old City walls of Jerusalem; one of
them was the *Leper Home*.

The German Baroness Keffenbrinck Ascheraden, who decided to devote
her life to charity, came with her husband on a pilgrimage to the Holy Land
in 1865. She saw the lepers living and begging at the city gates of Jerusalem
and instigated the establishment of an asylum to care for them. With the help
of the Anglican-German Bishopric in Jerusalem she established the first *Leper
Home* and was active in fundraising and establishing its operational infrastructure. She heard of the *Moravian Church*'s experience in caring for lepers in

---

11   Ibid., pp. 12–15.
12   79th AR 1950, pp. 2–3.
13   9,000 Muslims, Jews, and Christians lived within the walls of the Old City in densely
       populated and poorly ventilated dwellings under bad sanitary conditions. Epidemics of-
       ten erupted, causing many deaths. The harsh living conditions and the Ottoman author-
       ity's lifting of the prohibition of building outside the city walls encouraged the purchase
       of land and the erection of private and public buildings, thus creating the new city be-
       yond the walls. Competition between the European powers for influence over the area
       resulted in intensive activity and was reflected in significant changes in all facets of life:
       culture, education, economy, welfare, health, and religious life. In 1914, at the outbreak
       of World War I, there were around 70,000 inhabitants of a variety of ethnic groups in
       Jerusalem; see Ben-Arieh (1984), pp. 90, 184–189, 279, 396; Ben-Arieh (1986), p. 466.

South Africa since 1818 and sought their assistance.[14] "Ultimately the Moravian Church was called upon to engage in a service so consonant with its spirit and aim."[15] Brother Friedrich Tappe, who served as a missionary among Eskimos in Labrador, was chosen and sent to Jerusalem, arriving in 1867 with his wife Frederika to become "House Father and Mother" for the newly built home. In 1880, the *Moravian Church* assumed full responsibility for the asylum: funding it, running it, hiring staff, and eventually owning the property.[16] After the death of the House Father in 1908, this office was abolished and management of the home was taken over completely by the Matron and the sisters, an arrangement that continued until 1950.[17]

The *Leper Home* in Jerusalem was a highly regarded mission of the *Moravian Church* as a whole, with different degrees of involvement and control evolving over time, of the German, British, and American provinces. The Board of Directors was appointed to be accountable for its management, and a local committee, consisting primarily of members of the German-Lutheran congregation in Jerusalem, supervised it directly.

As the number of patients entering the first home increased, it became too small and a bigger one was inaugurated in 1887. It was designed as a walled, self-sufficient asylum with a capacity of 50–60 patients and staff, and was named *Jesus Hilfe*, although in practice people called it the *Leper Home*. It was surrounded by a large garden containing four water cisterns, livestock, a vegetable garden, and an orchard.

Initially, the *Leper Home* was based on the principle of segregation combined with good care of body and soul, which were thought at the time to be the best means of treating leprosy and its sufferers.[18] The patients living at the *Leper Home* were mostly Muslim men, women, and children of diverse social groups: villagers, farmers, Bedouins, and beggars. There were a few Christians and Jews too. The care the patients received was expected to ameliorate somewhat their physical suffering, enable them to experience some happiness, and heighten their spiritual awareness through Christian love.[19] The patients received the standards of care prevalent at the time: hygiene, fresh air, rich nourishment, physical activity, and spiritual guidance. They were expected to work in the house and garden and on the farm.[20]

Work in the *Leper Home* was carried out in accordance with three fundamental principles: "1. Every patient must come voluntarily. 2. The sexes must be separate. 3. No Mohammedan must be compelled to attend religious worship."[21] Those who broke the rules – patients who chose to marry, very awk-

---

14   Schwacke (1983), p. 605.
15   La Trobe (1907), pp. 20–21.
16   Ibid., pp. 20–26.
17   Schwake (1983), p. 622.
18   La Trobe (1907), pp. 8–9.
19   19th AR 1890, pp. 3–4; 44th AR 1915, p. 6.
20   Löffler (2007), p. 45.
21   41st AR 1912, p. 3.

ward patients who gave the sisters much trouble, and those who were a bad influence on the others – were sent away.[22] They could leave to visit their homes by permission and, from 1925 onwards, those who were cured were discharged.[23] Relatives could formally come and visit, but many of them did not, making the patients feel homesick and isolated.[24]

It was the only asylum of its kind in the Middle East and was considered a progressive institution and "a model of what such a place should be".[25] Experiments with new remedies were carried out there.[26] "It possesses all the essential requisites. It is a real Home and yet also a Hospital. It has staff nurtured in the tradition of leper nursing, and equipped with the knowledge of all that can be done and should be done."[27]

During the twentieth century the *Leper Home* in Jerusalem withstood many stormy events – both World Wars, and conflicts between Arabs and Jews – which affected the supply of basic provisions and staff and the ambience within the home. In 1948, following the establishment of the State of Israel, Jerusalem was divided between Israel and Jordan and the *Leper Home* remained on the Israeli side of the city. The *Moravian Church*, which had been concerned about its economic viability for some years, decided at last to give up the work in the *Leper Home*. The high costs of maintenance, the development of effective medical treatment, and the need to adapt to an influx of Jewish patients, which would demand changes in the running of the home, were behind the decision.[28] The entire compound was sold to the *Jewish National Fund* in 1950 and handed over to the *Israeli Ministry of Health*. From then on the home was officially named the *Hansen Government Hospital*, and work continued there until it closed for good in 2000.

The deaconesses' experiences at the *Leper Home* in Jerusalem

The first German sister arrived at the first *Leper Home* in 1874 to help the House Father care for the patients. "She proved the forerunner of a series of willing-hearted nurses from Moravian Congregations who, as need arose, have offered to go to the Leper Home."[29] From 1880 onwards, sisters were

---

22 23rd AR 1894, pp. 4–5; 42nd AR 1912, p. 3; 52nd AR 1923, p. 9; 53rd AR 1924, p. 11; 56th AR 1927, p. 17; 57th AR 1928, p. 12; 58th AR 1929, pp. 3, 6; 59th AR 1930, p. 4; 68th AR 1939, p. 4; 73rd AR 1944, p. 11.

23 54th AR 1925, p. 6.

24 53rd AR 1924, pp. 9–11; 54th AR 1925, pp. 7–11; 57th AR 1928, p. 5; 58th AR 1929, p. 12; 59th AR 1930, pp. 7, 10; 63rd AR 1934, pp. 8–9; 67th AR 1938, pp. 5–3; 68th AR 1939, pp. 6–9; 69th AR 1940, pp. 4–9; 71st AR 1942, p. 9; 72nd AR 1943, pp. 6–7; 73rd AR 1944, p. 7; 74th AR 1945, pp. 10–13; 77th AR 1948, pp. 10–13.

25 42nd AR 1913, p. 6.

26 36th AR 1907, p. 5; 40th AR 1911, p. 8; 54th AR 1925, p. 5.

27 34th AR 1905, p. 8.

28 Haas (1993), p. 149.

29 La Trobe (1907), p. 24.

sent by the EDI to the home regularly, in coordination with the Board of Directors, to care for the patients and eventually to manage the home. Except for the Matron, they received no special training prior to their voyage.[30] The Matron hired and managed the staff in accordance with the EDI, the Board of Directors and the local committee, and represented the sisters vis-à-vis these bodies at the same time.[31] Their wages were "mere pocket money".[32] They were entitled to a few days holiday each year, and a longer holiday after five years of service, during which they used to go home to Europe. At times these holidays had to be cancelled. Their health, a matter discussed and reported regularly, was also affected.[33]

The sisters faced a tremendous change in lifestyle and endured harsh physical conditions, as well as life-threatening situations in Jerusalem. The cultural gap was a great challenge both inside and outside the home. They had to use different languages and were confronted with other religions and different cultural behaviour in a land marked by political unrest. The Matron, who from 1908 assumed responsibility for the entire operation of the home, with the assistance of three to five sisters at a time, had to manage the allocated budget, hire suitable local staff, obtain supplies, maintain the buildings and the garden, communicate with the local government and municipal authorities, and report to the Board of Directors. Over and above all these, she and the other sisters had the task of caring for the physical and spiritual welfare of a diverse crowd of patients with a dreaded and incurable disease.[34]

Harsh physical conditions

The sisters came from Europe to Jerusalem, where the climate was hot and dry most of the year. The water supply depended on the rainfall during the four winter months. This water filled the cisterns and was used throughout the year for all the home's water requirements: drinking, washing, cooking, gardening and farming. The supply of water was a constant worry in the home.[35] Attempts were made to provide enough water, independently of the cisterns,

---

30 Löffler (2007), p. 71.
31 Löffler (2007), pp. 47–49.
32 49th AR 1920, p. 5; 50th AR 1921, p. 4.
33 51st AR 1922, p 3; 52nd AR 1923, p. 8; 53rd AR 1924, p. 7; 54th AR 1925, p. 7; 55th AR 1926, p. 6; Moravian Messenger (hereafter MM) Apr. 1927, p. 27, Sept. 1927, p. 69; 57th AR 1928, p. 3; 58th AR 1929, p. 4; MM Mar. 1931, p. 19; 61st AR 1932, p. 4; 62nd AR 1933, p. 4; 63rd AR 1934, p. 5; 64th AR 1935, p. 5; 65th AR 1936, p. 7; 67th AR 1938, p. 4; 68th AR 1939, p. 3; 69th AR 1940, p. 3; 71st AR 1942, p. 3; 72nd AR 1943, p. 3; 73rd AR 1944, p. 4; 75th AR 1946, p. 6; 78th AR 1949, p. 6.
34 42nd AR 1912, p. 4; 44th AR 1915, p. 5; 46th & 47th AR 1917 and 1918, p. 4.
35 39th AR 1910, p. 6; 54th AR 1925, p. 7; 55th AR 1926, p. 66; MM Feb. 1927, p. 10; 57th AR 1928, p. 3; MM Feb. 1928, p. 13, Nov. 1928, p. 82, Apr. 1930, p. 38; 62nd AR 1933, p. 5; 76th AR 1947, p. 6.

so the sisters "will be able to have a bath-room, a luxury that has hitherto been regarded as out of reach".[36]

Significant physical labour was required from the sisters. At times they had to do household work, such as cleaning, laundry and mending, repairs, kitchen and garden work, as well as their medical duties, which included changing bandages, giving injections, and caring for dying patients. All these tasks were performed while also trying to save money for the home.[37]

The language challenge

On arrival in Jerusalem the sisters encountered an Arabic-speaking society with which they were not acquainted. Arabic was essential not only in the *Leper Home* but also when making one's way outside it. After the British took Palestine from the Turks in 1917–1918, English became the next official language, so the sisters had to study both Arabic and English: Arabic for communicating with the patients, their families, and the general population, and English for dealing with the authorities, as well as for communicating with the Board of Directors, which by now was coordinated through the British Province.[38] Staff shortages and an increased workload made it difficult for the sisters to study the languages, but nevertheless they made the effort, sometimes taking the opportunity to be taught by a patient.[39] Before becoming Matron, Sister Elsa in 1922 and Sister Oggeline in 1924 were sent to England for a few months to study English and to get to know the members of the Board of Directors.[40] In her first report as Matron, Sister Oggeline writes: "Now we are all doing our best to perfect ourselves in Arabic, as it is so very important for the nurses to be able to make themselves understood by the patients, and if possible more than that."[41] In the 1937 annual report, Matron Margareta Ribbach welcomes a new sister:

> Dear friends, give a special thought to our new Sister, for what a change it is, to come from European conditions and get used to strange people with their native language and, to us, unaccustomed ways. Climate, food, surroundings, all are strange, and come hard to a newcomer who has to learn both languages.[42]

---

36   42nd AR 1912, p. 8.
37   41st AR 1912, p. 7; 42nd AR 1913, p. 6; 56th AR 1927, p. 12; MM Feb. 1927, pp. 10–11; 57th AR 1928, p. 3; MM Jul. 1933, p. 54; 47th AR 1919, p. 5; 50th AR 1921, p. 6; 52nd AR 1923, pp. 7–8; 53rd AR 1924, p. 7; 54th AR 1925, pp. 7–8; MM Feb. 1927, pp. 10–12; 57th AR 1928, p. 3; MM Apr. 1930, pp. 31, 38, Oct. 1931, pp. 75–80, Jul. 1933, p. 54.
38   Löffler (2007), p. 55.
39   39th AR 1910, p. 9; 53rd AR 1924, p. 7; 58th AR 1929, p. 3; 56th AR 1927, p. 13; MM Jan. 1927, p. 4, Apr. 1928, p. 25; 57th AR 1928, p. 3; 58th AR 1929, pp. 4–5; 62nd AR 1933, p. 4; 63rd AR 1934, pp. 5–6; 68th AR 1939, p. 3; 75th AR 1946, p. 6.
40   51st AR 1922, p. 4; 53rd AR 1924, p. 4.
41   53rd AR 1924, p. 7.
42   66th AR 1937, p. 4.

The patients as people of the East

The attitude of the sisters towards the patients as reflected in the annual reports was complex, and is expressed differently by each of them. Some sisters seem to be more critical and judgmental than others.[43] They regard the patients as human beings entitled to tender love and care, or as children who are in need of education, deserving motherly love. At the same time, they are referred to as inferior people of the East who are difficult to deal with. It is difficult to differentiate between the sisters' attitudes towards the patients as being 'natives' or Muslims, although sometimes an explicit reference to Islam as being the background for their behaviour is mentioned.[44]

As the Matron writes simply: "the Orientals are so different from us".[45] The patients' customs and conduct were very different from those of the European sisters: their diet, the way they ate, their personal hygiene, their attitude towards women, to mention just a few. Each patient is described in detail referring to his religious affiliation, state of health, behaviour, relationship with the other patients, and his attitudes towards the sisters. Patients are described as "undeveloped", "childish", "stubborn", "lazy", "sunk in superstition and unbelief", and "ungrateful". They are accused of loving unrestrained freedom, easily leaving their wives and treating them badly, being untruthful, fanatics, and lacking living hope. Some of them are described as trying patients who are violent, having a furious temper and cursing a sister who displeased them. These negative and critical descriptions, attributed to them being "Orientals", are combined with favourable and empathic expressions of kindness, consideration, and motherly emotions. When a patient shows signs of gratitude and a genuine will to help the sisters in their tasks, this is highly appreciated.[46]

An additional source of tension between the sisters and the patients was the patients' attitude towards the sisters as women. At the beginning it was difficult for the sisters to gain and maintain authority over the male patients, who were in the majority. When, in 1908, the Matron assumed charge of the Home,

> at first some of the men were discontented. They said they wanted a man over them, and did not want to be ruled by women. Considering the subordinate position women occupy in the East, this was not surprising, though it was unpleasant for the nurses and especially for the matron.[47]

---

43 AR 1923 written by Elsa Heinke, ARs 1924–1936 by Oggeline Nörgaard, ARs 1937–1938 by Margarete Ribbach, ARs 1939–1945 by Johanna Larsen, ARs 1946–1950 by Oggeline Nörgaard.

44 52nd AR 1923, p. 8; 54th AR 1925, pp. 7, 11; 56th AR 1927, p. 13l; MM Apr. 1928, p. 25; 58th AR 1929, p. 4; 72nd AR 1943, p. 8.

45 62nd AR 1933, p. 11.

46 52nd AR 1923, p. 8; 54th AR 1925, p. 12; MM Apr. 1926, p. 27; 56th AR 1927, pp. 13–17; 57th AR 1928, p. 6; 64th AR 1935, p. 7; 65th AR 1936, p. 12; 66th AR 1937, p. 5, 7; 67th AR 1938, p. 4; 69th AR 1940, p. 7; 75th AR 1946, p. 11.

47 38th AR 1909, p. 3.

In the 1924 annual report Matron Elsa writes:

> their behaviour to the nurses is also very satisfactory just now. This is a special source of gratification to us, for it is not always easy to know how to deal with the Mohammedan men, whose religion causes them to look upon all women, Europeans included, as inferior beings, and in this respect one man will often influence the whole company.[48]

It is difficult to draw conclusions from the annual reports about whether all male patients eventually accepted the sisters' authority. Generally it is indicated that most of them respected and appreciated what the sisters did for them, with the exception of the "difficult" patients. The sisters exercised discipline and kindness and tried to re-educate the patients, believing "the word of God" would change the patients for the better.[49] Matron Oggeline, who writes very detailed and vivid reports about each of the patients, states that "what pleases us is to see that their stay here does the patients good, not only outwardly, but above all inwardly".[50]

Spiritual work

The work among the lepers, in which the sisters played a major role, was driven by strong religious motives.[51] In the first report of the first *Leper Home* in Jerusalem in 1867, written by Bishop La Trobe and sent to members of the *Moravian Church* all over the world, he explains the reason for taking on the 'noble' work among the lepers in Jerusalem for a 'holy cause':

> Let all be helped, not only Hottentots, Chinese, widows and orphans [...], but also poor lepers in their mental and bodily wretchedness and degradation [...] leprosy is one of the most fearful disease of human body. The disease is and remains a malady which reveals the fruit of sin – death and corruption – in a frightful manner in the human body. [...] we are justified in regarding it as the ripe fruit of the greatest temporal and spiritual misery to which mankind can sink. [...] If little can be done for them physically, much may be to help them in a far higher sense. If Christian charity wills it they may be freed from the galling fetters of filth, nakedness and hunger [...] by recognizing their existence and their right to be treated. [...] In some sort the care of these sufferers may be regarded as a legacy of His to the Universal Church.[52]

The sisters, who grew up on this legacy, felt honoured and privileged to be sent to the *Leper Home* in Jerusalem. They were not expected to perform formal active religious teaching, "except that which could be given in conversation".[53]

According to the 1906 annual report, among the members of the *Moravian Church* there was a debate on how explicit the religious aspect of the work

48   52nd AR 1923 p. 8.
49   57th AR 1928, pp. 4–11; 65th AR 1936, p. 6.
50   57th AR 1928, p. 12.
51   MM Sept. 1917, p. 108, Oct. 1931, p. 77.
52   1st AR 1867, p. 5.
53   42nd AR 1912, p. 4.

should be in the everyday running of the home. The argument was whether the *Leper Home* was just a hospital, or "something more".

> Our hope must be that the Moslem may learn the power, truth, and grace of Christ, more from the consistency of our life and action, than from the frequency and urgency of religious speech. [...] What we do not do is to take advantage of sickness, in order that we may force our faith upon men who decline our spiritual ministrations.[54]

Under Ottoman rule, Christians were prohibited from preaching to Muslims. Until 1912, this prohibition was one of the fundamental principles on which the home was run. However, on the advice of the local committee, this was changed and different means were tried to get the patients to attend the meetings in the prayer room.[55] Most patients were apprehensive, rejected preaching or any attempt at persuasion, and did not attend the meetings in the prayer room.[56] This attitude among the patients gradually changed when Pastor Kurban, an Arabic-speaking pastor, was appointed.[57] The sisters did their best to influence the patients. They talked to them while bandaging their sores, asked them to come to the prayer room, gave them the New Testament, read it out to them, and sang and taught hymns.[58] The reports are filled with prayers and the hope of a greater Christian influence on the patients. The readers are asked to keep praying for a change in the patients, "that God will bring something into this otherwise empty life".[59] "When I think of our patients I must confess there is much misery for which there is no remedy, and there are many chains of sin; [...] We have the joy every now and then of seeing the working of God's spirit."[60] Although the sisters did their best, and at times even conducted the prayers, their success was rather limited and was criticised as a missionary failure.[61]

Caring for patients with an incurable disease

As mentioned above, leprosy was regarded as an incurable, degrading, and "repulsive" disease, affecting both body and soul. As patients would stay for many years, sometimes for a lifetime, the sisters witnessed their gradual worsening and increased suffering. Many suffered from sores on their limbs which often became infected and odorous. They suffered from fever and pain, and gradually became blind and severely disabled. "Much patience and love are

54 35th AR 1906, p. 4.
55 41st AR 1912, pp. 3–5; 43rd AR 1914, p. 5; 54th AR 1925, p. 11.
56 43rd AR 1914, p. 5.
57 41st AR 1912, p. 5; 42nd AR 1913, pp. 5–6; 57th AR 1928, p. 4. Kasis Farhud Kurban was the pastor of the *Leper Home* from 1912 to 1934. He and his work deserve a special study.
58 MM Sept. 1927, p. 69; 57th AR 1928, pp. 4, 8; 58th AR 1929, p. 8; MM Apr. 1929, p. 27, Oct. 1931, pp. 79–80; 66th AR 1937, pp. 7–13.
59 58th AR 1929, p. 10.
60 59th AR 1930, p. 11.
61 Löffler (2007), p. 71.

needed for this work, and must be given from above for each day afresh."[62]
One of the main tasks of the sisters was changing bandages. "It is indeed a
hard task at times, to bandage the same wounds day by day, year in and year
out, without seeing them heal."[63] Feelings of helplessness on the one hand,
and empathy, compassion and pity for the patients on the other are reflected
in most reports. But when reporting in detail on the individual patients and
detailing their suffering, the sisters' frustration and sorrow are accentuated.[64]
"What a sad experience it must be for our lepers, to be between hope and
disappointment, with the attainment of sound health before them as an un-
reachable land!"[65] In 1915 some hope of cure by aiouni oil seemed within
reach and the oil was administered with much enthusiasm by the sisters.[66] But
then the Matron writes that "in spite for [sic] all the improvements which we
are so grateful to have seen, leprosy remains a dismally insidious disease
which is immensely difficult to cure".[67]

Apart from the physical suffering of the patients, there was their detach-
ment from their families and community.[68] The sisters made an effort to give
the patients, especially the children, the feeling that they had a family in the
home. They celebrated their own birthdays with the patients and asked the
members and friends of the *Moravian Church* to send presents, especially for
Christmas, which was a great celebration in the home.[69] They used special
donations to take the patients on regular trips and picnics around the country.[70]

---

62 52nd AR 1923, p. 8.
63 66th AR 1937, p. 5.
64 15th AR 1886, p. 5; 50th AR 1921, p. 3; 51st AR 1922, pp. 6–7; 52nd AR 1923, pp. 9–11;
    53rd AR 1924, pp. 8–11; 54th AR 1925, pp. 8–13; 54th AR 1925, pp. 7–13; 56th AR
    1927, pp. 12–17; 57th AR 1928, pp. 4–12; 58th AR 1929, pp. 6–13; 59th AR 1930,
    pp. 4–11; 60th AR 1931, pp. 5–12; 61st AR 1932, pp. 6–11; 62nd AR 1933, pp. 5–11;
    63rd AR 1934, pp. 6–13; 64th AR 1935, pp. 5–13; 65th AR 1936, pp. 5–13; 66th AR
    1937, pp. 6–13; 67th AR 1938, pp. 5–13; 68th AR 1939, pp. 4–13; 69th AR 1940,
    pp. 4–9; 70th AR 1941, pp. 4–8; 71st AR 1942, pp. 4–10; 72nd AR 1943, pp. 4–10; 73rd
    AR 1944, pp. 6–13; 74th AR 1945, pp. 5–15; 75th AR 1946, pp. 7–15; 76th AR 1947,
    pp. 6–14; 77th AR 1948, pp. 7–13; 78th AR 1949, pp. 7–14; 79th AR 1950, pp. 5–12.
65 67th AR 1938, p. 5.
66 44th AR 1915, p. 5; 53rd AR 1924 p. 7.
67 53rd AR 1923, p. 3; 58th AR 1929 p. 6.
68 21st AR 1892, p. 6; 22nd AR 1893, p. 6; 64th AR 1935, pp. 5–6.
69 55th AR 1926, p. 6.
70 50th AR 1921, p. 6; 52nd AR 1923, pp. 11–12; 53rd AR 1924, pp. 7, 11–12; 53rd AR
    1924, p. 11; 58th AR 1929, p. 5; 59th AR 1930, p. 4; 61st AR 1932, pp. 4–5; 52nd AR
    1923, p. 12; MM Feb. 1927, p. 10; 57th AR 1928, p. 11; 58th AR 1929, pp. 5, 12; 61st
    AR 1932, p. 5; 63rd AR 1934, p. 5; 64th AR 1935, p. 6; 65th AR 1936, p. 6; 68th AR
    1939, p. 4.

Isolation and unrest in Jerusalem

The sisters were far from home, detached from a Moravian community. Communication with Europe was by means of letters and visits from *Moravian Church* friends and other paying guests who came to stay in the rest home – comprised of the sisters' spare rooms. The rest home provided them with "the change of society", which they welcomed in their state of homesickness and isolation. At times they were cut off from the world completely. This was especially stressful during times of war and when political restrictions prevented visitors from coming.[71] The sisters were acquainted with the Kaiserswerth deaconesses[72] and members of the *Lutheran Church* in Jerusalem, as well as with other Christians residing in Palestine, although it is unclear from the annual reports how close these contacts were and how they affected the sisters' isolation.[73]

At the outbreak of World War I, Jerusalem was declared to be under martial law and the home was completely cut off from direct communication with Europe for two years.[74] There was a shortage of food, clothing, bedding, fuel, and oil for lighting in the home. The farm, which supplied milk, had to be given up. Bullets and shells flew by during the fighting, and the walls grounds were pulled down for a military railway which was built across a piece of the land. Fortunately, the home itself suffered no damage.[75]

The situation became more stressful when the number of patients increased suddenly as lepers from the government shelter in Siloam came to seek help in the home.[76] The chairman of the local committee and Sister Elizabeth went together to the Mayor of Jerusalem and requested his help in supplying the home with wheat and lentils. Instead, he promised a daily supply of bread and some material for clothing, which enabled the home to cope with feeding and caring for the 11 new patients in addition to the 27 already there.[77] This grave situation not only prevented the Matron and the three sisters from taking the holiday they were entitled to, but they had to continue to manage the home in an unclear political situation in which the authorities demanded that the Matron submit monthly accounts of the home for inspection.[78]

---

71 51st AR 1922, p. 3; 52nd AR 1923, p. 7; 57th AR 1928, p. 4; 75th AR 1946, p. 6.
72 Jerusalem wurde mir zur Heimat (2008), p. 81.
73 Further research is needed to address the subject of social contacts and the relationships the sisters had with people and bodies outside the *Leper Home.*
74 47th AR 1917, p. 3.
75 45th AR 1916, pp. 2–4; 48th AR 1919, pp. 3–4.
76 The Siloam shelter was built by the Ottomans in 1874 to keep the beggars away from the city gates. They had to pay a fee and were supplied with a roof over their heads and a ration of bread and water, but received no care. Some asked to be admitted to the *Leper Home,* but could not comply with the strict discipline in the home and were sent back; see 4th AR 1875, p. 8; 23rd AR 1894, p. 6; MM Aug. 1917, p. 107; 64th AR 1935, p. 9; 67th AR 1938, pp. 6, 12; 68th AR 1939, pp. 7–8; 71st AR 1942, p. 3; 72nd AR 1943, pp. 4–5; 72nd AR 1943, pp. 9–10; 73rd AR 1944, p. 9; 75th AR 1946, p. 12.
77 45th AR 1916, pp. 2–3.
78 46th & 47th AR 1917 & 1918, p. 4.

In 1927, an earthquake shook Jerusalem. The sisters were terrified, and the damage caused to the massive building of the *Leper Home* required many repairs.[79]

At the outbreak of World War II all German citizens in Palestine were either imprisoned or expelled, and the *Leper Home* remained the only German Protestant institution that continued to function in Palestine. It became a meeting place for the few Germans who were not expelled,[80] and a religious service for them was held in the *Leper Home* every six weeks. The Matron, a German citizen who had gone home before the war, was not allowed to return. The remaining sisters, although also German citizens, were allowed to stay and run the home, but were placed under house arrest from May 1940. With special permission they were allowed to visit their German friends, the Kaiserswerth deaconesses in Sarona and Wilhelma.[81] Three nurses from the *Carmel Mission*[82] stayed in the home until they were released by an exchange deal in 1942. All others were set free in May 1945.[83]

In 1940, 18 patients were admitted to the home, taking the total number of inpatients to 33. Among them were five elderly women aged between 70 and 107, who required a great deal of attention and care to help them get used to their strange new surroundings. Staff shortages and illness caused anxiety and a risk of exhaustion. Sister Johanna, who replaced the missing Matron, had not had a holiday since 1935 and came close to suffering a physical and mental breakdown.[84] Friends and volunteers occasionally helped to bandage the patients and mend linen.[85] The home was able to supply food, clothing and treatment for all patients but "for the first time in the history of the Home further admissions had to be refused".[86] Despite all efforts to cut down expenses, the financial situation was reaching a critical stage.[87] In the fifth year of the war, Sister Johanna refers to the situation in Europe and her difficult responsibility in the home: "Whilst in the world abroad this war has been raging furiously, we too here in our Home have been having our struggle [...] it was with a sigh of relief that we came to the end of this particularly strenuous year."[88]

---

79 MM Sept. 1927, pp. 68–69; 57th AR 1928, p. 4.
80 Löeffler (2007), p. 79.
81 Sarona and Wilhelma were German Templer colonies established in Palestine during the nineteenth century. At the outbreak of WWII they were transformed into detention camps for German citizens; see Ben–Artzi (1996), pp. 12–17.
82 The *Carmel Mission* was established in 1904 on Mt. Carmel by German Protestants who separated themselves from the Templers. They set up a medical station in Haifa; see Eisler (1998), pp. 51–62.
83 *Jerusalem wurde mir zur Heimat* (2008), p. 81.
84 73rd AR 1944, p. 4; Löeffler (2007), p. 81.
85 69th AR 1940, pp. 3–4; 73rd AR 1944, p. 4.
86 70th AR 1941, p. 3.
87 71st AR 1942, p. 4; 59th AR 1943, pp. 3–4.
88 73rd AR 1944, p. 3.

Conflicts between Arabs and Jews

When the conflict between Arabs and Jews in Jerusalem became violent in 1929, it affected life in the home significantly. Sounds of shooting were heard in the home, causing anxiety among the sisters and the patients.[89] Later, when there was fighting in the Christian Arab neighbourhood around the home, many of the tiles were broken by splinters and rifle fire. The sisters were asked to put a red cross on the entrances, to try to protect them "if that means security".[90] Egyptian troops were stationed a mile and half away from the home, and the sisters were worried they would find themselves caught up in future fighting.[91] The more violent and restless the situation, the more anxious the sisters became. Visitors could not come, they could not send or receive letters, going into town became dangerous, and they felt imprisoned.[92] Eventually, when the neighbourhood became part of the Jewish city, the Arab helpers who lived in the Old City could not come to work at the home, and the sisters had to do everything by themselves.[93] The doctor, being an Arab, was unable to provide medical services, and the sisters had to seek help wherever it was available: from a first aid station, the *Health Department*, and the *Hadassah Hospital Dermatology Department*.[94]

Under these circumstances, the sisters had to provide the basic necessities of food and clothing for the patients. When buying in the market was forbidden, they baked their own bread and bought food from people who came to the door of the home selling fruit and vegetables.[95] Food was rationed and supplied by the government, and the *International Red Cross* brought provisions on a few occasions. Lack of fuel resulted in power cuts and the phone was out of order, forcing the Matron to walk long distances to reach people and the authorities. A patient who died during the clashes had to be buried in the grounds.[96]

The trouble outside the home was accompanied by tension within it, where both Arabs and Jews resided. The Jewish patients were nervous and feared they would be hurt by the Muslim patients.[97] In 1938, Sister Margareta writes that "during the troubles of last year our Moslem patients decided to kill our three Jewish patients. Our Christian patients told us so. What to do? We were very frightened!"[98] The patients became weary of the hatred, anxiety, and the constant dangers their families endured during the clashes.[99] The sis-

89   58th AR 1929, p. 3; 65th AR 1936, p. 5.
90   MM May 1948, pp. 34–35.
91   MM Dec. 1948, pp. 90–91.
92   MM Feb. 1939, p. 8; 68th AR 1939, p. 3; 77th AR 1948, pp. 5–6.
93   MM Dec. 1948, p. 91; 78th AR 1949, p. 5.
94   77th AR 1948, pp. 5–6.
95   65th AR 1936, p. 5; 77th AR 1948, pp. 5–6.
96   77th AR 1948. pp. 5–6.
97   65th AR 1936, p. 5.
98   Ibid.
99   67th AR 1939, p. 4; MM June 1938, p. 45.

ters managed to calm the patients down, and continued to write about the patients living like brothers and the home being an oasis of peace, or a "Home of Peace".[100] The Board of Directors, realising how strenuous and dangerous it was for the sisters, left it up to them whether to stay or leave the country. The sisters would not consider leaving the work and their patients.[101] They stayed until the *Moravian Church* decided to sell the compound. Sister Ogge-line, who retired as Matron in 1937 after 33 years of service, returned in 1945 after WWII, when urgent assistance was needed, and stayed until 1950. In the last annual report she writes:

> Is it true that I am going to write the annual report for the last time? I can hardly believe it is so; but the time is really coming near when our Mission withdraws. [...] When we look back on this past year and all the years, we must ask for God's forgiveness for the mistakes we have made; but we also have much to thank Him for he gave us the strength to do the work, and we had the privilege of the feeling of sympathy of the patients, when they realized we were really leaving.[102]

Conclusion

The 1950 annual report brings to an end the highly appreciated mission to the *Leper Home* in Jerusalem. During its 83 years of operation it required many resources to keep it going through difficult periods of instability in Jerusalem. It called for self-sacrifice, endurance, perseverance, and patience on the part of the sisters who came from Europe and spent many years in the *Leper Home*, playing a major role in the care of the patients and in the home's management. The vignettes of daily life, as presented in the annual reports, describe the nature of the work within the *Leper Home* as well as issues concerning the world outside it. These reports paint a picture of exceptional self-denying devotion, which was repeatedly accentuated through the multiple challenges the sisters faced while carrying out their mission.

Final remark: Further research is needed to investigate the relationship between the sisters and the EDI, the local committee and the Board of Directors, as well as the social contacts they had in Palestine and Europe. Private correspondence of the sisters as well as correspondence and other documentation of the EDI, local committee and Board of Directors need to be examined.

---

100 58th AR 1929, p. 3; 75th AR 1937, p. 7; 77th AR 1948, pp. 5–6; 78th AR 1949, pp. 5–6; MM May 1948, pp. 34–35.
101 76th AR 1947, p. 4; 77th AR 1948, pp. 5–6.
102 79th AR 1950, p. 3.

Bibliography

Literature

Ben-Arieh, Yehoshua: Jerusalem in the 19th century. Emergence of the New City. Jerusalem 1986.

Ben-Arieh, Yehoshua: Jerusalem in the 19th century. The old city. Jerusalem 1984.

Ben Artzi, Yossi: From Germany to the Holy Land. Jerusalem 1996 (Hebrew).

Eisler, Ejal Jakob: An outline of the Carmel mission (1904–1939). In: Ben Artzi, Yossi (ed.): Haifa: Local history. Haifa University Press / Zmora-Bitan 1998, pp. 51–62 (Hebrew).

Fries, Adelaide L.: Customs and practices of the Moravian church. (first edition Bethlehem, PA 1949) 3rd edition. Bethlehem, PA 2003.

Goldner, Christian: History of the deaconess movement in the Christian church. Cincinnati 1903.

Hartmut, Haas: Notizen aus Palästina. Basel 1993.

Heinke, Katharina: Die Diakonissenanstalt Emmaus. Aus der Geschichte. In: Welschen, Johannes; Schröter, Matthias; Rönsch, Sonja (ed.): Es gibt mehr als einen Anfang. Diakonissen erzählen aus ihrem Leben. Herrnhut 2008, pp. 11–16.

Hutton, Joseph Edmund: A history of the Moravian church. 2nd edition London 1909.

Biografische Porträts, Lebensgeschichten und ausgewählte Lebensläufe. Jerusalem wurde mir zur Heimat, Diakonisse Johanna Larsen erzählt. In: Welschen, Johannes; Schröter, Matthias; Rönsch, Sonja (ed.): Es gibt mehr als einen Anfang. Herrnhut 2008, pp. 78–95.

La Trobe, James: Work among lepers. (first edition Bristol 1878) 5th edition London 1907.

Löffler, Roland: Das Aussätzigenasyl Jesushilfe. Zur Geschichte einer Herrnhuter Wohltätigkeitsreinrichtung in Jerusalem. In: Unitas Fratrum 59/60 (2007), pp. 37–89.

Schattschneider, Allen W., Frank, Albert H.: Through five hundred years and beyond. A popular history of the Moravian church. (first edition Bethlehem, PA1956) fifth revised edition Bethelehm, PA 2009.

Schwake, Norbert: Die Entwicklung des Krankenhauses der Stadt Jerusalem vom Ende des 18. bis zum Beginn des 20. Jahrhunderts. Herzogenrath 1983.

Tobler, Titus: Beitrag zur medizinischen Topographie von Jerusalem. Krankenhäuser in Jerusalem. (First edition Berlin 1855) Haifa 2005 (Hebrew).

Yawalkar, S.J.: Leprosy for medical practitioners and paramedical workers (first edition Basle 1986). 7th edition Basle 2002.

Archives

Moravian Church Archive, London
– Annual reports of the Leper Home in Jerusalem (1867–1951) (AR)
– The Moravian Messenger, a Journal for the British Provinces (MM)

Websites

<http://en.wikipedia.org/wiki/Upper_Silesia>
<http://en.wikipedia.org/wiki/Niesky>

Scandinavia – A successful transfer of the German model

The deaconess movement and professional nursing. International demographics and Danish deaconess settlements at home and abroad 1836–1914

Susanne Malchau Dietz

The Protestant deaconess movement founded in Kaiserswerth, Germany, in 1836 is particularly well known in nursing history through Florence Nightingale's (1820–1910) writings. Nightingale briefly visited Kaiserswerth in 1850. She was impressed by the nursing standards and returned in 1851 to be trained as a nurse on equal terms with the deaconesses. The Nightingale pamphlet from 1850, *The Institution of Kaiserswerth on the Rhine, for the Practical Training of Deaconesses*, and her notes from 1851 serve as unique evidence of the deaconesses' nursing tradition and contribution to modern nursing.[1]

The majority of the history of the deaconess movement has been researched and documented through initiatives from within the movement itself or by theologians, and it is mostly restricted to local institutional history.[2] Exceptions to this include a few international approaches with statistics on the movement.[3] Recently, a number of current nurse historians have taken an interest in examining the significance of the deaconess movement in all historical periods.[4] These studies do not follow a statistical or demographic approach to the movement. However, they indicate that the deaconess movement was particularly successful in Scandinavia (Denmark, Norway and Sweden), and furthermore that immigrant communities from these countries were very significant for the introduction of the deaconess movement in the United States.[5]

This information was particularly interesting to me following my own research into the history of the *Danish Deaconess Foundation* and its contribution to Danish nursing curricula. The *Danish Deaconess Foundation* was founded 1863. It was the first Danish deaconess home and it was modelled after Kaiserswerth. The founder, Queen Louise of Denmark (1817–1898), appointed Miss Louise Conring (1824–1891) as the first superintendent of the home. She was educated and prepared for her position in deaconess homes in Sweden and Strasbourg and finally in Kaiserswerth, where she was consecrated by Pastor Theodor Fliedner (1800–1864). The *Danish Deaconess Foundation* was the first institution to introduce nursing education in Denmark, and it opened its own hospital for this purpose. The trained deaconesses were employed by public or Church authorities in district nursing, home nursing or hospital

---

1 Nutting/Dock (1935); McDonald (2004).
2 Disselhoff (1883); Hauge (1963); Köser (2006); Naumann (2008); Legath (2008); Kaiser/Scheepers (2010); Dietz (2013).
3 Bancroft (1889); Golder (1903); Büttner (2006).
4 Nelson (2001); Nolte (2009); Kreutzer (2010); Schweikardt (2010).
5 Nelson (2001); Kreutzer (2010).

nursing. In accordance with the Kaiserswerth model, Miss Conring shared the leadership function with a pastor (Dietz 2011 a and 2013).[6]

Within the framework of this study it became evident how important it is to investigate the deaconess movement in general and to identify the role that Scandinavia played in this aspect of history. Consequently, the first part of this article focuses on the demographic macrohistory of the deaconess movement: how did the deaconess movement develop and disseminate internationally in terms of numbers and nations? And what was the significance of Scandinavia to the movement? Part two takes a microhistorical approach and aims to identify how the nursing tradition of the deaconess movement has been formulated and practised. For this purpose, a case story of the foundation and nursing practice of the Danish deaconess motherhouse in Brush, Colorado, United States, in the period 1905 to 1909 is investigated. The source is previously unknown correspondence between the Danish deaconess Marie Hvidbjerg (1872–1925) and the superiors of the *Danish Deaconess Foundation*, found in the archives of the *Danish Deaconess Foundation* (A-DDF).

The period in question covers the foundation of the deaconess movement in 1836 to the outbreak of World War I in 1914, which changed the international political conditions and communication. The study only includes motherhouses that were members of the *Kaiserswerth General Conference*. The sources of the study are literature on the deaconess movement from 1860 to the present day and material from the archives of the *Danish Deaconess Foundation*.

The Kaiserswerth model and its transfer

German pastor Theodor Fliedner (1800–1864) and his wife Friederike, née Münster, (1800–1842) revived the office of the deaconess for Protestant women. In 1836, they founded the first deaconess motherhouse in Kaiserswerth near Düsseldorf, which was soon known as the 'grandmotherhouse', since it was from here that the movement rapidly spread across Germany and abroad. In 1861, Fliedner united the movement by establishing a worldwide organisation of motherhouses named the *Kaiserswerth General Conference*. The *Conference* was to meet every third year, and the success was soon evident: in the year of establishment, 27 motherhouses became members with a total of 1,197 sisters. In the decades to follow, membership increased rapidly. The *Conference* proved important for the future as it drew up the policies and rules for member houses and thus secured a shared international identity for the Kaiserswerth deaconesses.[7]

---

6   The second deaconess home in Denmark was *Saint Luke's Foundation*, established in 1900. However, it is not included in this article because it had very few deaconesses in the period in question (Malchau 2005).
7   Golder (1903); Naumann (2008).

The Kaiserswerth motherhouse was organised in accordance with the contemporary patriarchal family structure. This was of great importance, as a safe home for the deaconesses was essential for recruiting the desired daughters of the middle classes. The motherhouse was led by the pastor and the lady superintendent, called 'Mother'. They were the parents of the institution, and the sisters were regarded as their daughters. The superiors, the 'parents' had a duty to ensure the lifelong provision, protection and safekeeping of their deaconess 'daughters'.

The deaconesses entered as probationers, and after a period of training they were consecrated as deaconesses by approval of the sister community before they were given assignments. In contrast to the Catholic nuns, no vows were taken, and a deaconess was free to leave at any time e. g. to take care of aged or sick parents or to marry, which in fact happened frequently. Most of the educated deaconesses were sent to stations owned or administrated by the motherhouse, e. g. hospitals, district nursing, homes for elderly people, homes for 'fallen women', orphanages, schools for girls and parish work.[8]

As for the recruitment of deaconesses, daughters of pastors, physicians and schoolteachers were considered the most desirable candidates. The first deaconess at Kaiserswerth, Gertrude Reichardt (1788–1869), was the daughter of a physician, and she eventually became the iconic figure of the ideal deaconess. Florence Nightingale refers respectfully to her in 1851: "Deaconess Reichardt [...] is found invaluable in conducting the devotions of the male patients who look up to her as a mother, and in instructing and advising the probationers and younger deaconesses."[9] Yet it was not possible to realise this aspiration in the daily practice at the institution in Kaiserswerth. Nursing was regarded as a servant's job and thus no woman with a middle-class background would seriously consider joining the newly formed community of deaconesses. This work and life model was much more attractive for women from the lower classes.[10] This clash between ideals and reality also became apparent in Denmark:

In the 1880s, the pastor of the *Danish Deaconess Foundation*, Nicolai C. Dalhoff (1843–1927), gave a high priority to Danish recruitment strategies that followed the Kaiserswerth recommendations. In 1882, the Danish motherhouse was comprised of 80 deaconesses. However, regrettably, there was not a single schoolmaster's daughter among them. As for daughters of physicians, Pastor Dalhoff praised and envied Kaiserswerth for its Sister Reichardt, who was "highly regarded and deserves her place of honour in the Evangelical Lutheran Church [...], however she is an exception as only very few physicians' daughters have had a call to become deaconesses in Denmark. We only have two".[11]

---

8   Disselhoff (1883).
9   McDonald (2004), p. 497.
10   Schmidt (1998).
11   Quotation translated from the Danish. Dalhoff (1882), p. 79.

The recruitment of daughters of clergymen in Denmark was also depressingly low. Nearly 15 percent of the deaconesses in the German motherhouses in Hannover, Mecklenburg and Bavaria (Neuendettelsau) were daughters of pastors. In Denmark the number was four (less than half a percent). This contradicted Dalhoff's assumption that the daughters of pastors had by nature a call to become a deaconess, "the only office in the Church accessible to women".[12]

The statistics and Dalhoff's comments confirm that the deaconess motherhouses relied at first on recruiting daughters from the middle classes. These women had the desired prequalifications to be trained as responsible nurses. However, this recruitment strategy proved difficult, and in 1865 the Kaiserswerth motherhouse established a preparatory school for probationers aged between 14 and 18 years from the lower classes. The purpose of the school was to remedy deficiencies in their family upbringing or education. The Danish motherhouse followed the Kaiserswerth example in the 1880s.[13]

Demographics of the deaconess movement in Europe

The survival and growth of the deaconess movement depended on the demand for the deaconesses' qualifications and helping hands in the social and healthcare systems around the world, which were still in the early stages of development.[14] The available demographics provide evidence of an increasing demand for deaconesses in Europe.

Table 1: Number of motherhouses belonging to the *Kaiserswerth General Conference*, number of deaconesses and fields of activity 1861–1913[15]

Year	No. of motherhouses	No. of sisters	Fields of activity/ stations
1861	27	1,197	–
1864	30	1,592	368
1868	40	2,106	526
1872	48	2,657	648
1875	50	3,239	866
1878	51	3,901	1,093
1881	53	4,748	1,436

12 Quotation translated from the Danish. Dalhoff (1882), p. 78.
13 Disselhoff (1883); A-DDF: Records of deaconesses at the Danish Deaconess Foundation 1863–1943.
14 Porter (1997).
15 Golder (1903); Drexel Home (1913).

1884	54	5,653	1,742
1888	57	7,129	2,263
1891	63	8,478	2,774
1894	68	10,412	3,641
1898	75	12,935	4,519
1901	75	14,501	5,211
1913	87	21,965	7,923

Table 1 shows the growth of motherhouses belonging to the *Kaiserswerth General Conference*, the number of deaconesses and fields of activity that the motherhouses were involved in during the period 1861–1913. In 1864, 30 motherhouses had deaconesses working in 368 fields, and in 1913 the number had increased to 87 motherhouses with 7,923 fields of activity. An example of the priority given to nursing is the 'grandmotherhouse' in Kaiserswerth. In 1883, the house had 636 sisters working at 187 stations outside the mother-house (nine stations in Kaiserswerth and 178 stations in the rest of Germany and abroad). 113 of the stations were related to professional nursing (51 hospitals, 23 infirmaries and 39 district nursing stations).[16]

Table 2: Number of motherhouses and sisters belonging to the *Kaiserswerth General Conference* their distribution in Europe and religious dominance in 1901[17]

Country	No. of motherhouses	No. of sisters	Religious dominance in the country
Germany	47	12,367	Protestant/ Catholic
Switzerland	4	1,105	Protestant
Scandinavia: Denmark, Norway and Sweden	3	934	Protestant
The Netherlands	7	333	Protestant
Russia	8	288	Orthodox
France	2	100	Catholic
USA	2	99	Mixed
Austria-Hungary	2	82	Catholic
Total	**75**	**15,308**	

16   Disselhoff (1883).
17   Golder (1903).

Table 2 shows that in 1901 the 75 motherhouses belonging to the *Kaiserswerth General Conference* were distributed through Germany, neighbouring European countries and the United States. I will come back to the United States, but where the European deaconess settlements are concerned, the table demonstrates a significant connection between the dominant religion in a given country and the number of deaconess settlements. Even though the Kaiserswerth grandmotherhouse was established in a geographical area dominated by the *Roman Catholic Church*, the success of the movement was limited to the Protestant parts of Germany and neighbouring Protestant countries: Switzerland, Scandinavia (Denmark, Norway and Sweden) and the Netherlands, where the majority of motherhouses and deaconesses were situated.[18]

Table 3: 'Top nine' motherhouses belonging to the *Kaiserswerth General Conference* by number of deaconesses, 1913[19]

Motherhouses 1913	Country	No. of deaconesses
Kaiserswerth	Germany	1435
Bielefeld	Germany	1330
Stuttgart	Germany	980
Königsberg	Germany	927
Neuendettelsau	Germany	841
Dresden	Germany	777
Kristiania (Oslo)	Norway	539
Stockholm	Sweden	378
Copenhagen	Denmark	322

Table 3 depicts the 'top nine' motherhouses in 1913 by number of deaconesses. It shows that Germany was the leading country with the six largest motherhouses, closely followed by Norway, Sweden and Denmark in positions seven to nine.

In terms of growth, the European demographics document the fact that the deaconess movement was successful in the Protestant countries but did not cross the confessional borders of the Reformation that had been set in the

18   England is not included in the statistics even though "London was the first place Sisters were sent to outside of Germany. For eleven years (from 1846–1857) they gave their help in the German Hospital in Dalston." Disselhoff (1883), pp. 75–76. England became Anglican during the Reformation and, as argued by Mangion: "[Deaconesses] though generally supported by Church authorities [in England], were never enthusiastically embraced." They remained small in number in England and were mainly engaged in parochial work in the Anglican, Methodist and Scottish Presbyterian Churches. Mangion (2010), p. 72. See also the article by Mangion in this volume.
19   Der Armen- und Krankenfreund, April (1913), pp. 184 ff.

sixteenth century. This is in contrast to the European settlements of the Roman Catholic nursing congregations, which did cross confessional borders to a significant extent and successfully established themselves in Protestant countries, including Norway and Denmark, where a considerable number of Catholic nuns/sisters were engaged in nursing and hospital management.

In Denmark, the number of nuns was even higher than the number of deaconesses. In 1920, for instance, there were 700 nuns and 520 deaconesses.[20] This demonstrates the fact that the nuns were an important resource in the Catholic Church's missionary work policy in Protestant countries during the period in question. In fact, the Catholic congregations and orders came under the jurisdiction of the Propaganda Fide of the *Holy See* in Rome, today the *Congregation for the Evangelization of Peoples.*

Demographics of the deaconess movement in the United States

Nelson (2001) has argued that the establishment of the deaconess movement in the United States was due to the nineteenth century immigration patterns from Germany, Sweden, Norway and Denmark. Nationality, culture and religious affiliation were important factors in this process, and Protestant (Lutheran) congregations established deaconess motherhouses to serve the communities in their own language.

The idea of bringing the deaconess movement to America came from the Lutheran pastor William Alfred Passavant (1821–1894) from Pennsylvania. He visited Kaiserswerth in 1845, and there he "saw with astonishment what the Lord had done through Fliedner".[21] He persuaded Fliedner to send deaconesses to America, and in 1849 Fliedner arrived in person in Pittsburgh with four Kaiserswerth deaconesses to take charge of a hospital. This first initiative failed because of the anti-Catholic feeling at the time, which opposed anything resembling Roman Catholic institutions, and because of opposition to women in public functions, and the low importance attached to the education of women. However, in 1884, the German immigrant and businessman John D. Lankenau (1817–1901) successfully made a new attempt to establish a deaconess motherhouse in Philadelphia. The first seven deaconesses were recruited from an independent motherhouse in Iserlohn in Germany. In fact, an entire community of sisters agreed to go to America.[22]

20 Malchau/Nilsen (2004); Malchau (2005).
21 Golder (1903), p. 250.
22 Deaconess Work (1895); Golder (1903); Drexel Home (1913); Doyle (1929); Schweikardt (2010).

Table 4: Lutheran deaconess foundations and motherhouses in the United States[23]

	City & State	Station's existence	Foundation of motherhouse	Country of origin
1	Pittsburgh Pennsylvania	1849–c. 1891	Kaiserswerth station	Germany
2	Philadelphia Pennsylvania	1884–1966	1888	Germany
3	Baltimore Maryland	1895–1966	1895	Germany
4	Omaha Nebraska	1890–1966	1890	Sweden
5	St. Paul Minnesota	1896–1930	1902	Sweden
6	Brooklyn New York	1883–2001	1885	Norway
7	Minneapolis Minnesota	1890–1979	1890	Norway
8	Chicago Illinois	1897–1956	1897	Norway
9	Brush Colorado	1905–1995	1905	Denmark
10	Milwaukee Wisconsin	1893–1980	1893	Germany
11	Axtell Nebraska	1913–1988	1913	Sweden

Table 4 lists 11 Protestant (Evangelical Lutheran) deaconess foundations in America from 1849 to 1913, ten of which became independent motherhouses. Four foundations were inherited from Germany and seven from Scandinavia. The figures go some way to support the fact that Scandinavia helped the deaconess movement grow in America. However, the degree of success is questionable, since religious freedom and diversity evidently did not prove as conducive an environment as a purely Protestant society. In America the number of deaconesses remained limited. In 1913 there were 358 Protestant (Lutheran) deaconesses working in 78 fields of activity, including 14 hospitals and 12 homes for the elderly.[24] However, the American deaconesses gave a high

---

23 Deaconess Work (1895); Golder (1903); Augustana Synod (1910); Drexel Home (1913); Evangelical Lutheran Church in America (2011).
24 Drexel Home (1913).

priority to nursing and in the period after 1899 nearly all the deaconess hospitals opened schools of nursing for deaconesses as well as for lay women.[25]

The Danish motherhouse in the United States

In the 1880s, Lutheran immigrant congregations from Germany, Norway and Sweden successfully established their first deaconess motherhouses in America in cooperation with their home countries (Table 4). It took longer to establish a Danish motherhouse. An attempt was made in 1899 by Pastor M. N. Andreasen from the Danish congregation in Racine, Wisconsin. He inquired at the motherhouse in Denmark about the possibility of sending a deaconess. However, Rev. H. D. Frimodt Möller at the *Trinity Seminary* in Blair, Nebraska, interfered. He wrote a letter to Pastor Dalhoff in Denmark that questioned Pastor Andreasen's ability to carry out the project because of his young age and low position in the Church hierarchy. Frimodt Möller advised Dalhoff to wait and to take action only if the project was authorised by the *United Danish Evangelical Lutheran Church in America*. Dalhoff decided to wait and sent a reply to Andreasen saying that the conditions were too vague. This concluded the first attempt to establish a Danish motherhouse in America.[26]

The next attempt was made in 1903 by Lutheran pastor Jens Madsen (1869–1946). He succeeded, maybe because, unlike his predecessor, he was supported by the leading clergy in the Lutheran congregations.[27] Pastor Madsen was a former tuberculosis (TB) patient and was dedicated to helping people with this prevalent and often fatal disease. In 1903 he raised the initial funding for *Eben-Ezer*, a Danish deaconess home and sanatorium in Brush, Colorado. The founder of the Swedish motherhouses in America, Rev. Erik Alfred Fogelstrom (1859–1909), recommended in February of the same year that Dalhoff support the initiative.[28] In August, Madsen wrote to Dalhoff describing how the only provisions for Protestant TB patients in the state were two homes established for rich people belonging to the *Episcopal* and *Adventist Churches*. He outlined the scheme for a Danish deaconess home and sanatorium for poor people and ended by implying that a successful outcome depended on the request that "the motherhouse in Copenhagen will provide us

25 Doyle (1929); Nelson (2001).
26 A-DDF: Eben-Ezer USA: Letters from Andreasen (USA) to Dalhoff (Denmark) 8/2/1899 and 28/7/1899; letters from Andreasen (USA) to Zahrtmann (Denmark) 3/4/1899 and 20/5/1899, the latter with reply notes by Dalhoff; letter from Frimodt Müller (USA) to Dalhoff (Denmark) 18/5/1899.
27 A-DDF: Eben-Ezer USA: Letter from Fogelstrom (USA) to Dalhoff (Denmark) 9/2/1903; letter from Madsen (USA) to Dalhoff (Denmark) 6/8/1903. The letters reveal that Madsen was a graduate from the *Trinity Seminary* in Blair and was a personal friend of Frimodt Möller.
28 Augustana Synod (1910); A-DDF: Eben-Ezer USA: Letter from Fogelstrom (USA) to Dalhoff (Denmark) 9/2/1903.

with one or two deaconesses called to this deed and able to train other wom-
en".[29]

Dalhoff's reply must have been forthcoming as Madsen, in a letter dated
20 October 1903, was grateful for the answer. In this letter he introduced a
Danish immigrant, Marie Hvidbjerg, an experienced nurse, who was pious
and had a good reputation.[30] She had graduated as a nurse from the *Swedish
Lutheran Augustana Hospital* in Chicago and, in his opinion, was qualified to be
a leader. She had agreed to travel to Denmark to familiarise herself with the
life and spirit of the Danish motherhouse and would accompany a Danish
sister, or preferably two, to America, one of them destined to be appointed
Lady Superintendent. This letter apparently prompted Dalhoff to invite Marie Hvidbjerg to Denmark, but it also stopped any further discussion about
sending Danish deaconesses to Colorado. In fact, no one was ever sent. Dalhoff may have been reluctant because of Madsen's openly conservative approach to the deaconess movement, and his repeated complaints of poor
health.[31]

Sister Marie's education in Denmark

The Danish sister records document the fact that sister No. 792, Dorthea Marie Sörensen Hvidbjerg, was born in Denmark on 22 December 1872. She
was received into the Danish motherhouse on 7 January 1904 and admitted as
a probationer on 24 April 1904. Prior to her arrival she had lived in America
for ten years and had trained as a nurse in Chicago. The purpose of her stay
in Denmark was to be educated as a deaconess at the request of the Danish
Lutheran congregation in America, who had appointed her as a future sister
and co-leader of the new Danish deaconess motherhouse in Colorado.[32]

The written story of her life (obligatory for applicants) informs us that she
left for America at her mother's request to accompany a brother around 1888.
However, he moved on to California very soon after arriving and left her in
Chicago.[33] She then trained as a nurse in Chicago and later moved to Iowa to
work as a nurse in private homes.

---

29 A-DDF: Eben-Ezer USA: Letter from Madsen (USA) to Dalhoff (Denmark) 6/8/1903.
30 A-DDF: Eben-Ezer USA: Letter from Madsen (USA) to Zahrtmann (Denmark) 23/8/1904.
    In 1904, Madsen sent Zahrtmann the testimonial of conduct for Sister Marie that he reques-
    ted from clergymen and lay people: "Sister Marie was tireless in her commitment in her
    call. She was a light in her congregation and a precious centre figure for the young women."
31 A-DDF: Eben-Ezer USA: Letter from Madsen (USA) to Dalhoff (Denmark) 20/10/1903.
    One issue was the deaconess cap, and in this letter Madsen revealed a conservative view
    on the subject and on women; e.g. in referring to a new model of the deaconess cap he
    introduced at the Swedish motherhouse in Omaha. Madsen was opposed to the fact that,
    in his opinion, it looked as if it did not even cover the hair. Combing would be necessary,
    a lady of vanity would appear, and the pious deaconess would disappear.
32 A-DDF: Records of Deaconesses at the Danish Deaconess Foundation 1863–1943.
33 A-DDF: Marie Hvidbjerg – application and biography 1904.

Pastor Dalhoff agreed to organise a training programme at the Danish motherhouse tailored to Sister Marie's future work. The costs were paid for by the *Eben-Ezer Deaconess Home*. Lady Superintendent Sophie Zahrtmann (1841–1925) was in charge of the programme that had been heavily adapted to Madsen's requirements.[34] The programme lasted for 17 months and comprised from January to August 1904: housekeeping and cleaning, a theoretical course and hospital nursing (surgical ward and children's ward). From August 1904 to March 1905, Sister Marie was posted to external stations: a TB sanatorium and two congregational nursing stations (home nursing).[35] Sister Marie asked for Madsen's permission to complete her studies in America in the fall of 1904 at a relevant college, but he argued that it was of no use at her age (32). It would be better to remain in Denmark and practise nursing. In April 1905, Marie was admitted to a Danish missionary training school. Finally, before returning to America, she travelled in Europe, supposedly visiting other motherhouses.[36] There is no evidence that she took classes in ecclesiastical embroidery, which Madsen had asked to be arranged.[37] However, Marie was by now quite well trained.

Female power and struggle

Sister Marie was consecrated as a deaconess in Denmark on 10 September 1905, and on 20 September she began her return trip to America. She arrived at *Eben-Ezer* on 29 October 1905. Her correspondence with Lady Superintendent Sophie Zahrtmann in the years to follow reveals her great affection and attachment to the Danish motherhouse.[38]

In her first letter, written a week after she arrived, she admits to being very disappointed with *Eben-Ezer*: "The conditions are even more difficult than imagined." This disappointment was due to a conflict that cropped up on the return trip from Denmark. She had received a letter from Mrs Madsen asking her to replace the Danish deaconess cap with one designed and sewn by Mrs

34 A-DDF: Eben-Ezer USA: Letter from Madsen (USA) to Zahrtmann (Denmark) 23/8/1904.

35 A-DDF: Eben-Ezer USA: Letter from Madsen (USA) to Dalhoff (Denmark) 20/7/1904; letters from Madsen (USA) to Zahrtmann (Denmark) 23/8/1904 and 12/11/1904. In the letter dated 23/8/1904 Madsen asked for it to be arranged for Sister Marie to stay at the *Vejle Sanatorium* in Denmark as it would impress the medical profession in America. There are no records of such a stay.

36 A-DDF: Eben-Ezer USA: Letter from Madsen (USA) to Zahrtmann (Denmark) 18/7/1904. Sister Marie's European travel was recommended by Madsen, who wanted her to visit the grandmotherhouse in Kaiserswerth, other European motherhouses, and in America also the German *Mary Drexel Home* in Philadelphia, the German motherhouse in Milwaukee and the Swedish motherhouse in Omaha. There are no records of these visits.

37 A-DDF: Eben-Ezer USA: Letter from Madsen (USA) to Zahrtmann (Denmark) 23/8/1904; letter from Madsen (USA) to Dalhoff (Denmark) 2/7/1904.

38 A-DDF: Eben-Ezer USA and Records of Deaconesses at the Danish Deaconess Foundation 1863–1943.

Madsen. Sister Marie wrote: "You can imagine how disappointed I was at not being allowed to wear the Danish deaconess dress and cap, [and I did] reply that permission from the Danish motherhouse was needed." After this incident she was received in a 'freezing' atmosphere and confronted with the fact that Sister Maren (trained in Omaha) had been capped the day before with the 'ugly' *Eben-Ezer* cap. Sister Marie continued to wear the Danish dress and cap.[39]

This was the first sign of a female power struggle which eventually grew to unimaginable dimensions. The conflict centred on who should be regarded as Lady Superintendent at *Eben-Ezer*: Mrs Madsen or Sister Marie? Consequently, Pastor Madsen very soon found himself squeezed between the two parties. On the one side was his wife, who was very much involved in the development of *Eben-Ezer* and, prior to its establishment, had trained in housekeeping at the Swedish motherhouse in Omaha to qualify as a temporary superior until the Danish deaconesses took over.[40] On the other side was Sister Marie, who Pastor Madsen for unknown reasons never wanted to see appointed Superintendent, but regarded as a 'transitional leader'. Sister Marie's impression was that Mrs Madsen defined herself as Superintendent. That was fine with her, she claimed, if only they were in agreement. However, as a responsible nurse she needed to work in accordance with the standards of the Danish motherhouse. The problem was that Mrs Madsen contradicted any procedures she recommended.[41]

The first two months consolidated the conflict: Mrs Madsen, the first to be in power, ordered Sister Marie to clean and cook. On the advice of Sister Sophie Zahrtmann, provided long-distance from Denmark, Sister Marie consulted Pastor Madsen. He confided to her that Mrs Madsen wanted to be in charge but was unable to handle the responsibility – and that she was jealous. He had recommended to his wife to withdraw, advice that made her terribly angry. It was then arranged that Sister Marie leave the scene to nurse a sick man in his home, but she was called back after five days to chaotic conditions: "Mrs Madsen had left for the city in a furious state of mind, and the two young sisters and the patients welcomed me with open arms." Now Sister

39 A-DDF: Eben-Ezer USA: Letter from Hvidbjerg (USA) to Zahrtmann (Denmark) 5/11/1905. Quotation translated from the Danish.
    In 1905, Madsen told Dalhoff that he preferred Sister Marie to wear the Danish deaconess habit and that it could eventually be adapted to the American climate (Letter from Madsen (USA) to Dalhoff (Denmark) 24/5/1904). However, in 1907, Madsen asked Sister Marie to wear the Eben-Ezer habit like the other sisters. It was now an issue of power, and she refused. Zahrtmann advised on the matter, but there are no records of her answers (Letter from Hvidbjerg (USA) to Zahrtmann (Denmark) 14/3/1907).
40 A-DDF: Eben-Ezer USA: Letter from Madsen (USA) to Dalhoff (Denmark) 6/8/1903.
41 A-DDF: Eben-Ezer USA: Letters from Hvidbjerg (USA) to Zahrtmann (Denmark) 5/11/1905 and 26/1/1906.

Marie was in power. In this way the conflict rose to such a pitch that even the patients began to interfere.[42]

In July 1906, Sister Marie wrote: "Pastor Madsen blames me for the conditions and I do feel incompetent. It would be easier to give up, but my heart is in this work." However, a much-needed intermission arose: due to Pastor Madsen's fragile health, Sister Marie accepted the assignment of fundraising for *Eben-Ezer*, and for six months she enjoyed visiting Lutheran congregations in the surrounding states. She reported to Dalhoff that the very positive result was due to her wearing the Danish deaconess dress.[43]

The nursing standards

In 1905 there were only a few (six to ten) patients at *Eben-Ezer*, and they did not come from Colorado but from remote places in neighbouring states.[44] The construction of the home was at this early stage limited to two buildings: one with the patients' rooms and the other with a kitchen, dining room and accommodation for the staff. Sister Marie was not pleased with the standard of nursing and she especially criticised the hygiene conditions. She found the institutions filthy and was shocked to observe TB patients being allowed to help themselves to food in the kitchen. Although she did not consider cleaning to be part of her work, she felt obliged to do it for the safety of the patients.[45]

However, the physician's rounds and prescriptions every other day were managed conscientiously, and bedside nursing was practised round the clock. For instance, Sister Marie reported on the care of a newly admitted insane woman in a poor state: "I sleep in the same room as her, and during the day I have to look after her. I was so worried about her condition, but she has calmed down a bit by now. It is not as hopeless as presumed."[46]

No doubt Sister Marie felt powerless, but she fought hard in the never-ending conflict of interests caused by unclear leadership and vague and unprofessionally formulated standards of nursing care. She lost the battle. In 1909, the *Eben-Ezer* board finally decided to appoint Mrs Madsen as Lady Superintendent and they immediately ordered Sister Marie to wear the *Eben-Ezer* deaconess dress and cap. Mrs Madsen was now in power and demonstrated it by

---

42 A-DDF: Eben-Ezer USA: Letters from Hvidbjerg (USA) to Zahrtmann (Denmark) 5/11/1905, 26/1/1906 and 16/12/1906, 14/3/1907. Quotation translated from the Danish. (Letter from Hvidbjerg (USA) to Zahrtmann (Denmark) 15/1/1906).

43 Dalhoff (1907); A-DDF: Eben-Ezer USA: Letter from Hvidbjerg (USA) to Zahrtmann (Denmark) 14/3/1907.

44 A-DDF: Eben-Ezer USA: Letter from Madsen (USA) to Zahrtmann (Denmark) 23/8/1904.

45 A-DDF: Eben-Ezer USA: Letters from Hvidbjerg (USA) to Zahrtmann (Denmark) 5/11/1905 and 26/1/1906.

46 A-DDF: Eben-Ezer USA: Letter from Hvidbjerg (USA) to Zahrtmann (Denmark) 5/11/1905.

withholding the prescribed eggs that Sister Marie needed for the TB patients' diet and cure. Sister Marie felt lonely and socially excluded from the community, which had by now expanded to four deaconesses.[47]

Return to Denmark

It was evident that Sister Marie had to resign. However, how this was to be arranged was a reputation issue for *Eben-Ezer*, and obviously the only way to avoid losing face was for Sister Marie to return to Denmark. The Danish superiors were already involved in the conflict as the long-distance advisers of both Pastor Madsen and Sister Marie, who each presented their own version of events.[48]

The problem was that Sister Marie had been consecrated in Denmark as a gesture of friendship. She was not considered to be a member of the Danish motherhouse, and the superiors did not have the power to call her home. Pastor Madsen had advised Sister Marie to discontinue her contact with Denmark as she could not serve two masters, and he also had a duty to provide for her for the rest of her life. However, from 1908 onwards, Pastor Madsen and Sister Marie both begged the superiors in Denmark to help them to a solution, and in August 1909 Dalhoff finally wrote a letter granting Sister Marie full membership of the *Danish Deaconess Foundation*. She arrived in Denmark on 26 October 1909. The superiors of the Danish motherhouse continued to correspond with Pastor Madsen and to keep track of developments at *Eben-Ezer*, however there was not a single word about Sister Marie in their letters.[49]

Today, the single photo of Sister Marie on the *Eben-Ezer* website presents a mystery. She is wearing neither Mrs Madsen's 'ugly cap' nor the Danish cap for consecrated deaconesses. She is wearing the Danish probationer cap.[50]

Epilogue on Sister Marie

The narrative presented here, based on the sources in the A-DDF, concerning the departure of Sister Marie from *Eben-Ezer* both complements and contradicts the story as it is presented today on the websites of the *Evangelical*

---

47 A-DDF: Eben-Ezer USA: Letter from Hvidbjerg (USA) to Zahrtmann (Denmark) 9/5/1909. In the letter, Sister Marie gave a harsh and probably not entirely fair description of her fellow sisters: Sister Maren was given notice every two months due to conflicts, Sister Sine was spoilt and only committed to playing the organ, and Sister Ingeborg was feeble.

48 A-DDF: Eben-Ezer USA: Letter from Madsen (USA) to Dalhoff (Denmark) 15/9/1909. Dalhoff's draft letters to Madsen and Sister Marie Aug. 1909.

49 A-DDF: Eben-Ezer USA: Letter from Hvidbjerg (USA) to Zahrtmann (Denmark) 14/3/1907; Dalhoff's draft letters to Madsen and Sister Marie Aug. 1909; letters from Madsen (USA) to Dalhoff and Zahrtmann (Denmark) 1909–1918.

50 Eben Ezer. Lutheran Care Center (2011).

Lutheran Church in America and the *Eben Ezer Lutheran Care Center*.[51] Here it is stated that Miss Marie Hvidbjerg, a Danish sister from Cedar Falls, served at *Eben-Ezer* until 1909, when she "became ill and returned to the motherhouse in Denmark". However, there is no evidence that Sister Marie was sick. In fact, the letter of recommendation provided by the house doctor of *Eben-Ezer*, Dr A. E. Lusby, written in 1909, refers to Sister Marie as a competent nurse and a sound and healthy woman.[52] It is also a fact that Pastor Dalhoff would never have granted her full membership of the Danish motherhouse if there was any indication of her being sick. It would have been far too risky, as the Danish motherhouse, by admitting her, took over the obligation of providing for her for the rest of her life. It is important to bear this in mind when I reveal the tragic story of the last years of Sister Marie's life.

In Denmark, Sister Marie was head nurse at the *Danish Deaconess Foundation's* TB sanatorium for a couple of years, and later served at different congregational nursing stations. She was apparently contented until 1915, but then she slowly but steadily fell out with everyone: her fellow sisters and her superiors. It became increasingly difficult to find suitable work for her. In 1918 she was diagnosed as being mentally ill, and in 1924 paranoia took over. She refused treatment and declined to move to a home for disabled people owned by the motherhouse. Instead, and to the great embarrassment of her superiors, she drifted between the missionary hotels in Copenhagen, always wearing her beloved Danish deaconess dress. In summer 1924 she was admitted to *Frederiksberg Hospital*. She refused to eat and was nourished through a feeding tube. She died on 19 May 1925 at the age of 53.[53]

Conclusion

Focusing on the roots of the deaconess movement, nursing tradition and demographic statistics, this study adds to our knowledge about the contribution of the deaconess movement to the nursing profession. It argues that the success and dissemination of the movement depended on religious conditions and on the grandmotherhouse in Kaiserswerth setting international standards. The most prosperous deaconess settlements were situated in Protestant countries in Europe, which explains the success of the movement in Scandinavia and areas in the United States with immigrant populations from these countries.

51 The life story of Sister Marie is presented from a Danish perspective and still needs to be scrutinised further by studying any material that may exist in the archives of the *Eben Ezer Lutheran Care Center* and the *Evangelical Lutheran Church in America*, USA.

52 A-DDF: Eben-Ezer USA: Letter from Lusby, Brush Colorado (USA) to Dalhoff (Denmark) 23/11/1909.

53 A-DDF: Marie Hvidbjerg – letters and notes about Sister Marie's illness and death 1915–1925, biography 1904.

The case story of Sister Marie and the establishment of a Danish mother-house in Colorado provides evidence of the introduction of professional nursing within the deaconess movement, which opened up new opportunities for women. Women were given the opportunity to leave the family home and to be trained and work professionally and, most importantly, still live in accordance with the contemporary patriarchal structure and norms for female conduct.[54] Sister Marie bowed to these expectations, but as an independent character she certainly also questioned them. Her personal story was not a success. She failed in Colorado. But her ordeals provide a unique source of evidence concerning the introduction of professional nursing in a vast country and a newly established community. She stood for nursing practice that aimed to comply with the Kaiserswerth standards. However, in trying to uphold this standard of nursing she found herself caught between a professional approach and the domestic work of women at the time. The case also emphasises the importance of transparency in leadership for ensuring a high standard of nursing.

The result of the study indicates the importance of continuing research into the significance of the deaconess movement for the nursing profession. This applies to studies of individual motherhouses and comparative studies in a European and U.S. American context. It is also important to keep in mind that deaconesses introduced professional nursing in the secular sector; this perspective of the development of professional nursing also needs further investigation.[55]

Bibliography

[A-DDF] Archives of the Danish Deaconess Foundation, Frederiksberg, Denmark.

[Augustana Synod] The Augustana Synod. A brief review of its history 1860–1910. Rock Island 1910.

Bancroft, Jane M.: Deaconesses in Europe and their lessons for America. New York; Cincinnati 1889.

Büttner, Annett: Das internationale Netzwerk der evangelischen Mutterhausdiakonie. In: Ariadne. Forum für Frauen- und Geschlechtergeschichte 45 (2006), pp. 64–71.

Dalhoff, Nicolai Christian: Fra Diakonissestiftelsen. In: Føbe 5 (1882), pp. 77–79.

Dalhoff, Nicolai Christian: Fra Diakonissestiftelsen. In: Føbe 3 (1907), p. 16.

[Deaconess Work] The deaconess work in the Evangelical Lutheran Church in the United States. Report of the committee on deaconess work. Presented to the General Council at Easton, Pa, 1895.

Der Armen- und Krankenfreund, April 1913, pp. 184–186.

Dietz, Susanne Malchau: Køn, kald og kompetencer. Diakonissestiftelsen kvindefællesskab og omsorgsuddannelser 1863–1955. Copenhagen 2013.

---

54 Mangion (2010).

55 My sincere gratitude to consultant Gunilla Svensmark for commenting on and proof-reading the manuscript.

Dietz, Susanne Malchau: The dilemma of female modesty and professional nursing. Conflicts in the leadership of the Danish Deaconess Foundation in the late 19th century. Paper presented at the International Conference on Nursing History, Berlin May 2011 a.

Dietz, Susanne Malchau: Women religious and nursing in the Renaissance. Kolding 2011 b.

Disselhoff, Julius: Kaiserswerth. The deaconess institution of Rhenish Westphalia, its origin and fields of labour. Translated from the German by A. N. London 1883.

Doyle, Ann: Nursing by religious orders in the United States. Part IV – Lutheran deaconesses, 1849–1928. In: The American Journal of Nursing 10 (1929), pp. 1197–1207.

[Drexel Home hand book] Hand book of the Mary J. Drexel Home and Philadelphia Motherhouse of Deaconesses, 1883–1913. Philadelphia 1913.

Eben Ezer. Lutheran Care Center. Online available www.ebenezer-cares.org/index.php?s= 14552 (Accessed 23/7/2011).

Evangelical Lutheran Church in America. Online available www.elca.org/Who-We-Are/ History/ELCA-Archives/Exhibits/Lutheran-Deaconess-History.aspx (Accessed 10/4/2011).

Golder, Christian: History of the deaconess movement in the Christian church. Cincinnati; New York 1903.

Hauge, Svend: I troskab mod kaldet. Den Danske Diakonissestiftelse 1863–1963. Copenhagen 1963.

Kaiser, Jochen-Christoph; Scheepers, Rajah (ed.): Dienerinnen des Herrn. Beiträge zur weiblichen Diakonie im 19. und 20. Jahrhundert. Leipzig 2010.

Kreutzer, Susanne: Nursing body and soul in the parish. Lutheran deaconess motherhouses in Germany and the United States. In: Nursing History Review 18 (2010), pp. 134–50.

Köser, Silke: Denn eine Diakonisse darf kein Alltagsmensch sein. Kolletive Identitäten Kaiserswerther Diakonissen 1836–1914. Leipzig 2006.

Legath, Jennifer Anne Wiley: The Phoebe phenomenon. The Protestant deaconess movement in the United States 1880–1930. Unpublished thesis. University of Princeton 2008.

McDonald, Lynn (ed.): Florence Nightingale's European travels, Volume 7 of the collected works of Florence Nightingale. Waterloo; Ontario 2004.

Malchau, Susanne: Romersk-katolske sygeplejeordner i Danmark efter reformationen. In: Kvinder, køn & forskning. 1–2 (2005), pp. 88–105.

Malchau, Susanne; Nilsen, Else-Britt: Appendix: Tables and Figures. In: Werner, Yvonne Maria (ed.): Nuns and sisters in the Nordic countries after the Reformation. Uppsala 2004, pp. 419–36.

Mangion, Carmen M.: Women, religious ministry and female institution-building. In: Morgan, Sue; Vries, Jacqueline de (ed.): Women, gender and religious cultures in Britain, 1800–1940. London; New York 2010, pp. 72–93.

Naumann, Cheryl D.: In the footsteps of Phoebe. A complete history of the deaconess movement in the Lutheran Church – Missouri Synod. St. Louis 2008.

Nelson, Sioban: Say little, do much. Nursing, nuns, and hospitals in the nineteenth century. Philadelphia 2003.

Nolte, Karen: Dying at home. Nursing of the critically and terminally ill in private care in Germany around 1900. In: Nursing Inquiry 2 (2009), pp. 144–154.

Nutting, M. Adelaide; Dock, Lavinia Loyd: A history of nursing. (First edition 1907) 9th edition 1935. New York; London 1935.

Porter, Roy: The greatest benefit to mankind. A medical history of humanity from antiquity to the present. London 1997.

Schmidt, Jutta: Beruf: Schwester. Mutterhausdiakonie im 19. Jahrhundert. Frankfurt/Main; New York 1998.

Schweikardt, Christoph: The introduction of deaconess nurses at the German hospital of the city of Philadelphia in the 1880s. In: Nursing History Review 18 (2010), pp. 29–50.

Stein, Harald: Nogle blade af den kristne kvindes historie. Et bidrag til diakonissesagens fremme. Copenhagen 1872.

Archives

Archives of the Danish Deaconess Foundation, Frederiksberg, Denmark (A-DDF).
Eben-Ezer USA, letters
– Andreasen to Dalhoff 8/2/1899, 28/7/1899
– Andreasen to Zahrtmann 3/4/1899, 20/5/1899
– Dalhoff draft letters to Madsen and Sister Marie Aug. 1909
– Frimodt Müller to Dalhoff 18/5/1899
– Fogelstrom to Dalhoff 9/2/1903
– Hvidbjerg to Zahrtmann 5/11/1905, 15/1/1906, 26/1/1906, 16/12/1906, 14/3/1907, 9/5/1909
– Lusby to Dalhoff 23/11/1909
– Madsen to Dalhoff 6/8/1903, 20/10/1903, 24/5/1904, 2/7/1904, 20/7/1904, 15/9/1909, 1909–1918
– Madsen to Zahrtmann 18/7/1904, 23/8/1904, 12/11/1904

Records of Deaconesses at the Danish Deaconess Foundation 1863–1943
– Marie Hvidbjerg – application and biography 1904
– Marie Hvidbjerg – letters and notes 1915–1925

Deaconesses in the history of nursing in Finland, 1890s to 1960s

Pirjo Markkola

In 1936, Finland marked the centenary of deaconess education with a commemorative publication. None of the Finnish deaconess institutes was one hundred years old, but the leaders of deaconess education who contributed to the publication wanted to emphasise the fact that they belonged to a transnational movement initiated in Kaiserswerth in 1836. Deaconess education in Finland is described as a daughter of the German deaconessate. The director of the *Helsinki Deaconess Institute*, Pastor Edvin Wirén, also emphasised the female diaconate's contribution to the history of nursing:

> Thinking about the past hundred years, we have a good reason to commemorate the role of diaconate (*diakonia*) in creating and improving the general education of nurses. While nursing was previously provided by uneducated women, the diaconate pioneered the education of trained nurses in many countries. Furthermore, the diaconate has indirectly initiated significant social services in many other fields.[1]

Pastor Wirén summarises an essential feature of female diaconate, not only in Finland but in many other countries as well. The first deaconess institute founded in Kaiserswerth in 1836 became an explicit model for other institutes throughout Europe and beyond. Not surprisingly, the movement gained a foothold in the Nordic countries where Lutheranism was an official denomination. In addition to Kaiserswerth, some other Central European deaconess institutes served as models for the Nordic institutes. Their main line of work was to nurse the sick and needy, but deaconesses were also involved in education and social work among the poor. Deaconess education provided new challenges and new experiences for young Protestant women, who were given the chance to join a deaconess institute and devote their entire lives to the service of God. The churches claimed repeatedly that deaconesses were not Protestant nuns, but the similarities were striking. Deaconesses were single women whose vocation was to serve the poor and the sick. *Diakonia (service)* represented a clearly marked choice to follow God: deaconesses belonged to the community of a deaconess institute; they wore a deaconess habit and were not paid for their work. The community took care of their daily needs and provided social security in case of illness and old age. In contrast to the Catholic orders, deaconesses were allowed to leave the community if they got married or found that the deaconessate was not their calling.[2]

---

1   Wirén (1936 b), p. 20.
2   On Lutheran theology relating to the calling in the nineteenth century, see Hammar (1999); Hammar (2000), pp. 37–67; on nursing as a religious calling, see Kreutzer (2008), pp. 181–183; on deaconess education, see Prelinger (1986), pp. 215–225; De Swarte Gifford (1987); Baumann (1992), pp. 45–56; Schmidt (1998); Nolte (2008), pp. 120–123; Nolte (2009), pp. 145–146; Kreutzer (2010), pp. 134–150; Soine (2013), pp. 20–41; on

Deaconesses were the first educated nurses in nineteenth-century Finland. Education for deaconesses was introduced in the 1860s, whereas secular training for nurses was not introduced until the 1880s.[3] Nursing in the hospitals of the deaconess institutes was the deaconesses' primary field of work, but deaconesses were also sent to work in the wider community. Deaconesses were educated to serve with Lutheran parishes, charitable associations, municipal hospitals and poor relief, and social institutions run by the state. The hospitals of the deaconess institutes often provided the best medical care available. Education was based on a hierarchical system and it took several years to become a fully trained deaconess. Students who passed their classes in the first year were promoted to probationary deaconesses, who were qualified to work in the hospital or in the wider community, but they had to amass considerable working experience before they were consecrated as deaconesses. Deaconesses were also pioneers in the field of public health nursing. The first visiting nurses in Finland were sent by the deaconess institutes, and it was not until much later that the state took over this work and deaconesses were gradually replaced by public health nurses.[4]

In this article, my focus is on deaconess education and the work of deaconesses in the fields of parish nursing and public health nursing in Finland. I examine the role of Finnish deaconesses in nursing from the 1890s to the 1960s. Public health nursing, I argue, was a field in which deaconesses continued to play an important role alongside other visiting nurses. In the 1890s, the state provided support for public health nursing and the work of deaconesses expanded. As late as 1930, deaconesses and their work in parish nursing formed a substantive part of public health nursing in rural Finland. In 1944, a law was passed on municipal public health nursing, but deaconesses continued to play an important, complementary, role until the 1960s. The 1972 law on public health excluded deaconesses from public health nursing.[5]

My material consists of the archival sources and publications of the Finnish deaconess institutes. The *Helsinki Deaconess Institute* has extensive records at the *National Archives* in Helsinki, including correspondence, student records and annual reports. The first pamphlets and leaflets about deaconess education were published in the 1860s and an increasing number of publications are available from the 1880s onwards. Periodicals published by the Finnish deaconess institutes were launched in the 1890s. Moreover, national health statistics, committee reports, legislation and published histories of deaconess institutes and nursing schools have been used to set the context of the female diaconate in Finland.

         the first deaconess institutes in the Nordic countries, see Kansanaho (1967); Ekmund
         (1973); Martinsen (1984); Koivunen Bylund (1994); Markkola (2000), pp. 107–118;
         Markkola (2013), pp. 70–88.
3   Sorvettula (1998).
4   Markkola (2000), pp. 107–118; cf. Kreutzer (2008).
5   Malkavaara (2002), pp. 225–226.

When it comes to terminology in the field of parish nursing and social work of the church, the concept of *diakonia* (service) is slightly problematic and difficult to translate into English. I have chosen to use the terms 'deaconessate', 'female diaconate' and 'deaconess movement' interchangeably. However, the term 'deaconess movement' is also associated with attempts to organise the deaconessate. I also use the term 'diaconate' when I refer both to male and female diaconate.

The deaconessate in a changing society

Deaconess education was part of a transnational awakening and reform movement of the nineteenth century. In Finland it was rooted in the social and political context: an era of social questions that brought about a shift from the old, ordered society to a new civil society.[6] The *social question* in Europe was usually perceived as deriving from the complications of industrialisation, as a labour issue. In Finland, the issue of the emerging industrial working classes was intertwined with the problems of rural poverty. Until the twentieth century, Finland was an agrarian country in which the vast majority earned their livelihood from agriculture. In 1900, about two-thirds of the population was agrarian. Poverty was a common problem in rural areas, as almost half of the agricultural population were farm labourers and other landless people, who suffered both from underemployment and seasonal unemployment. Moreover, despite late industrialisation, the industrial working class was increasing. The number of urban workers in 1910 was four times higher than in 1870. The 1890s in particular saw a steep growth in the urban population.[7]

Another political issue of the late nineteenth century was a growing nationalist movement and the *Russian question*, which referred to relations between Finland and Russia. Having been a part of Sweden for centuries, Finland formed a Grand Duchy within the Russian Empire from 1809 to 1917. The social structure and legal system remained Scandinavian during this period, as the Emperor recognised the Swedish laws, including the official Lutheran confession and the status of the *Evangelical Lutheran Church* as a state church. At the turn of the twentieth century, the status of Finland within the Russian Empire became an issue for both the Finnish and the Russian side, as the Finns favoured nationalistic interpretations of sovereignty and the Russian aim was a coordinated adminitrative structure, in which matters concerning the whole Empire would be ruled according to Russian legislation. In this context, people became organised into civic associations, such as the nationalist movement, temperance associations and the labour movement, among oth-

---

6   Heininen/Heikkilä (1996), pp. 162–163. On Finnish history, see Kirby (2006); Lavery (2006); Meinander (2011); on women in Finland, see Manninen/Setälä (1990).

7   Haapala (1992), pp. 232–233; Markkola (1990), p. 18. The population of Finland in 1900 was 2.9 million. The majority were Finnish-speaking, but until the end of the nineteenth century the language of administration was Swedish.

ers. The strengthening of civic society, in turn, contributed to the establishment of new religious and charitable organisations. Moreover, the official status of the Lutheran church did not change or deteriorate, in spite of the conflicting tendencies in the relationship between Finland and Russia. In 1917, in the aftermath of the Russian revolution, Finland gained independence and the strong position of the Lutheran church continued.[8]

While developing the deaconessate in Finland, the active members of the Lutheran church were challenged by a certain amount of pressure towards secularisation. Secularisation appeared not only in the form of a growing tendency to neglect church doctrine but, more importantly, in a redefinition of the social division of labour. The role of the Lutheran church in local administration was affected by the separation of parishes and municipal authorities in the 1860s. In the new division of labour, responsibility for the organisation of poor relief and popular education was transferred from parishes to municipal authorities.[9] The development of municipal poor relief system, in particular, challenged the churchmen to reconsider the role of Christian charity in a changing society.

The diaconate developed in this changing society. A social order based on households, in which the head of the household was responsible for the well-being and discipline of his household members and servants, did not fit in with an industrialising and urbanising world, nor was it seen as attractive by the emerging middle classes, who saw promising opportunities in the ideas of a free labour market and capitalist economy. The old patriarchal system of care was ruled out, but the local authorities and the state were not willing to assume responsibility for everyone in need of care. Moreover, new ideas about hygiene, preventive health care and public health were challenging Finland's modest health care system. The wide gap between family care and public care created a vacuum and a need for voluntary social work, philanthropy, diaconate and new political initiatives. This vacuum inspired the Finnish leaders of the deaconess movement to propose a liberalist model, in which philanthropic and religious organisations would share responsibility for the well-being of needy people with a public poor relief system, which was to play a residual role as a last resort.[10] The model allowed the deaconess movement to find a meaningful purpose solving social problems.

Economic changes and political tensions combined with ideological and religious changes to pave the way for the individualisation of citizens. The revivalist movements typically emphasised Christianity as a choice guiding the deeds and minds of people, a choice which had both social and individual repercussions. Faith was no longer seen as the collective, self-evident cornerstone of a Christian worldview. The Pietist movement of the eighteenth and

---

8   Heininen/Heikkilä (1996), pp. 162–163; Kirby (2006); Lavery (2006); Meinander (2011).
9   Kansanaho (1960), pp. 110–113, 192–204.
10 The vacuum idea is presented by the Swedish historian Roger Qvarsell (1993), p. 217; Markkola (1999), pp. 169–170. On health policy in Finland, see Harjula (2007); Helén/ Jauho (2003).

early nineteenth centuries accentuated service and benevolence as Christian obligations towards fellow human beings. These ideas manifested themselves in a home mission movement, which formed a wider context for the organisation of the diaconate in Finland. One of the most direct models for the organised *Nordic home mission* was the German *Inner Mission* established by Protestant pastor Johann Hinrich Wichern. The goal of the *home mission*, according to the German model, was to solve the *social question* through the renewal of popular piety. Home missions worked for the benefit of the poor; nevertheless, the ultimate goal was to save souls.[11] The role of women was understood to be crucial in promoting these goals. Women's active social role was both promoted and opposed by referring to the authority of the Bible.

Lutheran Christianity was also challenged by evangelicalism and other new revivalist movements. During the last quarter of the nineteenth century, the Free Church revivalism and the *Salvation Army* reached Finland and found support in urban areas. Both movements were active in social work and managed to recruit many women.[12] These challenges, too, were met by developing church-based charitable work and establishing home mission societies which worked in close co-operation with the Lutheran clergy. In Finland, home mission societies recruited deaconesses primarily for urban settings, whereas in rural areas it was often the diaconate committee established by the parish that organised the employment of deaconesses in their municipality.

Introduction of deaconess education in Finland

The first deaconess institute in Finland was founded with the economic and moral support of Aurora Karamzin (1808–1902), a benevolent widow who promoted philanthropy in Helsinki. Karamzin was very familiar with the *Evangelische Hospital* (*Evangelical Deaconess Institute*) in St. Petersburg and, during a visit to Kaiserswerth in 1866, she became impressed by the work of German deaconesses. In 1867, an exceptionally severe famine in Finland prompted her to donate funds for the foundation of a deaconess institute in Helsinki. Karamzin invited the Finnish deaconess Amanda Cajander (1827–1871) from the *Evangelische Hospital* to lead the emerging institute and to carry out the practical work. She appeared to be a good choice. After being widowed at the age of 29, Amanda Cajander had joined the deaconess institute in St. Petersburg and pursued nursing studies at the hospital. Moreover, her late husband had been a medical doctor, with whom she had made an excursion to some of the German home mission institutes in the 1850s. As the first deaconess in Finland, she became a pioneer in the field of nursing.[13]

11 Kansanaho (1960), pp. 7–10; Murtorinne (1992); Hope (1995), pp. 409–417; Prelinger (1987); Nolte (2008), pp. 116–121.
12 Helander (1987), pp. 33–35; Holm/Sandström (1972); Markkola (2000), pp. 123–131.
13 The first Finnish woman to complete a deaconess education was Laura Calonius, who was consecrated at the *Evangelische Hospital* in St. Petersburg in 1860, but she did not return to Finland. Kansanaho (1967), p. 25.

During its early years, the *Helsinki Deaconess Institute* founded a small hospital with eight beds, an orphanage, and an asylum for female servants. In the wintertime the institute also ran a soup kitchen. The primary groups served by the deaconesses were women and children. Until Sister Amanda's untimely death, Aurora Karamzin offered her both mental and material support. While travelling abroad, for example, she often acquired modern instruments for the hospital. However, Karamzin's most visible contribution to the development of nursing and deaconess education in Finland was the house she bought for the institute in Helsinki.[14] These two women were driving forces behind an attempt to introduce formalised nursing education, and they managed to start a new era in the field of Christian charity in Finland.

Despite the brave start, the deaconess institute remained small during its first decades. In the early 1880s there were only ten deaconesses, who primarily worked in the hospital of the institute. In 1883, the Finnish deaconess Lina Snellman (1846–1924) was recruited from Stockholm to lead the institute. During the early years, due to a lack of support, she even planned to close the institute and turn it over to a hospital, but gradually she managed to turn the deaconessate into a potential choice for young women and succeeded in ensuring the continuation of deaconess education in Finland. In contrast to her predecessors, who had emphasised humble service in silence, Sister Lina made the deaconessate visible among young women, partly by publishing a good number of articles, booklets and books in Swedish and in Finnish. Women's movements and some revivalist movements disseminated information about deaconess education.[15] As women's other educational opportunities remained limited, Finland formed a fertile ground for deaconess education in the late nineteenth century. Lina Snellman's good contacts with the Swedish deaconess leaders were an additional asset; moreover, her family background gave credibility to her efforts to promote deaconess education.[16]

In 1895, Sister Lina had 33 deaconesses and deaconess students in her institute, and in the next ten years the number of deaconesses and probationary deaconesses increased to 88. Deaconess education was also gathering more support from the clergy, and the pastor who ran the institute alongside the female director, was active in promoting the deaconess movement and informing parish pastors about deaconess education. The growth continued in the twentieth century. In 1935, the motherhouse in Helsinki housed over 400 women: 216 deaconesses, 127 probationary deaconesses and 66 students. A couple of years later, the number of deaconesses and students had increased

---

14 Amanda Cajander's letters to Aurora Karamzin, 1867–1870. Aurora Karamzin's Records. National Archives (KA), Helsinki; Kansanaho (1967), pp. 27–36; Ramsay (1993), pp. 70–71, 105; Tallberg (1989), p. 274.

15 For example, the *Women's Association*, the first women's rights organisation in Finland, published a call for deaconess students in its journal in 1894. Diakonissoiksi. In: Koti ja yhteiskunta 5 (1894).

16 Mustakallio (2001), pp. 33–39; Markkola (2012), pp. 237–238. Lina Snellman's father was the first cousin of Senator J. V. Snellman, one of the most remarkable statesmen and political theorists in nineteenth century Finland.

again to 439.[17] In the 1950s, the institute attracted even more students than before, partly because young women with a primary school education were eligible to attend deaconess institutes, whereas nursing schools prioritised students with a secondary school diploma. In 1960, the total number of deaconesses and students was 634, of whom 505 were consecrated deaconesses.[18]

The second deaconess institute in Finland was founded in 1869. It was initiated by the *German Evangelical Congregation* in the city of Viborg (*Viipuri* in Finnish), which was a lively and multicultural town in eastern Finland, only about 140 kilometres north-east of St. Petersburg. The German congregation had close contacts with Evangelical churches in Russia, the eastern Baltic region and Germany. The influential and wealthy Hackman family, who originated from Germany and were involved in Finnish industry and commerce, played a key role in establishing deaconess education in Viborg. The main figure was the young Olga Hackman (1839–1865). She joined the deaconess institute in Dresden in the early 1860s, but did not live long enough to finish her studies. When she passed away at the age of 26, she left a legacy to the motherhouse in Dresden. After some consultation, her family decided to use her legacy and some other resources in Finland to set up a deaconess institute in Viborg.[19] Legislative restrictions meant it was easier to import the idea of deaconess education to Finland than to transfer Olga Hackman's inheritance to Dresden.

In terms of deaconess education, the institute in Viborg drew inspiration both from the *Evangelische Hospital* in St. Petersburg and the deaconess institute in Dresden.[20] Dresden seemed to be pursuing the 'deaconess crusade' in eastern and north-eastern parts of Europe, committing itself to the Kaiserswerth objective of establishing daughter institutes throughout Europe and on other continents. Nursing and childcare constituted the core of the deaconesses' work in Viborg. The small institute could not send out deaconesses to serve in parish nursing; instead, they were employed in the hospital founded by the institute. The first parish nurse was not sent out until 1896. In 1921, the total number of deaconesses and students was 69. Only 24 of them were deaconesses, 34 were probationary deaconesses and 11 were students. However, in the 1920s and 1930s, the number of deaconesses increased and new students were actively recruited.[21] In the mid-1930s, the institute reported higher figures, indicating that the motherhouse had experienced a remarkable growth. In 1935, the total number of deaconesses and students was almost 200: 60 consecrated deaconesses, 98 probationary deaconesses and 35 students.[22] In World War II, Finland lost the city of Viborg and the institute was

---

17 Wirén (1936 a), pp. 21–28; Diakonissanstaltens i Helsingfors verksamhet år 1940. In: Från Diakonissanstalten i Helsingfors 5–6 (1941), p. 68.
18 Kansanaho (1967), p. 278; Erkamo (1969), p. 208.
19 Betel (1919), pp. 3–7; Vappula (2009), p. 15.
20 Betel (1919), pp. 6–8; Vappula (2009), pp. 12–15.
21 Markkola (1999), pp. 178–179.
22 Korpijaakko (1936), p. 36; Vappula (2009), pp. 39–42.

evacuated to the town of Lahti in southern Finland, where deaconess education was continued after the war.

The expansion of the deaconessate in the 1890s

While deaconess education was introduced in two cities in the south of Finland in the 1860s, it was not until 30 years later that the deaconess movement
reached other parts of the country. In the 1880s and 1890s, deaconess education and the diaconate were actively debated in public and private arenas, and
several books and pamphlets were published. Some philanthropic women,
Lutheran pastors and medical doctors dedicated themselves to the deaconess
cause. One of the most remarkable results of the lively debate was the diaconate regulations (instructions) issued by the church. The diocese of Kuopio
in northern Finland had its diaconate regulations approved by the Senate in
1893. According to the regulations, parish nursing and parish poor relief were
to be led by the pastor, organised by a voluntary committee and implemented
by deaconesses or deacons. The poor, the sick and poor children were the
primary groups to be cared for. The Archdiocese of Turku in western Finland
started following the regulations concerning deaconesses the same year,
whereas the diocese of Porvoo in the south decided to rely on Fliednerian
motherhouses in their parish nursing and poor relief.[23] Nevertheless, in spite
of the differing regional solutions, the diaconate became an established part of
Lutheran parish work in the 1890s, and so the foundations were laid for parish
nursing.

Two deaconess institutes were founded in eastern and northern Finland at
around the same time. The new educational institutions, however, did not follow the motherhouse model. Instead, the deaconess school of Sortavala, established in 1894, and the deaconess institute of Oulu, established in 1896, provided shorter 'parish sister' training courses, following the elementary nursing
model developed at the *Lovisenberg Deaconess House* in Norway. Education at
Lovisenberg was divided into a traditional motherhouse track, offering longer
deaconess training, and a shorter training track for parish sisters. This model
impressed the founder of the Sortavala institute, teacher Jenny Ingman (1854–
1921), who embarked on a grand tour at the beginning of the 1890s, visiting
12 deaconess institutes in the Nordic countries and continental Europe. It was
her conclusion that the longer training courses offered by the Fliednerian
motherhouses were too expensive and time-consuming for the needs of remote rural parishes.[24] A deaconess school was established to train 'parish sisters'. Although the school became a deaconess institute, it did not adopt the
motherhouse model. Women who graduated from the institute were sent to
parishes as salaried employees. Nursing education was provided at a local

23   Kansanaho (1967), pp. 93–95; Mustakallio (2002), pp. 206–207.
24   Markkola (1999), pp. 181–182. Ivalo, Jenny: Hvilken är diakonissans förnämsta uppgift?
     In: Betania (1913), pp. 145–146; Kanervo (1936), pp. 46–54; Kilström (1987), pp. 65–71.

hospital until the institute was able to build its own hospital in 1901. Originally, the education of parish sisters lasted only nine months, but this period was gradually extended to three years. By 1935, a total of 252 deaconesses had been trained in Sortavala and 80 women were continuing with their deaconess studies. As a result of World War II, Finland lost parts of Karelia to the Soviet Union and the institute was evacuated. In 1945, the institute relocated to Pieksämäki, a small town in eastern Finland, which was to become its permanent home in the post-war era.

The Norwegian model was also favoured by church activists in northern Finland. In the town of Oulu, several pastors and philanthropic women were particularly interested in deaconess education, but they found the Fliednerian system too complicated, whereas the Lovisenberg institute in Norway seemed to provide appropriate answers to local social problems. Correspondence between pastors in Oulu and the pastor of the *Lovisenberg Deaconess House* led to a decision to send a 26-year-old teacher, Selma Stenbäck (1869–1951), to study nursing in Oslo. Like many other female deaconess leaders, she came from a Lutheran clergyman's family. After a training period of one year, she became the first female director of the *Oulu Deaconess Institute* in 1896. She left the institute, but was later replaced by a competent nurse, Ms Elin Smarin (1870–1929), who served as the institute's female director and as a nursing teacher for many years. In 1902, the nursing education provided by the *Oulu Deaconess Institute* was recognised by the state authorities, and trained parish sisters were licensed to work as visiting nurses. Parish sisters lacked a formal tie to their training institution; instead, they served parishes, municipal authorities and voluntary organisations as salaried employees. In the 1920s, the *Oulu Institute* adopted the Fliednerian motherhouse model, thus joining the traditions of the European deaconessate. This was partly due to increasing cooperation between the Finnish deaconess institutes and the national diaconate committee, which was set up in 1921, and partly due to practical attempts to provide old age security for the women trained by the institute. By 1935, the *Oulu Deaconess Institute* had trained 342 deaconesses. Many of them worked either in parish nursing or as visiting nurses hired by the public sector.[25]

The four institutes in Helsinki, Viborg, Sortavala and Oulu were the major training institutions for deaconesses until after World War II. The objective of the deaconessate was not only to alleviate physical and material needs; mental and spiritual distress needed addressing too. To meet these challenges successfully, deaconesses were trained in diverse areas. Newcomers were provided with practical training in household chores, such as cleaning, sewing, darning, doing laundry and preparing meals. Theoretical and practical classes in nursing were arranged at the institute's hospital. Nursing and health care were taught by physicians and professional nurses (deaconesses). Theoretical education, in addition to anatomy, physiology, pathology, nursing and health

25 Berättelse över Diakonissanstaltens i Helsingfors verksamhet under år 1920. In: Betania (1921), p. 79; Mustakallio (2001), pp. 102–105, 313–314; Markkola (1999), p. 182; Mustakallio (2002), p. 211.

care, consisted of tuition in Christianity, language, mathematics, history, geography and general diaconate knowledge. Other teachers were usually pastors and school teachers.[26]

Some institutes paid more attention to nursing; others preferred to see deaconesses as Christian sisters who offered spiritual comfort to their patients. Those deaconess institutes that followed the Fliednerian model expected a longer period of instruction than the younger institutes founded in the 1890s that trained women to serve in rural parishes as parish sisters. As a deep personal faith in God was understood to be the most important quality of a deaconess, all institutes instructed their students in 'character building'.[27] Nevertheless, the role of deaconesses in nursing and public health was to become more professional in the twentieth century. Owing to increasing state intervention, the institutes were obliged to upgrade their classes in nursing and public health issues.[28] The tensions between professionalism and character building, in fact, reveal the dual nature of the deaconess role that prevailed from the very beginning. A deaconess was simultaneously a professional nurse and a voluntary fellow human being serving 'out of love for her Saviour',[29] as one Finnish pastor put it in the early twentieth century.

Parish nursing

Initially, the deaconess institutes preferred to recruit educated women from middle-class homes rather than daughters of working-class or rural families, who were suspected of wanting to join the institution in pursuit of social upward mobility.[30] One of the most welcome students at the *Helsinki Deaconess Institute* was a sea captain's daughter, Cecilia Blomqvist (1845–1910), who became the Finnish pioneer in parish nursing. She entered the institute in the 1870s, when it was still in the process of formation and suffering from a lack of human and material resources.[31] Sister Cecilia's work included both nursing and social work. At the deaconess institute she was soon in charge of the hospital, and she visited working-class neighbourhoods, nursed the sick, pro-

26   Betel (1919), pp. 23–26; Miettinen (1936), pp. 70–78; Heikinheimo (1946), p. 33; Kansanaho (1967), pp. 129–130.

27   This emphasis was not without problems. The dropout figures at the *Helsinki Deaconess Institute* in the early twentieth century indicate that an overwhelming majority of students left the institute before they were consecrated. The Roll of Deaconesses 1. HDL Ba:1. KA, Helsinki.

28   Ivalo (1920), pp. 82–91; Markkola (2000), p. 111.

29   The goal of the deaconess institutes was "to educate women, who, out of love for their Saviour have voluntarily chosen [as] their calling in life the nurturing of the suffering, the sick and the fallen". Virkkunen (1909), p. 477.

30   Cf. Nolte (2009), p. 145.

31   Cecilia Blomqvist. The Roll of Deaconesses 1. Deaconess Institute of Helsinki (HDL) Ba:1. KA, Helsinki.; Kansanaho (1967), pp. 41–42, 50–51, 64. In practice the institutes attracted rural and working-class women. The Roll of Deaconesses. HDL, KA, Helsinki.

vided teaching for children and rescued needy children, sending them to foster homes and to the orphanage founded by the institute. In 1879 she was sent to the small town of Rauma to initiate parish nursing among the urban poor. Sister Cecilia's work in Rauma is generally regarded as the beginning of parish nursing in Finland,[32] although opinions may differ about the definition of parish nursing as a new, separate field. In Rauma, Cecilia Blomqvist continued work that was similar to the work the deaconesses were pursuing in Helsinki. With the motherhouse as their base, deaconesses contributed to parish nursing in their neighbourhood. The *City Mission* of Helsinki was set up in 1883 with the explicit aim of continuing the nursing services and social work initiated by the deaconess institute in working-class districts.[33]

Cecilia Blomqvist's example was soon followed by other deaconesses. Parish nursing was to become the most far-reaching arm of the female diaconate, especially in the twentieth century. In 1895 there were only five deaconesses involved in parish nursing, while the majority of deaconesses worked in the hospitals and shelters run by the institutes. Gradually the number of sisters working outside the walls of the motherhouses increased. More extensive work in rural parishes became possible once the deaconess institutes in Sortavala and Oulu were established in the 1890s. The shorter training period to become a parish sister made the occupation a viable option for young women, and the fact that the new institutes were Finnish-speaking contributed to their sudden growth and the expansion of their education services. The predominant language at the *Helsinki Deaconess Institute* was Swedish, and the Viborg institute was founded by the small but influential German-speaking minority. There was a need for education in Finnish, as almost 87 per cent of the Finns were Finnish-speaking. About 13 per cent spoke Swedish as their mother tongue, while the other languages remained marginal.[34] The new institutes educated an expanding number of women to serve rural parishes. The old institutes became more open to the majority language and the *Lutheran Church of Finland* defined *diakonia* as an integral part of parish activities. On the whole, these trends created better conditions for parish nursing.

In the 1890s, health conditions in rural areas and urban working-class districts were regarded as a severe social problem, and the *Diet of Four Estates* took steps to combat it, passing new legislation and issuing new regulations. From 1899 onwards, municipal authorities and voluntary organisations in rural areas could obtain financial support from the state to employ visiting nurses. In the first five to ten years, they were entitled to public support that covered half of the salary paid to the visiting nurse. Deaconesses employed as visiting nurses had their education recognised by medical authorities. When

32   Kansanaho (1967); Mustakallio (1999), pp. 94–101.
33   On the *City Mission of Helsinki*, see the files of Cecilia Blomqvist. The Roll of Deaconesses 1. HDL Ba:1. KA, Helsinki; Kansanaho (1960), pp. 201–204.
34   Markkola (1999), pp. 190–191. Mustakallio (1999), pp. 94–101; SVT VI. Väestötilastoa (population statistics) 37. Helsinki 1905, pp. 68–78.

the system was launched, only municipalities and voluntary associations were eligible for the state support, but after a while parishes were included as well.[35]

Rural nursing and deaconess education were tightly intertwined in the late 1890s and early 1900s. The first visiting nurses hired by municipal authorities were parish sisters trained at the *Oulu Deaconess Institute*, and the physician of the institute, Dr Konrad Relander, promoted health legislation in the *Diet of Four Estates*. Moreover, in 1903 he published the first Finnish-language textbook on nursing targeted at rural deaconesses, visiting nurses and rural families. In the textbook he encouraged women from rural families and urban working-class and lower-middle-class homes to enter nursing schools, as he believed these women were better suited to the demanding conditions of rural nursing than women from the educated classes.[36] In the course of the twentieth century, Dr Relander's vision was realised in the deaconess institutes, where an increasing number of rural women and working-class women pursued deaconess studies.

The importance of parish nursing increased in other institutes as well. As early as 1908, the annual report of the *Helsinki Deaconess Institute* explained that the most important part of nursing was the work in which deaconesses were engaged as visiting nurses.[37] The state support encouraged not only municipal authorities and parishes but also voluntary organisations to hire visiting nurses. Diaconate associations and women's sewing circles, tuberculosis associations and other health organisations employed deaconesses and funded the part of the salary not covered by the state subsidy.[38] Local arrangements to provide health care and nursing were often based on a complicated network in which municipal authorities, parishes and civil society associations worked in close cooperation and received substantial funding from the state to maintain their services.

At the turn of the twentieth century, the work of deaconesses in parishes was divided into poor relief and nursing. Both fields were regulated by their educational institutions. The *Sortavala Deaconess Institute* published its revised regulations in 1903 and the *Helsinki Deaconess Institute* followed suit in 1908.[39] Although the Helsinki Institute was a Fliednerian institution following the Kaiserswerth motherhouse model, and Sortavala was established to train parish sisters who would be employed in rural parishes, the similarities between the two sets of rules were striking.

---

35 Keisarillisen Majesteetin Armollinen Kirje 21.2.1899. Asetuskokoelma (As. kok.) 9 (1899); Mustakallio (2001), pp. 220–223.

36 Relander (1903); Mustakallio (2001), pp. 220–223; Markkola (1999), pp. 192–193.

37 Berättelse om Diakonissanstaltens i Helsingfors verksamhet år 1908. In: Betania (1909), p. 90.

38 Markkola (1999), pp. 192–193.

39 Instruktion för församlingsdiakonissa, då hennes hufvuduppgift är sjukvård. Utarbetad af Diakonissanstalten i Sordavala. In: Betania (1903), p. 71; Anvisningar för församlingsdiakonissan, då hennes hufvuduppgift är sjukvård. In: Betania (1908), pp. 39–42.

A deaconess who was hired to concentrate on nursing was advised to nurse the sick and needy. She was to provide sick people with care, hygiene and – if necessary – access to a physician or a hospital. As a nurse, the deaconess had to follow carefully the instructions given by a doctor. She was also obliged to prepare appropriate food for the sick, provided that groceries were available. One important task was to teach the family and the community how to take care of the sick. If material help was needed, the deaconess was instructed to source support from the municipal poor relief or from charitable individuals. Additionally, she was expected to be responsible for public health in her community. If there were contagious diseases, the deaconess had to undertake all necessary measures against them. Although nursing and health care were the primary fields, the role of a deaconess as a visiting nurse also included a spiritual dimension. She was expected to promote the distribution of Bibles and read religious texts to those who did not have a chance to attend religious gatherings.[40]

Instructions for those deaconesses who worked in poor relief and social services were slightly different. Here there was an emphasis on spiritual support. Moreover, deaconesses were expected to look after neglected children, released prisoners and other morally endangered groups, and the sick and needy. It was also their duty to urge poor people to help themselves and to introduce the principles and practices of philanthropy to those who were better off. When doing social work, they were explicitly advised to avoid conflict with municipal poor relief systems.[41]

In this context it is not surprising that a deaconess was expected to work in close cooperation with the clergy. In parishes, deaconesses were supervised by the pastor. In their role as nurse, deaconesses were also instructed by doctors. In the event of conflicting instructions and assignments, the deaconess was obliged to contact the head of the diaconate committee, usually the pastor, and follow his instructions. The importance of obeying clerical authorities was further clarified in correspondence between deaconesses and their motherhouses, and in journals published by deaconess institutes. Regardless of the importance of nursing, deaconesses were expected to look after souls. Hierarchies of care were made explicit and earthly well-being was subordinate to spiritual, eternal well-being.[42] Other hierarchies were instituted: between fe-

40   Instruktion för församlingsdiakonissa, då hennes hufvuduppgift är sjukvård. Utarbetad af Diakonissanstalten i Sordavala. In: Betania (1903), p. 71; Anvisningar för församlingsdiakonissan, då hennes hufvuduppgift är sjukvård. In: Betania (1908), pp. 39–42.

41   Instruktion för församlingsdiakonissa, då hennes hufvuduppgift är att vårda församlingens fattiga. Utarbetad af Diakonissanstalten i Sordavala. In: Betania (1903), pp. 25–26; Anvisningar för församlingsdiakonissan, då hennes hufvuduppgift är att vårda församlingens fattiga. In: Betania (1908), pp. 38–39.

42   E. g. Snellman, Lina: Något om diakonisskallets förmåner och faror. In: Betania (1908), pp. 121–124; Brax, Greta: Huru kunde vi inom systergemenskapen bevara medvetandet därom, att vi tjäna Herren och icke människor? In: Betania (1908), pp. 183–184; Ivalo, Jenny: Hvilken är diakonissans förnämsta uppgift? In: Betania (1913), pp. 145–149; Wennerström, Elsa: Vilka särskilda faror medför diakonissans uppgift för utvecklingen av

male and male servants of God, as well as between the laity and the clergy – deaconesses were subordinate to churchmen.

In 1906–1909 a survey on the deaconessate was conducted in Finland. The survey revealed that in 1909 the total number of deaconesses, parish sisters and students was 280. Almost 40 per cent of them were employed in parishes and 40 per cent served in various institutions, including hospitals, orphanages and other institutions.[43] The status of the diaconate was further strengthened in 1913, when the *General Synod*, in its capacity as the highest decision-making body of the Lutheran church, proposed an amendment to the church law (*Ecclesiastical Act*). According to the amendment, the vicar of the parish was expected to promote diaconate in his parish and to attempt to hire competent deacons and deaconesses to serve the parish. The amendment to the *Ecclesiastical Act* came into effect in 1918.[44] The diaconate was defined as an official, yet voluntary, part of the church institution in Finland.

Consequently, the role of parish nursing, as an important part of the deaconessate, was strengthened. According to statistics presented by the Finnish clergy, every second parish employed a deaconess in 1922. The number of parishes was 571, and more than 400 deaconesses were involved in nursing or social work in parishes. Some parishes had hired two or even more deaconesses. In 1935, a total of 409 women belonged to the community of the oldest deaconess institute in Finland and 168 of them were employed in nursing or poor relief outside the institute. Table 1 presents total figures for all deaconess institutes from 1900 to 1940.

Table 1: Deaconesses working outside the deaconess institutes in Finland, 1900–1940.

Year	1900	1910	1920	1930	1940
Parish nursing	30	121	314	434	408
Nursing	18	30	55	93	130
Other	5	48	114	85	161
Total	53	199	484	612	699

Source: Markkola (1999), p. 190. Based on annual reports of the deaconess institutes, the Betania journal (1911, 1921) and Från Diakonissanstalten i Helsingfors journal (1931, 1941).

Table 1 suggests that the work of deaconesses was growing in all fields, but parish nursing was clearly dominant. In 1940, however, several deaconesses were transferred from parish nursing to military nursing. We know, for exam-

hennes personlighet. In: Betania (1914), pp. 9–13; Nordström, U.: Diakonisskallet och förberedelsen därtill. In: Betania (1914), pp. 79–85; Villkoren för församlingsdiakonin. In: Betania (1915) 1; Vennerström, Elsa: Diakonisskallet. In: Betania (1916), pp. 134–141; Sjukvårdens plats och betydelse i diakoniarbetet. In: Från Diakonissanstalten i Helsingfors (1926), pp. 117–122.

43   Diakoniarbetets nuvarande tillstånd i Finland. In: Betania (1909), pp. 68–72, Betania (1909), pp. 85–87, Betania (1909), pp. 100–104.

44   Mustakallio (2002), pp. 215–216.

ple, that more than 80 deaconesses from the *Oulu Deaconess Institute* who are not included in Table 1, worked in the institute's hospital. Another reservation concerning the categories has to be made. Deaconesses who were employed by the municipal poor relief system or by charitable or religious organisations, such as city missions, are included in the 'Other' category. City missions, for example, employed deaconesses both in childcare institutions and as visiting nurses. The same can be said about municipal authorities where deaconesses worked as nurses and social workers. In other words, a good number of deaconesses grouped under the category 'Other' were involved in nursing work that was comparable to parish nursing.[45] These difficulties in categorising the work of deaconesses are in fact revealing. They indicate that the work of deaconesses was both flexible and diffuse by nature.

Increasing state intervention

In the twentieth century, "nurturing of the suffering, the sick and the fallen"[46] had to adapt to comply with the criteria set by the Finnish medical authorities. In general, it seems deaconess institutes were willing to modify their nursing education to accommodate the increasing state intervention. The *Oulu Deaconess Institute*, for example, expanded its training period from two years to three years in 1921 and simultaneously restructured and formalised its theoretical teaching.[47] As a result of the reforms, the deaconess institutes were able to meet national standards for nursing education. However, attempts to provide a more thorough education for nurses and to harmonise the education provided by national, regional, local and private hospitals were promoted throughout the early twentieth century, in particular by nurses' associations and medical organisations.[48] Deaconess institutes had to adapt the training they provided in an environment that was constantly changing.

In 1929, the legislation governing nursing and the qualifications of nurses was revised. According to the new legislation, the state was to maintain nursing schools and provide nursing education. Private nursing schools, such as deaconess institutes, had to be approved by the medical authorities, meet the standards set by them and be subjected to state supervision. The new law allowed deaconesses to work as licensed nurses in hospitals owned by the deaconess institutes and, with special permission from the authorities, as visiting

45   Sisarten vuosikertomukset (annual reports from the sisters). Deaconess Institute of Helsinki (HDL), Ea1 1902–1929. KA, Helsinki; Berättelse över Diakonissanstaltens i Helsingfors verksamhet år 1930. In: Från Diakonissanstalten i Helsingfors (1931), p. 81.

46   Virkkunen (1909), p. 477.

47   Heikinheimo (1946), pp. 33–34.

48   Sorvettula (1998), pp. 69–77, 144–153. The main nursing associations were the Swedish-speaking *Sjuksköterskeföreningen i Finland*, founded in 1898, and the Finnish-speaking *Suomen Sairaanhoitajatarliitto*, founded in 1925. The former, in particular, was active in providing education for nurses.

nurses.[49] The Fliednerian deaconess institutes, with their long training periods, found it relatively easy to adapt to the new requirements, although the institute in Viborg was obliged to improve its theoretical and practical nursing classes to meet the higher qualification standards. The *Oulu Deaconess Institute* was prepared for the legislative changes well ahead of time, but the deaconess institute in Sortavala was still struggling with the content of nursing education in the 1930s. The other deaconess institutes had their nursing education recognised by the medical authorities in the 1930s, but the nursing courses started in Sortavala were not formally recognised until 1947. Before the formal recognition, deaconesses trained in Sortavala were not licensed to work as nurses, nor was their parish work supported by the state, but they could provide simple health care in parishes. Another alternative for Sortavala sisters was to work in the areas of poor relief and childcare.[50]

The introduction of public health nursing added another new dimension to parish nursing. Visiting nurses and deaconesses were just expected to be competent nurses, whereas public health nurses had to acquire additional skills. Voluntary associations played a key role in the introduction of further education for public health issues. The *Finnish Association for the Prevention of Tuberculosis* started organising specialised training courses for nurses in 1914. In 1920, the *Mannerheim League for Child Welfare* initiated special courses in childcare. These classes were merged in 1924 into a six-month course in public health nursing. Moreover, one voluntary organisation offered training in school nursing following the German example. All these courses were attended both by nurses and by deaconesses. Since nursing education had been taken over by the state in 1929, it was expected that education in the area of public health nursing would soon become a state responsibility as well. Voluntary associations turned their attention to other activities and were ready to hand over their training courses to public authorities. Not surprisingly, the state took over this type of training in 1931 and established a new school for nurses specialising in public health nursing.[51]

49 Laki sairaanhoitajattarien koulutuksesta 9.11.1929. As.kok. 340/1929; Asetus sairaanhoitajattarien koulutuksesta 21.12.1929. As.kok 424/1929; Asetus sairaanhoitajattaren- ja sairaanhoitajatoimen harjoittamisesta 21.12.1929. As.kok. 426/1929; Sorvettula (1998), pp. 218–219.
50 Systrarnas sjukvårdsutbildning. In: Från Diakonissanstalten i Helsingfors (1930), pp. 106–107; Erkamo (1969), pp. 157–160; Malkavaara (2002), p. 228; Huhta (2005), p. 95.
51 Maaseudun terveydenhoito-olot ja niiden kehittäminen. Komiteanmietintö 1939:9. Helsinki 1939, pp. 21, 47–48; Sorvettula (1998), pp. 35–36; Larsson (1945), pp. 19–24.

Table 2: Public health nurses in Finland in 1930, 1935 and 1938.

Year	1930	1935	1938
Visiting nurses	545	496	497
Public health nurses	52		
Tuberculosis nurses	172		
School nurses	120		
All public health nurses*		413	486
Total	889	909	983

* Public health nurses, tuberculosis nurses and school nurses
Source: Official statistics of Finland XI. Health statistics 1930, 1935 and 1938.

In 1930, the official statistics of Finland showed that the number of visiting nurses was 545. At the same time, deaconess institutes reported that 434 deaconesses worked in parish nursing. This could mean that up to 80 per cent of visiting nurses were deaconesses sent by the deaconess institutes. Again, however, these figures are problematic, because only those deaconesses whose employers received state support were included in the statistical category of visiting nurse. Moreover, if public health nurses, school nurses and tuberculosis nurses are added to the picture, the share of deaconesses falls to 49 per cent. As school nurses were not visiting nurses like the other groups, they can be excluded, and the estimated share of deaconesses could then be around 56 per cent. More reliable information can be found in a report by a committee tasked with investigating health conditions in rural areas in the 1930s. In 1937, there were 289 public health nurses, 198 visiting nurses and 238 deaconesses working in the Finnish countryside providing nursing services.[52] Deaconesses accounted for 33 per cent of all nurses involved in visiting and public health nursing. Despite the increasing number of public health nurses, deaconesses represented an important group of rural nurses in Finland in the 1930s.

In general, rural health issues were topical in the latter part of the 1930s and several meetings were held to discuss them. Governors discussed health legislation in May 1936, representatives of rural municipalities agreed on a health care resolution in November 1936; in 1937, agricultural societies made several proposals to improve rural sanitary conditions, and several other meetings were held by voluntary associations, medical doctors, health care organisations and public health nurses. Consequently, in July 1937, the government set the above-mentioned committee the task of investigating measures to improve health conditions in rural areas. The committee published its report in 1939.[53] The nursing education provided by the deaconess institutes of Helsinki and Oulu was mentioned in the report. The courses provided by nursing

52   Maaseudun terveydenhoito-olot ja niiden kehittäminen. Komiteanmietintö 1939:9. Helsinki 1939, p. 48.
53   Komiteanmietintö 1939:9, pp. 3–4.

schools lasted three years, but the deaconess institutes were reported to provide slightly longer courses.

During World War II, the administration and provision of public health services, social care and relief were reorganised. War losses brought issues of physical and material need to the fore. Social policies and family policies were developed to support people whose family members had been killed or disabled in the war or who were suffering from material losses. Lack of food and worsening health on the home front were other challenges that needed to be met. As a consequence, new social legislation was passed. In 1944, a system of compulsory district health care was established, and public health nursing was made a compulsory part of municipal health care. Every municipal authority was entitled to hire public health nurses. Other health reforms included improved maternity and infant care, as child welfare clinics were made mandatory. At the same time, the *Ecclesiastical Act* was amended and the diaconate was made a mandatory component of the parish, which meant that each parish had to employ deaconesses. Two parallel sets of reforms – municipal and ecclesiastical – were carried out to improve health services. As deaconesses were allowed to continue their work as educated nurses, the Church continued to play an important role in Finnish health care.

The post-WWII era

In the period following World War II, there were many problems caused by the war that needed to be solved. The housing problem in Finland was urgent: more than ten per cent of the housing stock had been lost in the war, and about 12 per cent of the population – from the areas ceded to the Soviet Union – had no homes to return to.[54] As mentioned earlier, two deaconess institutes were among the institutions evacuated. In the reconstruction era, the input of deaconess institutes was urgently needed in health care and public health. Human and material losses, broken families, poor health and traumatised war veterans formed a mental and physical landscape in which health authorities, social workers and educational institutions needed to build decent social conditions for the Finnish people. Relatively comprehensive health care statistics reveal that deaconesses played an important complementary role in public health nursing until the 1970s, when the Finnish health care system was reformed.

---

54   Roiko-Jokela (2004), pp. 27–28; Malinen (2014), pp. 75–78.

Table 3: Public health nurses, district nurses and deaconesses in Finland, 1945–1971.

	Public health nurses	District nurses	Deacon-esses	Total number	Share of Deaconesses
1945	688	158	318	1164	27.3%
1950	967	174	343	1484	23.1%
1955	1296	175	393	1864	21.1%
1960	1726		533	2259	23.6%
1965	2060		501	2561	19.6%
1970	2280		701	2981	23.5%
1971	2335		784	3119	25.1%

Sources: SVT XI: 56–74. Public health and medical care 1945–1971. Helsinki 1957–1972. In 1959, statistics were changed and the category of district nurse lost its significance in the total number of public health nurses.

The share of deaconesses remained high until the early 1970s, when the 1972 *Public Health Act* excluded deaconesses from public health nursing. Municipalities built their welfare services and parishes sought a new emphasis for their diaconate. Since the *Ecclesiastical Act* of 1944 made the diaconate obligatory for parishes, the deaconesses employed by parishes represented a remarkable resource for parish social work and services among the elderly population.

According to the original idea of the female diaconate, nursing represented only one aspect of the work performed by deaconesses. It was noted by the deaconess institutes that the increase in parish nursing and the deaconesses' involvement in public health care, together with a proper nursing education, spelled an emphasis on health care, while the deaconesses' traditional role in social and spiritual care was receiving less attention.[55] In the early 1950s, the deaconess education provided by the *Helsinki Deaconess Institute* was reformed. Students from a primary school background had to attend preparatory classes before starting their actual training. The ordinary deaconess training took four years. Introductory courses lasted six months, followed by nursing education over two years and nine month. The remaining nine months were reserved for social and spiritual care. Already by 1957, more attention was being given to social work and other skills not related to nursing. The other deaconess institutes were also looking for new tasks. The former institute of Viborg, now based in Lahti, was involved in caring for disabled children and adults and the elderly.[56] Educators of deaconesses attempted to adjust the original deaconess concept to the changing circumstances and a society in the process of modernisation. The original idea of targeting the most vulnerable groups and people was applied both explicitly and implicitly in post-war society.

55   Kansanaho (1967), p. 269.
56   Kansanaho (1967), pp. 276–277; Erkamo (1969), pp. 218–220.

Moreover, the motherhouse system faced several challenges. Some deaconesses started to criticise the lack of freedom embedded in the system.
Labour relations, in particular, became an issue. Deaconesses were not allowed to choose their work, part of their salary was still paid to the institute
and, depending on their behaviour, they were at risk of being dismissed from
the motherhouse community, which would mean losing the pension benefits
provided by the deaconess institutes. Changes to the motherhouse organisation were made in the 1940s, and deaconesses were gradually entitled to their
own salaries and brought into line with other waged workers on the labour
market. In 1958, the *General Synod* incorporated deaconesses in the church's
pension system, thus solving some of the biggest problems inherent in the
motherhouse system. Deaconess institutes changed their constitutions and the
motherhouse system was abolished.[57] Deaconesses were no longer a special
group tied to and supported by the motherhouse: they became salaried employees in the service of parishes and health care authorities.

Concluding remarks

In 1936, when the centenary of deaconess education was celebrated in Finland, parish nursing and the role of deaconesses were topical for a number of
reasons. The organisation of rural health care, in particular, was on the political agenda and this concern did not go unnoticed by the deaconess leaders.
While the state, municipal authorities and voluntary organisations were struggling with poor sanitary conditions in rural areas and a lack of health care
services, the directors of the deaconess institutes were able to refer to their
own tradition, dating back to Kaiserswerth in 1836. It was not a coincidence
that Pastor Wirén emphasised the role of the diaconate in the education of
nurses.

Nursing education in the deaconess institutes was closely related to the
needs of Finnish society. In the nineteenth century no other nursing was provided in rural Finland, and the nursing provided by deaconesses was extremely limited as well. In the course of the twentieth century, health care was
gradually developed and nursing education became more regulated. However,
the Finnish state, and the public sector in general, was dependent on non-state
actors such as deaconess institutes. Deaconess institutes were willing to col-
laborate with the public sector and even to adjust to the increasing state intervention from the 1920s onwards. Moreover, state intervention involved some
obvious advantages, such as state support for parishes and municipalities to
recruit deaconesses to work in parish nursing. The collaboration with ecclesiastical and secular actors was not without tension, and some deaconesses and
their leaders feared that the female diaconate would turn into a plain nursing
profession and lose its special character. The deaconess institute of Sortavala,

---

57 Erkamo (1969), pp. 210–214; Kansanaho (1967), pp. 266–274, 279–280; Vappula (2009),
    pp. 170–171.

later based in Pieksämäki, was the most sceptical towards nursing. As early as 1919 its leaders complained that sisters were spending too much time in the service of public health care, carrying out duties that should be the responsibility of the municipalities.[58] Nevertheless, until the 1960s, a good proportion of deaconesses, in particular from the other deaconess institutes, were involved in public health nursing, and they accounted for a significant proportion of all public health nurses by the time they were excluded from the field in 1972.

An obvious strength, and sometimes a weakness, was the dual nature of the deaconessate as a provider of both physical and spiritual care, caring for both body and soul. Every time new public health services were introduced and the work of the deaconesses was discussed, an emphasis on spiritual nurturing was presented as the specialist field of a female diaconate. In their daily work, deaconesses employed in parish nursing were expected to achieve a balance between health care and caring for the soul. When working with their secular employers, their work ethics reflected this dual role. For the deaconess leaders, this duality turned out to be strength. When one door closed, for instance in health care, other doors opened in social care and parish work, with new groups in need of care.

Bibliography

Literature

Baumann, Ursula: Protestantismus und Frauenemanzipation in Deutschland 1850 bis 1920. Frankfurt/Main; New York 1992.
De Swarte Gifford, Carolyn (ed.): The American deaconess movement in the early twentieth century. New York; London 1987.
Ekmund, Gunnel: Den kvinnliga diakonin i Sverige 1849–1861. Uppgift och utformning. Lund 1973.
Haapala, Pertti: Työväenluokan synty. In: Pertti Haapala (ed.): Talous, valta ja valtio. Tutkimuksia 1800-luvun Suomesta. Tampere 1992.
Hammar, Inger: Emancipation och religion. Den svenska kvinnorörelsens pionjärer i debatt om kvinnans kallelse ca 1860–1900. Stockholm 1999.
Hammar, Inger: From Fredrika Bremer to Ellen Key. Calling, gender and the emancipation debate in Sweden, c. 1830–1900. In: Markkola, Pirjo (ed.): Gender and vocation. Women, religion and social change in the Nordic countries, 1840–1940. Helsinki 2000.
Harjula, Minna: Terveyden jäljillä. Suomalainen terveyspolitiikka 1900-luvulla. Tampere 2007.
Heininen, Simo; Heikkilä, Markku: Suomen kirkkohistoria. Helsinki 1996.
Helander, Eila: Naiset eivät vaienneet. Naisevankelistainstituutio Suomen helluntailiikkeessä. Helsinki 1987.
Helén, Ilpo; Jauho, Mikko (ed.): Kansalaisuus ja kansanterveys. Helsinki 2003.
Holm, Nils G.; Sandström, H.: Finlandssvensk frikyrklighet. Åbo 1972.
Hope, Nicholas: German and Scandinavian protestantism 1700–1918. Oxford 1995.
Huhta, Ilkka; Malkavaara, Mikko: Suomen kirkon sisälähetysseuran historia. Vuodet 1940–2004. Helsinki 2005.

---

58   Tervehdys Sortavalan Diakonitarlaitoksesta 16 (1919), p. 34.

Kansanaho, Erkki: Sata vuotta kristillistä palvelutyötä. Helsingin Diakonissalaitos 1867–1967. Porvoo; Helsinki 1967.

Kansanaho, Erkki: Sisälähetys ja diakonia Suomen kirkossa 1800-luvulla. Pieksämäki 1960.

Kilström, Bengt Ingmar: Kyrka och diakoni I–I. Åbo 1987.

Kirby, David: A concise history of Finland. Cambridge 2006.

Koivunen Bylund, Tuulikki: Frukta icke, allenast tro. Ebba Boström och Samariterhemmet 1882–1902. Stockholm 1994.

Kreutzer, Susanne: "Before, we were always there – Now, everything is separate". On nursing reforms in Western Germany. In: Nursing History Review 16 (2008), pp. 180–200.

Kreutzer, Susanne: Nursing body and soul in the parish. Lutheran deaconess motherhouses in Germany and the United States. In: Nursing History Review 18 (2010), pp. 134–150.

Lavery, Jason: The history of Finland. Westport; London 2006.

Malinen, Antti: Perheet ahtaalla. Asuntopula ja siihen sopeutuminen toisen maailmansodan jälkeisessä Helsingissä 1944–1948. Helsinki 2014.

Malkavaara, Mikko: Sodasta laman kynnykselle. Köyhyys ja diakonia hyvinvointivaltiota rakennettaessa. In: Virpi Mäkinen (ed.): Lasaruksesta leipäjonoihin. Köyhyys kirkon kysymyksenä. Jyväskylä 2002.

Manninen, Merja; Setälä, Päivi (ed.): The lady with the bow. The story of Finnish women. Helsinki 1990.

Markkola, Pirjo: Deaconesses go transnational. Knowledge transfer and deaconess education in nineteenth-century Finland and Sweden. In: Fleischmann, Ellen; Grypma, Sonya; Marten, Michael; Okkenhaug, Inger Marie (ed.): Transnational and historical perspectives on global health, welfare and humanitarianism. Kristiansand 2013, pp. 70–89.

Markkola, Pirjo: Diakonissan mellan det privata och det offentliga. Kvinnlig diakoni i Sverige och Finland 1880–1940. In: Janfelt, Monika (ed.): Den privat-offentliga gränsen. Det sociala arbetets strategier och aktörer i Norden 1860–1940. Copenhagen 1999.

Markkola, Pirjo: Lina Snellman (1846–1924). Helsingin diakonissalaitoksen johtajatar. In: Mustakallio, Hannu (ed.): Kirkollisia vaikuttajia Pyhästä Henrikistä nykyaikaan. Helsinki 2012, pp. 237–238.

Markkola, Pirjo: Promoting faith and welfare. The deaconess movement in Finland and Sweden, 1850–1930. In: Scandinavian Journal of History 25 (2000), Nos. 1–2, pp. 107–118.

Markkola, Pirjo: Women in rural society in the 19th and 20th centuries. In: Manninen, Merja; Setälä, Päivi (ed.): The lady with the bow. The story of Finnish women. Helsinki 1990.

Martinsen, Kari: Freidige og uforsagte diakonisser. Et omsorgsyrke voxer fram 1860–1905. Oslo 1984.

Meinander, Henrik: A history of Finland. London 2011.

Murtorinne, Eino: Suomen kirkon historia 3. Autonomian kausi 1809–1899. Porvoo; Helsinki; Juva 1992.

Mustakallio, Hannu: Emansipaatiota, diakoniaa ja filantropiaa. Pohjoispohjalaiset naiset diakoniaa ja hyväntekeväisyyttä edistämässä 1900-luvun alkupuolelle saakka. In: Teologinen Aikakauskirja 104 (1999), pp. 94–101.

Mustakallio, Hannu: Palvelun poluilla Pohjois-Suomessa. Oulun diakonissakoti 1896–1916. Oulu 2001.

Mustakallio, Hannu: Köyhät, sairaat ja kirkko. Suomalaista diakoniaa 1800-luvulta 1940-luvulle. In: Mäkine, Virpi (ed.): Lasaruksesta leipäjonoihin. Köyhyys kirkon kysymyksenä. Jyväskylä 2002.

Mustakallio, Hannu: Palvelun poluilla Pohjois-Suomessa. Oulun diakonissakoti 1896–1916. Oulu 2001.

Nolte, Karen: Dying at home. Nursing of the critically and terminally ill in private care in Germany around 1900. In: Nursing Inquiry 16 (2009), 2, pp. 144–154.

Nolte, Karen: "Telling the painful truth". Nurses and physicians in the nineteenth century. In: Nursing History Review 16 (2008), pp. 115–134.

Prelinger, Catherine M.: Charity, challenge, and change. Religious dimensions of the mid-nineteenth-century women's movement in Germany. New York; Westport; London 1987.

Prelinger, Catherine M.: The nineteenth-century deaconessate in Germany. The efficacy of a family model. In: Joeres, Ruth-Ellen B.; Maynes, Mary Jo (ed.): German women in the eighteenth and nineteenth centuries. A social and literary history. Bloomington 1986.

Qvarsell, Roger: Välgörenhet, filantropi och frivilligt socialt arbete. En historisk översikt. In: Frivilligt socialt arbete. Kartläggning och kunskapsöversikt. Rapport av socialtjänstkommittén. Statens offentliga utredningar 82 (1993), Stockholm 1993, pp. 217–241.

Ramsay, Alexandra: Huvudstadens hjärta. Filantropi och social förändring i Helsingfors – två fruntimmersföreningar 1848–1865. Helsingfors 1993.

Roiko-Jokela, Heikki: Asutustoiminnalla sodasta arkeen. In: Markkola, Pirjo (ed.): Suomen maatalouden historia 3. Helsinki 2004.

Schmidt, Jutta: Beruf: Schwester. Mutterhausdiakonie im 19. Jahrhundert. Frankfurt/Main 1998.

Soine, Aeleah: The motherhouse and its mission(s). Kaiserswerth and the convergence of transnational nursing knowledge, 1836–1865. In: Fleischmann, Ellen; Grypma, Sonya; Marten, Michael; Okkenhaug, Inger Marie (ed.): Transnational and historical perspectives on global health, welfare and humanitarianism. Kristiansand 2013, pp. 20–41.

Sorvettula, Maija: Johdatus suomalaisen hoitotyön historiaan. Helsinki 1998.

Tallberg, Marianne: Nursing and medical care in Finland from the eighteenth to the late nineteenth century. The background for the introduction of nurses' training in Finland in 1889, with some comparisons with developments in Sweden. In: Scandinavian Journal of History 14 (1989), p. 274.

Vappula, Kari: Rientäkää, älkää pysähtykö. Laitosdiakoniaa 70 vuotta Viipurissa ja 70 vuotta Lahdessa. Lahti 2009.

Primary sources

Periodicals

Betania 1903–1925.
Från Diakonissanstalten i Helsingfors 1926–1941.
Koti ja kirkko 1911.
Koti ja yhteiskunta 1894.
Tervehdys Sortavalan Diakonitarlaitoksesta 1919.

Official records

Asetuskokoelma 1899, 1929 (Annual collection of passed legislation).
SVT VI: 37 Väestötilastoa (Population statistics) 37. Helsinki 1905.
SVT XI: 56–57 Lääkintöhallituksen kertomukset vuosilta 1939–1954 (Annual reports of medical authorities). Helsinki 1955–1956.
SVT XI: 58–74. Yleinen terveyden- ja sairaanhoito 1955–1971 (Public health and medical care). Helsinki 1957–1972.
Maaseudun terveydenhoito-olot ja niiden kehittäminen. Komiteanmietintö (Committee report on rural sanitary conditions) 1939, 9. Helsinki 1939.

Published material

Betel. Piirteitä Viipurin Diakonissalaitoksen toiminnasta 1869–1919. Viipuri 1919.

Heikinheimo, A. I.: Pohjois-Suomen kirkollisen rakkaudentyön kehto. Oulun Diakonissakoti 1896–1946. Oulu 1946.

Heikinheimo. A. I.: Oulun diakonissakodin vaiheista. In: Palvelevan rakkauden askeleissa. Sata vuotta diakoniatyötä. Helsinki 1936.

Ivalo, Jenny: Diakonian lukukirja. Sortavala 1920.

Kanervo, O.: Sortavalan Diakonissalaitos. In: Palvelevan rakkauden askeleissa. Sata vuotta diakoniatyötä. Helsinki 1936.

Korpijaakko, O.: Viipurin Diakonissalaitos. In: Palvelevan rakkauden askeleissa. Sata vuotta diakoniatyötä. Helsinki 1936.

Larsson, Sigrid: Sairaanhoitajattarien oppikirja XVI. Terveydenhoitajatartoiminta. Porvoo; Helsinki 1945.

Miettinen, Aino: Diakonissakasvatuksesta. In: Palvelevan rakkauden askeleissa. Sata vuotta diakoniatyötä. Helsinki 1936.

Oulun diakonissakoti 1896–1921. Oulu 1922.

Relander, Konr.: Lyhyt sairaanhoitajan opas. Maaseutu-diakonissoja ja -sairaanhoitajia sekä kodin sairaanhoitoa varten. Helsinki 1903.

Wirén, Edvin: Helsingin Diakonissalaitos. In: Palvelevan rakkauden askeleissa. Sata vuotta diakoniatyötä. Helsinki 1936 a.

Wirén, Edvin: Nykyaikaisen diakonian synty ja kehitys. In: Palvelevan rakkauden askeleissa. Sata vuotta diakoniatyötä. Helsinki 1936 b.

Virkkunen, Paavo: Uskonnolliset ja hyväntekeväisyysyhdistykset. In: Oma maa. Helsinki 1909.

Archives

National Archives (KA), Helsinki. Aurora Karamzin's Collection.

National Archives (KA), Helsinki. Deaconess Institute of Helsinki (HDL).

Limits of transfer – Cultural and societal contexts

"No nurses like the deaconesses?" Protestant deaconesses and the medical marketplace in late-nineteenth-century England[1]

Carmen M. Mangion

> There are no nurses like the deaconesses. Other nurses, however well prepared in the best of training-schools, do not have the same high motive that lifts the service on the plane of religious duty, where the question of self-interest is wholly lost sight of.[2]

This excerpt, written by American Methodist and ardent deaconess promoter Jane M. Bancroft (1847–1932) in her *Deaconesses in Europe and their Lessons for America* (1889), pitted the 'high motive' of the religious vocation of the nurse deaconess against the 'self-interest' of the non-deaconess nurse. Bancroft also suggests, in the title and body of her text, the growing and dynamic nature of the deaconess movement as it spread throughout Europe and the United States. The articles in this volume attest to this vibrancy. The deaconess movement in England, however, was an anomaly of sorts. Though deaconess life had its place in England from 1861, its growth in terms of numbers of deaconesses was not substantial. The role of the deaconess, though attractive to many religious women and men, was constrained by its perceived similarity to community-centred religious life (that of both Anglican and Roman Catholic sisters and nuns). Links with Kaiserswerth were important to the early beginning of many deaconess communities, but the need to distance the movement from 'foreign' elements echoed the societal undercurrents and limited its growth and influence. Deaconesses in England worked in the parish, taught in schools, managed orphanages and nursed in hospitals. Institutional deaconess nursing was an important early means of ministerial outreach but, in some quarters, its importance waned by the end of the nineteenth century. The marginalisation of deaconess nursing, particularly in its institutional forms – the core concern of this article – was a result of the interplay between the religious mission of deaconesses and the developing sophistication of the medical marketplace.

Much of the modern historiography of English deaconesses has revolved around the deaconess movement itself or the authority and autonomy of the deaconess. The historiography of the 1970s and 1980s examined the authority of the deaconesses, with Catherine Prelinger charting the gendered hierarchy of the diaconate and Janet Grierson focusing on the twentieth-century struggle for equality between deacon and deaconess.[3] Brian Heeney and Sean Gill, in

---

1   I am grateful to several archivists for their guidance, including Theresa Joan White of the Community of St Andrew, Annett Buettner of Kaiserswerth and the archivists at Haringey Archives. Thanks also to Barbra Mann Wall for casting an eye over the text. All errors, of course, are my own.
2   Bancroft (1889), p. 127.
3   Prelinger (1986); Grierson (1981).

their volumes, have pointed to the connections between the deaconess and women's ministry in the Anglican church.[4] Martha Vicinus, interested in nineteenth-century women's authority, declared that deaconesses, while independent in their work, were likely to be under the authority of the clergy.[5] Jenny Daggers disagreed, arguing that deaconesses had little autonomy.[6] The most recent substantive work, the 2004 PhD dissertation of Henrietta Blackmore, examined in a more extended and nuanced way, the tensions of both the community and the parochial approach of the deaconess movement within the *Church of England*.[7] This article adds another dimension to this historiography, looking at nursing and medical care provided by deaconesses and examining their contribution to England's medical marketplace.

Despite the institutional nature of numerous deaconess communities, archives are a rarity and the dearth of primary source material has made research on deaconesses difficult. The most fulsome records can be found for the *London Diocesan Deaconess Institution* (the present *Community of St Andrew*), the *Rochester Diocesan Deaconess Institution* and the *Evangelical Protestant Deaconesses' Institute and Training Hospital*. Even the *German Hospital*, where nursing care was provided by Lutheran deaconesses, and which contains a rich archive, has very little material about their deaconesses. Only the *London Diocesan Deaconess Institution* contains a deaconess register – not the original, but one painstakingly compiled by a prodigious archivist. Much of the material used in this article was gleaned from the archives of the *Community of St Andrew* and the *Haringey Archives*, which hold the records of the *Evangelical Protestant Deaconesses' Institution and Training Hospital*. The material used includes committee meeting books, annual reports, some correspondence, promotional magazines, leaflets and reports. A further substantive source was printed material from local and national newspapers and journals. Most of these are institutional sources, meant to encourage donations or record meetings, but these documents also offer a means of interrogating the relationship of the nurse deaconesses to the medical marketplace.

This article will begin by examining the constraints limiting the growth of the deaconess movement in England. Then, through the analysis of two communities of Protestant deaconesses, one belonging to the *Church of England* and the other evangelical,[8] it will examine deaconess nursing. England's competitive medical marketplace was a dynamic, diverse and shifting arena. There were numerous purveyors of medical care: orthodox and unorthodox medical

4   Gill (1994), pp. 163–168; Heeney (1988), pp. 68–74.
5   Vicinus (1985), p. 66.
6   Daggers (2001), pp. 656–657.
7   Blackmore (2004).
8   David Bebbington's (1989) definition of nineteenth-century evangelicalism links it to understandings of conversionism, activism, Biblicism and crucicentrism. Though not denominational specific, evangelicals were often affiliated with nonconformist (so not conforming to the state church, the *Church of England*) religious denominations such as Unitarianism, Congregationalists, Baptists and Methodists. Evangelical deaconesses, then, were more likely to belong to nonconformist Protestant religious groups.

practitioners as well as nurses trained through experience and those trained in hospital-run nurse training schools. Medical care was still found most often in the home, but the numbers of voluntary (both general and specialist) and state-run hospital beds were increasing exponentially.[9] The management of the voluntary hospital, administered by philanthropic bodies, was growing in complexity as the costs of running such institutions increased. The medicalisation of these institutional spaces, increasingly populated with new and changing medical technologies and the resultant needs for improved technical training of the medical practitioner and the nurse, provided substantial barriers to entry. This essay suggests too that the place of religion in voluntary hospitals, which were increasingly being seen as public institutions, was being rethought.

Deaconesses in England

Much of the historiography on nineteenth-century nursing in England contrasts a coarse and aged 'Sairey Gamp', the caricature of the supposedly poorly-trained nurse of the early nineteenth century, with the youthful, modern hospital-trained nurse of the later nineteenth century.[10] What is sometimes disregarded is the influence of religious nursing. As an antidote to the 'Gamps', philanthropists such as Quaker Elizabeth Fry (1780–1845) created the *Protestant Sisters of Charity* (later renamed the *Institution of Nursing Sisters*) as Christian nurses for the sick and poor.[11] Ellen Ranyard's (1810–1879) Protestant Biblewomen nurses in 1868 were sent out to nurse and Christianise the poor.[12] Anglican sisterhoods which emerged out of the Oxford Movement[13] nursed at some of London's major voluntary hospitals, *King's College Hospital, Charing Cross Hospital* and *University College Hospital,* from the 1860s to the end of the century.[14] The prevalence of religious nursing waned by the end of the century and was replaced by the hospital-trained nurse, whose role was im-

---

9   Institutional medical care in the nineteenth century came in broadly two forms: voluntary hospitals, which were managed by philanthropic bodies, and state-run hospitals, which were typically associated with the New Poor Law (1832).

10 Sairey Gamp was a fictional nurse from The Life and Adventures of Martin Chuzzlewit (1844) by Charles Dickens, and is the pejorative name for untrained nurses. See Summers (1989).

11 Huntsman, Bruin and Holttum (2002), p. 358.

12 Ducrocq (1984); Prochaska, (1987); Williamson, (1996).

13 This movement initiated by Edward B. Pusey and John Henry Newman sought to re-catholicise the *Church of England* through a shift in doctrinal thinking and liturgical practices. Anglican sisterhoods developed out of this movement. They took vows of poverty, chastity and obedience, lived a community life in convents under the day-to-day authority of a Mother Superior and were either contemplative (leading a life of prayer within an enclosure) or mixed (also involved in charitable works such as nursing or teaching). For more on Anglican sisterhoods see Mumm (1998).

14 See Mangion (forthcoming 2016). Historians Anne Summers (1991) and Carol Helmstadter and Judith Godden (2012) have argued persuasively that these groups were influential to early nursing practice.

bued with a sense of morality, but without the denominational emphasis.[15]
The historiography of nursing has tended to overlook the efforts of deaconesses, perhaps due in no small part to their small numbers and their short-
lived efforts in England's medical marketplace.

The preoccupations of late twentieth and twenty-first-century historians of
the English deaconess movement correspond closely to the tensions of the
nineteenth century: concerns over the authority and autonomy of the deaconess were ever-present. Much of the historical research on the nineteenth-century Anglican deaconess movement suggests that their establishment resulted
in part from the opposition to Anglican sisterhoods, whose homosocial form
of religious life relied to a great extent on women's ministry directed by wom-
en.[16] Feeling the pressure from unfavourable linkages with Anglican sisterhoods, who were seen as 'autonomous' and renegade, Anglican deaconesses
and their supporters reiterated time and again that the deaconess was derived
from Scriptures and that, as church workers, they were under the authority of
the clergy. Deaconesses were meant to be bound to their bishop and associated with a parish, and their parish work came under the authority of the
parish clergy.

Deaconess supporters such as J. M. Ludlow were well aware of these concerns about the role of deaconesses. He challenged deaconess antagonists in
his *Edinburgh Review* article of 1876:

> And now comes the question – Is an Institute of Deaconesses required; is it practicable
> in England, on any truly effective and extensive scale? There will be indifference to over-
> come in some, the dislike to novelties in others. But we know, that we have the charity; we
> hope, that we have the religious feeling. We do not fear reason nor inquiry. But what we
> do fear – we confess it – is a cry; a cry, against which neither reason nor charity not reli-
> gion are of the slightest service. Protestantism may be in danger! The Papists are coming!
> Because a certain number of single women have agreed to live in one house, put on one
> dress, and join their earnings and efforts into one common stock for the relief of certain
> acknowledged social evils, the whole Apocalypse is likely enough to be ransacked for the
> millionth time, to prove that the mark of the beast is upon them! Grant, that it were a
> new thing in Protestantism to form a female community; is that a reason for condemning
> it?[17]

He articulated the concerns of those opposed to deaconesses: that the deaconess was a novelty; that she endangered Protestantism; and that a life in community was considered too close an association to Catholic religious life. And more
to the point was the fear that these women would be managed by women:

> I believe that for Sisterhoods of Mercy or Deaconesses' Institutes to be really honest and
> healthy, to preserve their due relation to the family order of the Church, to strengthen
> instead of weakening it, it is absolutely necessary that they should be under the direction
> of a man, and that one who is, or at least has been, a husband. Left to the direction of an
> unmarried woman, it seems absolutely impossible they should not gradually merge into

---

15 Bashford (1998), p. xv.
16 For a greater explanation of the differences between Anglican sisterhoods and Protestant
    deaconesses see Mangion (2010).
17 Ludlow (1876), p. 446.

ascetic celibacy, – Romish celibacy, – that celibacy which is an insult to marriage, to motherhood, and which sooner or later only sustains itself by the polygamous figment of a special union of the individual Sister with Christ.[18]

Female community life managed by women was an integral component of the development of both sisterhoods and the early deaconess institutions such as Elizabeth Ferard's (1825–1883) *London Diocesan Deaconess Institution* founded in 1861.[19] Perhaps influenced by this critique, the deaconess movement's structural basis shifted from 1887 with the introduction of Isabella Gilmore's *Rochester Diocesan Deaconess Institution.* Gilmore supported a more parochial approach to deaconess life. Her institution functioned more as a training centre, rather than a community; her deaconesses were expected to reside in a parish rather than in a motherhouse.[20] The work of these parish deaconesses was directly managed by the clergy of the parish in which they worked and where they lived.

Also an issue, as can be read in social commentator Elizabeth M. Sewell's apologia of the *Church of England* deaconess movement, was the importance of national identity and Englishness, which she imbricated with the functioning of the state religion. She pointed to the 'distinctly Anglican' nature of the deaconess movement in the *Church of England.* She contended:

> The Deaconesses of the English Church are, then, it must be remembered, distinctly Anglican; and the strength of the Institution will surely be found in the steadfast maintenance of Anglican principles as distinct from all extremes either of Ritualism or Puritanism, because with these principles the English Church itself must either stand or fall.[21]

Sewell was specifically addressing *Church of England* concerns, but similar debates about the dangers of deaconess life were heard in other Protestant denominations. Here too, defenders pointed to their deaconesses as 'Protestant-looking' nurses, contrasting them to Catholic nuns and noting that deaconesses did not take life-long vows.[22]

In England the deaconess movement was not as popular an option of religious life as Anglican sisterhoods, much to the dismay of many of the Anglican prelates and clergy who supported the deaconess institution as a potential replacement for the supposedly errant sisterhoods. Figures for religious sisters and deaconesses are bound to understate both cohorts but it is likely that for every Anglican deaconess 'set apart' there were ten Anglican sisters who were 'professed'. Approximately 4,000 women professed lifelong religious vows as Anglican sisters from 1845 to 1900 and only 431 Anglican deaconesses were set apart from 1860 to 1919.[23] Scholars have suggested that community life

---

18   Ludlow (1865), p. 301.
19   Mangion (2010).
20   Blackmore (2007), p. xxxiii.
21   Sewell (1873), p. 464.
22   "A Community of Deaconesses", Daily News (3/05/1869).
23   Blackmore (2007), Appendix 2; Allchin (1958), p. 120.

and religious vows were attractive to religious women who wanted a public and tangible commitment to a life of church service.[24]

As can be seen from Table 1, the *Church of England* had the greatest numbers of deaconess institutions, with 16 religious institutes by 1919. Other Protestant denominations, such as the Methodists, had four groups by 1901; the Lutherans and Baptists had one group each. A third grouping of evangelical Protestant deaconesses included communities such as the *Mildmay Deaconesses* and the *Evangelical Protestant Deaconesses' Institute and Training Hospital.* Both communities were open to evangelical members of any Protestant denomination.[25]

Within these communities of deaconesses there were some common features: they wore a form of religious dress and they were trained in a community (though once a deaconess, some remained in the community motherhouse whilst others lived in the parish). Deaconesses often promised to commit themselves for a fixed period of time, although for many women this was a lifelong vocation. Women could leave deaconess life as their personal circumstances dictated. Training included both theological as well as occupational training, although the length and extent of both varied from one deaconess community to another and over time.

Deaconess life in England frequently centred on parish work. This included pastoral work and a wide range of social care in the home, from providing nutritious meals to nursing the sick. Some communities took on the management of nursing in both voluntary and state hospitals. These hospital affiliations have helped in identifying some trends and patterns relating to deaconesses and their contribution to the medical marketplace. As can be seen from Table 2, six deaconess communities managed the nursing in 26 medical institutions over the course of the nineteenth century. The nursing in at least 14 of these institutions was managed by a deaconess matron and staffed by deaconess nurses, although the *Mildmay Hospitals* and probably the *Evangelical Protestant Deaconesses' Institute and Training Hospital* included nurse probationers and nurses who were not deaconesses. As will be discussed in the next section, the deaconess management of nursing in the majority of these institutions was short-lived. For example, *St Catherine's Convalescent Home,* managed by the *London Diocesan Deaconess Institution,* operated for only 11 years. By the end of the nineteenth century, the evangelical Protestant deaconesses had virtually disbanded and the Anglican deaconesses were only managing the nursing of *St Michael's Home* and possibly *All Saints. The Home* and the majority of the *Mildmay institutions,* however, were still in existence. This general shift away from institutional nursing work is important and reflects the ambiguous role of the deaconess and the complexities of the English medical marketplace. These complexities will be teased out in the following two case studies.

---

24 Mumm (1998), pp. 3–4, 33; Mangion (2010), p. 88.
25 See Footnote 8.

Table 1

DEACONESS INSTITUTIONS ESTABLISHED IN ENGLAND

DATE	DEACONESS INSTITUTE	TRAINING STRUCTURE	DENOMINATION
1860	Mildmay Deaconesses	Community	Evangelical Protestant
1861	London Diocesan Deaconess Institute	Community	Church of England
1865	Evangelical Protestant Deaconesses' Institute and Training Hospital	Community	Evangelical Protestant
1869	Ely Deaconess Home	Community	Church of England
1869	Chester Deaconess Institution	Community	Church of England
1874	Canterbury Church Deaconess Home	Parochial	Church of England
1875	Salisbury Diocesan Deaconess Institution	Parochial	Church of England
1879	Winchester Diocesan Deaconess Home	Community	Church of England
1880	East London Deaconess Institute	Community	Church of England
1882	St Andrew's Deaconess Home, Bath & Wells	Community	Church of England
1884	Llandaff Diocesan Deaconess Institution	Parochial	Church of England
1887	Durham Diocesan Mission House	Community	Church of England
1887	Rochester Diocesan Deaconess Institution	Parochial	Church of England
1887	Sisters of the People (Primitive Methodist)	Community	Methodist
1889	Lichfield Deaconess Institution	Parochial	Church of England
1890	Exeter Diocesan Deaconess Home	Parochial	Church of England
1890	Baptist Deaconesses	Community	Baptist
1890	Wesleyan Deaconesses (Sisters of the Children)	Community	Methodist
1891?	Liverpool Deaconess Association	Not known	Church of England
1891	United Methodist Free Church Deaconesses	Community	Methodist
1895	Primitive Church Deaconesses	Community	Methodist

Source: Blackmore, Appendix 1; Mangion (2010), p. 74.

Table 2

DEACONESS INSTITUTE	HOSPITAL	LOCATION	FOUNDATION DATE
Kaiserswerth/Darmstadt Deaconesses	German Hospital	Dalston, London	1842-1945
London Diocesan Deaconess Institute	Home Wards	Burton Crescent; Tavistock Crescent	1862-1882
London Diocesan Deaconess Institute	Great Northern Hospital	London	1863-1868
London Diocesan Deaconess Institute	St Catherine's Home	Finchley; Dorking; Redhill	1872-1883
London Diocesan Deaconess Institute	St Michael's Home	Westgate	1876-1973
London Diocesan Deaconess Institute	St Andrew's Cottage Convalescent Home	Deal, Kent	1890
London Diocesan Deaconess Institute	All Saints Convalescent Home for Children	Highgate	1888-1924
East London Deaconesses	Malvern Deaconess and Convalescent	Malvern	
Winchester Diocesan Deaconess Institute	Home of Comfort	Southsea	1896-1956
Evangelical Protestant Deaconesses' Institute and Training Hospital	Tottenham Hospital	Tottenham, London	1865-1898
Evangelical Protestant Deaconesses' Institute and Training Hospital	Cork Infirmary	Cork	
Evangelical Protestant Deaconesses' Institute and Training Hospital	Perth Infirmary	Perth	
Evangelical Protestant Deaconesses' Institute and Training Hospital	Sunderland Infirmary	Sunderland	
Evangelical Protestant Deaconesses' Institute and Training Hospital	Enfield Cottage Hospital	Enfield	
Evangelical Protestant Deaconesses' Institute and Training Hospital	Protestant Home for Incurables	Cork	
Evangelical Protestant Deaconesses' Institute and Training Hospital	Herbert Convalescent Home	Bournemouth	
Evangelical Protestant Deaconesses' Institute and Training Hospital	Doncaster General Infirmary	Doncaster	
Mildmay Deaconesses	Mildmay Cottage Hospital/ Memorial Hospital	Mildmay Road	1874-1978
Mildmay Deaconesses	Mildmay Invalid House		
Mildmay Deaconesses	Mildmay Mission Hospital	Shoreditch	1877-1948
Mildmay Deaconesses	Ossulston Convalescent Home	Ossulton, Barnet	
Mildmay Deaconesses	Enfield Cottage Hospital	Enfield	
Mildmay Deaconesses	General Infirmary	Doncaster	
Mildmay Deaconesses	Mildmay Home for Incurables	Torquay	
Mildmay Deaconesses	Medical missions	various	

DEACONESS NURSED MEDICAL INSTITUTIONS IN ENGLAND, 1846-1900

Source: Various sources

London Diocesan Deaconess Institution

The most well-documented of the Anglican deaconess communities is the *London Diocesan Deaconess Institution* founded by Elizabeth Ferard, the first Anglican deaconess to be 'set apart' in England. Ferard trained in Kaiserswerth and this experience was relevant to the development of her deaconess institution.[26] She maintained her relationship with Kaiserswerth by attending the 1865 *Kaiserswerth Conference* and, in 1863, other members of her London community interacted with "a highly gifted and thoroughly skilled deaconess" who was sent from Kaiserswerth to help temporarily in hospital work. The *Deaconess Institution's* chaplain from 1861–1868, Reverend Thomas Pelham-Dale (1821–1892) also visited Kaiserswerth and reflected that he gained much from his contact with Kaiserswerth founder Theodor Fliedner (1800–1864), pointing to the "inestimable advantage of personal communications with one whose experience of the working of Deaconesses' Institutions now extends over a period of thirty years".[27] Fliedner's Kaiserswerth was a model extolled and utilised by other nascent deaconess communities. The Chester deaconesses, founded in 1869 under Sarah Emma Aldred or Minna FitzMaurice, began with the help of two deaconesses trained in Kaiserswerth and Strasbourg. Early nursing promoters Elizabeth Fry, Florence Nightingale (1820–1910), Agnes Jones (1832–1868) and Florence Lees (1840–1922) visited or trained in Kaiserswerth, seeing it as an archetypal training ground for women's nursing and ministerial work.[28] What these interactions reflect is the significance of Kaiserswerth as a hub to a transnational deaconess movement. It was a centre of knowledge and ideas that were transferred across national boundaries.[29] This English example shows the networks of common interests, and the shared objectives of a form of women's ministerial work. The physical movement of deaconesses, to and from Kaiserswerth, was vital to this knowledge exchange.

The link to Kaiserswerth was frequently lauded in published reports but, significantly, its influence was anglicised. The author of the 1868 annual report reminded readers that the institute was "founded upon the model of Kaiserswerth, and adapted to the Church of England".[30] This reference to adaptation was imperative to asserting an English identity; an identity that was connected (at least for these commentators) to the state church. Essayists frequently acknowledged that deaconess life, though associated with Kaiserswerth, was reconceived to reflect English ways and values. These attributes were rarely articulated, but what was apposite was that their religious principles were linked to the national church, the *Church of England*. Notably, ref-

---

26 It was originally called the *North London Deaconess Institution* until 1869, when it was renamed in an effort to link it to its diocesan imprimatur. In 1943, it was renamed the Deaconess Community of St Andrew. For more on Ferard see Blackmore (2007), pp. xvi–xvii.

27 Community of St Andrew (henceforth CSA): Annual Report, 1863, p. 8.

28 Bancroft (1889), pp. 146–147; Lees (1874), p. xvi.

29 Iriye (2004), p. 213; Clavin (2005), p. 422.

30 CSA: Annual Report, 1868, p. 5.

erences to and interactions with Kaiserswerth seem to dissipate, particularly after Ferard retired in the 1870s, reflecting perhaps a new generation of leadership's confidence in steering the *London Diocesan Deaconess Institution*.

Institutional nursing

The objective of the *London Diocesan Deaconess Institution* was prominently noted on the front of each annual report from 1863: its purpose was "promoting organised women's work". A few years later the additional aim of "the renewal of the ancient and primitive Order of Deaconesses" was added.[31] Nursing was always considered a component of this 'women's work' and was considered integral to this religious ministry: Ferard advocated that deaconess nursing ought to be directed towards "the Glory of God in the salvation of souls".[32] Perhaps because of her experience at Kaiserswerth, Ferard valued hospital nurse training.[33] The 1863 annual report indicated that "the Sisters should become sufficiently experienced in nursing to take charge of the sick, either in hospitals or in their own homes".[34] That year, she contacted the *Great Northern Hospital's Medical Committee*,[35] suggesting that the London deaconesses manage the nursing of the then 25-bed hospital.[36] They committed two deaconesses, who worked free of charge, and managed the paid nursing staff.[37] This was an important training ground for probationer deaconesses. Medical care of the body was also taken seriously: deaconesses were expected to apply "the utmost diligence for their [patients'] bodily welfare and restoration of health".[38] The work must have been challenging – the hospital was located in a poor neighbourhood where, according to one commentator, "helpless creatures from all quarters in every stage of disease are being carefully and skilfully nursed by the noble-minded ladies". By 1865, they were nursing over 1,100 patients weekly, both on the wards and as outpatients.[39] But their

31 CSA: Annual Report, 1863, cover on this and subsequent annual reports. Annual Report, 1865, p. 5.
32 CSA: Ferard, "Directions for Sisters Nursing in Hospitals".
33 Blackmore (2007), pp. 3–37. Ferard's diary documenting her time in Kaiserswerth is also included in this volume.
34 CSA: Annual Report, 1863, p. 6.
35 The *Great Northern Hospital* was founded in 1856 by Dr Sherard Freeman Statham at 11 York Road (renamed York Way). The hospital relocated several times until it was rebuilt in Holloway Road in 1888 with 68 beds and renamed the *Great Northern Central Hospital*.
36 London Metropolitan Archives (henceforth LMA): Great Northern 1869 Annual Report, p. 8. This and future mentions of the 'London deaconesses' will refer to deaconesses belonging to the *London Diocesan Deaconess Institution*.
37 LMA: H33/RN/A2/1 Great Northen [sic] Hospital Minute Book Medical Committee, Vol I, Minutes dated 13/03/1863.
38 CSA: "Directions for Sisters Nursing in Hospitals", p. 1.
39 LMA: H33 RN/Y11/1 "Cuttings Book, 1860–1872": "The Great Northern Hospital" To the Editor by Frederick Bincks, Secretary, no journal name, no date, p. 143; "A Cry from North London" by George Reid, Standard (09/12/1865).

time at the *Northern Hospital* was short-lived. In 1868, the deaconesses left the hospital, forced out, it appears, by a disagreement between Ferard and the chaplain, Pelham-Dale (who was also on the hospital management committee), over the community structure of the deaconess institution – something that, at the time, Pelham-Dale was deeply opposed to.[40]

The second institutional setting for deaconess training was the *Home Wards*, opened in the deaconess motherhouse on Burton Crescent under the medical superintendence of Dr Webb as Honorary Physician.[41] The 1863 annual report noted:

> The small hospital, if only it can be maintained, will prove of great advantage. First, as a refuge for the patients themselves; being especially intended for those who have seen better days. Cases are considered eligible in exact proportion to the nursing they require, and that which often prevents admission to the general hospital – that the case is quite hopeless – is here not considered an objection.[42]

This deaconess-managed institution nursed 'hopeless' patients, including those in the last stages of cancer and tuberculosis. These patients fell outside the remit of the voluntary hospitals.[43] Voluntary hospitals were competitive institutions; their reliance on benefactors and donors meant that their efficiency, the economising of the process of diagnosis and treatment, was an important factor to their success.[44] 'Hopeless' patients were detrimental to this rationalising process. First, chronically ill patients who needed long-term care took up valuable resources of time, space and nursing. Second, dying patients were not seen as a success. Hospital statistics publicised the numbers 'cured' in the hospital; high death rates were a sign of failure. By offering their nursing services to this cohort of patients, the deaconesses were not competing directly with voluntary hospitals.

The deaconesses also accepted into the *Home Wards* a 'better class' of patient, such as nursery governesses, reduced gentlewomen, upper servants or wives of artisans.[45] These persons were seen as "above those who are admitted into public hospital" who "shrink from entering large hospitals and cannot afford to hire a nurse".[46] The *Winchester Diocesan Deaconess Home*, an offshoot of the London deaconesses, managed by Deaconess Emma Mallet Day, operated a similar entity. The *Home of Comfort in Southsea* was also meant for a 'better class' of patient: patients "who are unable to provide for themselves the necessary comforts during a long and expensive illness. Hospitals are not

---

40 LMA: Great Northern Annual Report, p. 8. Pelham-Dale had joined the hospital committee in 1863. Dale also resigned as chaplain of the *London Diocesan Deaconess Institution*.
41 CSA: Annual Report, 1863, pp. 6–7.
42 CSA: Annual Report, 1863, p. 7.
43 CSA: Annual Report, 1864, p. 7; Annual Report, 1865, p. 7. See also Mangion (2013), pp. 239–262. One article noting the value of the work of the *Home Wards* indicated there were few institutions willing to "receive a poor person only to die!". Clarke, 1872, p. 54.
44 Granshaw (1992), p. 212.
45 CSA: Annual Report, 1863, p. 6; Annual Report, 1865, p. 8.
46 CSA: Annual Report, 1865, p. 8; Annual Report, 1869, p. 7; Annual Report, 1872, p. 7.

available for cases where treatment can only alleviate not cure".[47] These institutions purposefully met the needs of a patient cohort outside the remit of the voluntary hospital. There were practical reasons for this. Voluntary hospitals, being charitable institutions, were intended for the respectable but poor working classes. The more well-to-do had medical care in their homes. Those in between these two social classes had fewer options. Not all members of the middle classes could afford private nursing care in their homes. In this way the deaconess institution did not compete with the voluntary hospitals. Importantly, this was fulfilling an unmet need in the medical marketplace. Financially too, there would be advantages: this class of patient was more likely to pay fees or offer small donations.

When the motherhouse moved to larger premises at 12, Tavistock Crescent in Westbourne Park in 1873, the *Home Wards* moved also. A letter in *The Times* framed as a plea for potential benefactors complained that nursing was "most seriously impeded by the inadequate accommodation". There was room for ten patients in four rooms but they were hoping to build spacious wards, a dispensary and a chapel.[48] The funding for this never materialized. By 1882, the Home Wards were closed down "as funds were insufficient to maintain so costly a work".[49] Sarah Flew's research on the financing of Anglican home missionary associations argues convincingly that the committed cohort of benefactors that were funding institutions such as Ferard's deaconesses were dying out, and not being replaced.[50] Her analysis of the annualised revenues of the London deaconesses from 1861 to 1914 point to a "high degree of steadiness" but also reveal that dwindling subscriptions and donations were offset by increased donations from the deaconesses and the parishes themselves.[51]

Nurse training was an important component of the deaconesses' education. The *Home Wards* were meant to be a centre of training for deaconesses. In 1875, the Honorary Physician of the *Home Wards*, Mr H. Cripps Lawrence gave a six-month course of lectures on nursing and this was a practice continued by later honorary medical practitioners.[52] Honorary Physician Mr Edmund Owen ran an "admirable school for the training of Probationers in

---

47 Portsmouth History Centre: CHU 1/90/3/1/4, Winchester Diocesan Deaconess Home, Portsmouth Annual Report, 1898, p. 9. From White, (2011), Appendix A, we learn that Day was trained at the London Diocesan Deaconess Institution. She was set apart on 3 December 1874 and was Head Deaconess of the Winchester Diocesan Deaconess Home in 1876.

48 Day (1873), p. 12.

49 CSA: Ancilla Domini, 03/1887, p. 3; Finance Committee Notes 1881–1942, 03/11/1881, 01/12/1881, 13/01/1882, and finally on 9/02/1882 honorary medical staff told of impending closure.

50 Flew (2014).

51 Flew (2013), pp. 438–439.

52 CSA: Annual Report, 1875, p. 7; Inner Council minutes, 6/10/1875. Mr Lawrence's suggestions for nursing lectures were approved; subsequent minutes note additional approval for nursing lectures.

surgical nursing".[53] Dr Friend gave a course of Ambulance Lectures in the winter of 1888.[54] After the closing of the *Home Wards*, probationers obtained nurse training in voluntary hospitals. One probationer deaconess, writing in *Ancilla Domini* in 1889, observed that her three months of nursing experience in a 144-bed hospital in a country town "was especially valuable, as the nurses did what is usually done by the medical students in a larger hospital". She took temperatures, prepared dressings and attended to wounds in both the men's and women's wards. In the children's ward she treated a child who had been badly scalded and another who had hip disease and she dressed children's wounds daily.[55] Other deaconess probationers were trained in *St Mary's Hospital* in the surgical as well as the casualty ward, where "one gains great and varied experience".[56] Some deaconesses trained for six months at the *Liverpool Workhouse Infirmary* and *Reading County Hospital.*[57]

Ferard's intention in both the *Northern Hospital* and the *Home Wards* was to provide deaconesses with the 'practical nursing' skills needed in their work as parish visitors. By the 1890s, nurse training had evolved in many London hospitals into a three-year training programme.[58] Deaconess nurse training did not provide the education meant for a professional hospital nurse; often deaconess nurses were 'paying probationers' and received an abbreviated course of training of six months, rather than the full three years. One probationer nurse deaconess commented to this effect that "although in our special work as Deaconesses, we have very little time for much actual nursing, we are often glad to be able to give a few hints about it, and then we find the value of this practical experience gained in the hospital".[59] Though the work of a parish deaconess involved visiting members of the parish and tending to their spiritual and corporal needs, nursing care according to this probationer was limited to 'practical nursing'. It seems the deaconesses were not involved in long-term home nursing in their role as parish deaconesses.

Convalescent care

Institutional nursing care continued as a part of the London deaconesses' concern, but within convalescent institutions. There is less archival evidence for three of the four convalescent homes managed by the deaconesses, perhaps because the first three developed in an ad hoc manner, unlike the targeted development of the sought-after work at the *Great Northern Hospital* and the *Home Wards*. The first of these convalescent homes was opened by Elizabeth Ferard. After she resigned as head deaconesses in 1874, she moved to Finch-

53 CSA: Annual Report, 1872, pp. 7–8.
54 CSA: Annual Report, 1888, p. 77.
55 CSA: Ancilla Domini, 10/1889, pp. 141–142.
56 CSA: Ancilla Domini, 04/1900, p. 29.
57 CSA: Finance Committee Notes 1881–1942, 04/04/1884 and 08/05/1885.
58 Hawkins, p. 105.
59 CSA: Ancilla Domini, 10/1889, p. 142.

ley, where she opened *St Catherine's Home* as a summer convalescent / holiday home catering to small groups of children in poor health. Each year, forty children returned home 'strengthened and improved, both in mind and body, by the fresh country air, good food and watchful care there bestowed upon them'.[60] Ferard personally financed the home and managed it along with one or two deaconesses; it also operated as a training centre for deaconesses.[61] When she moved to Dorking in 1874, and then to Redhill in 1878, the convalescent home relocated also. When Ferard died in 1883, the home was closed down. The second convalescent home, opened in 1888 by Miss Boys in Deal, was *St Andrew's Convalescent Home* for new mothers and their babies. It was managed by one of the deaconesses and housed six to seven convalescent mothers and their infants during the summer months.[62] During the fifteen weeks of the first year, thirty women and six infants convalesced there. It was thought that the 'bracing air' at Deal along with wholesome food, including locally donated fruit, vegetables, fowls, cakes and eggs, put "vigour into the hearts and bodies of the convalescent".[63] It is likely this was the only year of operation, as no further mention was made of it in the London deaconesses' house publication, *Ancilla Domini*. The third short-lived (for the deaconesses) nursing venture was the *All Saints Convalescent Home for Children* on Talbot Road in Highgate. This home had been opened by the vicar of All Saints in 1880, and by 1884 had been extended over the schoolrooms.[64] In 1888, two deaconesses were assigned to All Saints as parish workers but also with responsibility for the *Convalescent Home*.[65] The last reports on this home are dated January 1891; it seems likely the deaconesses left this work, although the convalescent home did not close until 1924.[66]

The most long-lived convalescent home under deaconess management was *St Michael's Convalescent Home* in Westgate-on-Sea. It opened to female convalescents in 1876 and in 1882, after renting the three-story villa next door, accepted male convalescents.[67] The earliest figures indicate that in 1884 ninety men and 125 women convalesced at *St Michael's*.[68] Convalescents could stay for four weeks. Some patients were repeat convalescents, coming year after year, whilst others came for only one year.[69] Unfortunately, patient records are not extant and annual reports tell us more about who was not a patient. Convalescents excluded the chronically ill, those that required specific medical treatment, those in the latter stages of pulmonary consumption, those with

---

60 CSA: Annual Report, 1872, pp. 7–8; Annual Report, 1875, p. 8.
61 CSA: Annual Report, 1883, p. 10.
62 CSA: Ancilla Domini, 05/1888, p. 63.
63 CSA: Ancilla Domini, 10/1888, p. 78.
64 The convalescent home occupied the upper floor of the mission house from 1880 and was extended over the schoolrooms in 1884. Baggs et al. (1980), pp. 172–182.
65 CSA: Ancilla Domini, 01/1889, p. 89.
66 CSA: Ancilla Domini, 01/1891, p. 209.
67 CSA: Ancilla Domini, 11/1888, pp. 73–74.
68 CSA: S. Michael's Home for Men and Women, 1885 [no page numbers].
69 CSA: Annual Report, 1878, p. 10.

ulcers and abscesses with discharges or with any type of infectious or contagious disease. In addition, helpless persons or those of unsound mind were excluded.[70] Like other convalescent hospitals, this institution was intended for those who had been in hospital care, and needed extra time to recuperate. Importantly, the type of care needed did not seem to necessitate expensive medical technology. Patients included schoolmistresses and pupil teachers[71] as well as domestic servants, although by the end of the nineteenth century, *St Michael's* catered mostly to those of the artisan classes.[72] In 1884, the London deaconesses considered the development of a special local committee which would be responsible for fundraising[73] and three years later the 1887 annual report announced this committee was in place and that *St Michael's* was no longer a financial 'burden' to the deaconesses. This suggests they were finding it difficult funding such a large institution. The local committee followed the model of the subscriber-funded voluntary hospital, where subscribers were given tickets to distribute to potential patients. The local committee was eager to construct a custom-built convalescent home, and was successful in funding this expansion. In 1900, when the new building opened, it accommodated 91 men and 122 women.[74] The deaconess community retained legal possession of the convalescent home, with two deaconesses responsible for the nursing and day-to-day management. The local committee remained an important partner and secured the operation of the convalescent home, which remained in existence until 1973.[75]

So what can we learn about the institutional nursing work of the *London Diocesan Deaconess Institution*? The management of nursing at the *Great Northern Hospital* and the development of the *Home Wards* were a means of ministering to body and soul as well as a vehicle for training deaconesses for parish work. After these institutions closed down, deaconesses were trained as paying probationers in the nurse training schools in voluntary hospitals. Their training was structured to meet the ailments they would tend to as parish deaconesses. The institutions managed by the London deaconesses addressed the needs of patients outside the traditional cohort of voluntary hospitals. They attended to 'hopeless' cases and a 'better class' of patient. They avoided competing directly with voluntary hospitals but, despite this differentiation, they were unable to generate enough funding to operate these institutions. Their reliance on a charitable model tied to an individual funder was not effective. *St Michael's Convalescent Home* was the exception; but it followed more closely the subscriber model used by most voluntary hospitals in the 1890s, where finances were managed by a committee.[76]

70   CSA: Annual Report, 1887, p. 9.
71   CSA: S. Michael's Home for Men and Women, 1885 [no page numbers].
72   CSA: S. Michael's Home for Men and Women, 1894, p. 2.
73   CSA: Finance Committee Notes 1881–1942, 04/04/1884.
74   CSA: S. Michael's Home for Men and Women, 1894, p. 7.
75   White (2011), p. 172. *Charing Healthcare* is now operating *St Michaels Nursing Home* in these buildings.
76   Morris (1990), pp. 412–413. Waddington (2000), pp. 141–143.

The next case study examines another facet of deaconess involvement in the medical marketplace. It identifies the changing role of the deaconess nurse in hospital management, pointing to the influence of gender in the medical marketplace.

Evangelical Protestant deaconesses

Medical man and German-born Jewish convert to Christianity Michael Maximilian August Heinrich Laseron (1819–1894) and his wife, Clara von Porchwitz Rolls, were not dissimilar to numerous other founders of voluntary hospitals in nineteenth-century England.[77] Their personal experience, in their case the death of their first child Hannah in 1855 and their religious faith, provided the impetus for their philanthropy. They sought to meet the needs of the poor in and around Tottenham, north-east London, where they lived.[78] They organised several charitable ventures, including a ragged school for boys and girls, an orphan home for girls, Sunday schools and soup kitchens.[79] In 1865, they responded to the many requests for nursing care by setting aside two rooms in the *Girls' Orphanage* as hospital wards for six patients. This proved to be an unconducive recuperative environment, so Laseron rented a former chapel and schoolroom in nearby Snell's Park, Upper Edmonton, and created an infirmary with twelve beds.[80] Laseron's dream of a free hospital became more tangible with the donation of £6,000 from a wealthy nonconformist patient, John Morley (1807–1896), a woollen manufacturer. Morley's brother Samuel, Liberal Member of Parliament for Nottingham, also invested in the venture.[81] This led to the opening of the *Evangelical Protestant Deaconesses' Institution and Training Hospital* on the south-east side of Tottenham Green in 1868. At its inauguration in 1869, the fifty-bed hospital contained two large wards for men and women and a smaller ward for children.[82] It was expanded in 1881 and again in 1887 to contain 100 beds. By 1895, patient numbers were reported at 559 inpatients and 9,834 outpatients.[83]

The Laserons' evangelical faith was intricately linked to their philanthropy. Kaiserswerth-trained deaconess Libussa von Schmeling began working in the orphanage sometime after its opening in 1855 and perhaps encouraged Laseron's interest in deaconesses. Laseron travelled to Berlin in 1867 to the *Betha-*

---

77 "Evangelical Protestant Deaconesses' Institution and Training Hospital", The Christian: A weekly record of Christian life, Christian testimony and Christian work (1870), p. 373. For more on the development of voluntary hospitals see Granshaw (1992), p. 201.

78 Haringey Archives Service (henceforth: HAS): Michael Laseron, A Narrative of the Origin and Progress of the Girls' Industrial Orphan Home, and the Evangelical Protestant Deaconesses' Institution and Training Hospital (1875), pp. 1–2.

79 "Community of Deaconesses", Liverpool Mercury (04/05/1869).

80 HAS: Laseron, A Narrative, pp. 32–33.

81 Fisk (1923), pp. 188–189.

82 "Community of Deaconesses", Liverpool Mercury (04/05/1869).

83 "The Tottenham Deaconess Institution", Daily Mail (17/07/1896).

nien Haus, which had been founded by Theodor Fliedner, and returned to London with a deaconess to train three aspiring nurses, probably older girls from the *Home for Girls*.[84] The hospital was acknowledged as being modelled upon the principles of Kaiserswerth.[85] During the 1887 opening of the hospital extension, several significant deaconess personages were present, including Theodor Fliedner with two pastors and three deaconesses from Berlin and Copenhagen.[86] But hereafter, just as in the example of the *London Diocesan Deaconess Institution*, evidence of regular (or even irregular) contact with Kaiserswerth disappears.

From the beginning, the role of the deaconess was important for the religious ethos of the hospital, the medicalised nursing care and the management of the hospital. Deaconess von Schmeling, noted for her "very likeable German notions of home-comfort" became the first Lady Superintendent of the hospital from 1868 to 1873.[87] Scottish-born Elizabeth C. Dundas (known as Christian or Christiane) began nursing at the hospital in 1872, and when von Schmeling left for health reasons in July 1873, Dundas replaced her.[88] The deaconesses were represented as 'medical missionaries' fulfilling "a need of higher Christian influences at the bedside"[89] with a mission of healing a man's wounds and relieving his sufferings' in order to find 'ready access to his heart'.[90] Deaconess recruits were plentiful in the early years. Candidates were required to bring a pastor's recommendation and hold 'evangelical principles'. Denominationally speaking, they were likely to be nonconformists or Low Church Anglicans. In the early years, deaconesses were trained for one year (extended to two years in 1894) and then 'set apart'. Although they did not take vows, deaconesses were asked to promise to remain for five years after their initial formation.[91] Even so, not all deaconesses stayed the course and not all probationers completed their training. The year 1887 included an unusually large number of departures. Two deaconesses left "on account of error, having imbibed views contrary to the fundamental principles of our Institution" (one suspects either high Anglican or Roman Catholic beliefs); another two were asked to leave because of "grave faults which could not be overlooked". But also, more typically, there were two deaconesses and two probationers who left for family reasons and another three probationers and two

84 HAS: Laseron, A Narrative, p. 37. Libussa von Schmeling remains a bit of a mystery. Her name does not appear in the Kaiserswerth or Bethanienhaus archives. I am grateful to Annet Buettner, Sabine Langenfaß and Helga Rosemann for responding to my email queries about von Schmeling.

85 "Community of Deaconesses", Liverpool Mercury (04/05/1869).

86 This would likely be Theodor Fliedner's son Fritz Fliedner (1845–1901). After Fliedner's death, Kaiserswerth was managed by the husband of Louise Fliedner (Theodor Fliedner's daughter), Julius Disselhoff (1827–1896).

87 "Community of Deaconesses", Liverpool Mercury (04/05/1869).

88 Fisk (1923), p. 191.

89 HAS: Christopher Crayon, "The Protestant Deaconesses" (25/05/1872).

90 "The Tottenham Deaconess Institution and Hospital", Daily News (08/10/894).

91 "A Community of Deaconesses", Liverpool Mercury (04/05/1869).

deaconesses whose health did not stand up to such physically demanding work.[92] Despite these departures, on 6 July 1887, eight women were 'set apart' in the presence of Laseron and a nonconformist minister and joined the ranks of the Tottenham evangelical deaconesses. By 1894, there were 74 deaconesses, 46 of whom were in Tottenham; the remainder nursed in one of 14 outstations.[93] There were seven deaconesses at the Sunderland Infirmary, five in the *South Dublin Union Infirmary* and the remainder in ones and twos at district posts, convalescent homes and small hospitals.[94] Some deaconesses nursed in the Franco-Prussian War and the Turco-Servian campaigns and were awarded the German Grand Cross of Merit in 1870 and the Tuscova Order of Service in 1876.[95]

Laseron's death in 1894 uncovered a financial crisis that had probably been festering for years. He had been an adept fundraiser; the hospital had prominent supporters, and received visits from the Prince and Princess of Wales (later King Edward VII and Queen Alexandra) in 1887, and again in 1894.[96] But his ill health in later years slowed his fundraising exertions and hospital costs were increasing. By 1898, the hospital had a debt of £2,500 and reduced expenditures by leaving fifty hospital beds unoccupied. The hospital's *Medical Council* applied to the *Charity Commission* for financial aid, but was refused because the hospital management was not placed in the hands of the subscribers. The model of the voluntary hospital with a management committee and medical council and subscriber-based funding had become the expected form of hospital management.[97] The old model of charismatic founder benefactor, as this case reveals, became a liability on the death or illness of the founder.

There is little documentation on nurse training in extant records. One source deriving from the *Royal College of Nurses* indicates that by 1890, deaconess nurses were trained on a two-year course which included bandaging, anatomy and physiology along with some surgery.[98] The nursing work on the ward required specialist nursing knowledge. Acute care was a regular feature of the hospital case load; by 1877, 20–25 per cent of the inpatients were accident victims. By this time, the hospital had already begun using antiseptics in the surgical treatment of wounds, and wards were washed daily with diluted carbolic acid.[99] Nurse training appears to have been done on the wards and through lectures by medical men. Despite this evidence of nurse training, it

92   "The Prince and Princess of Wales at Tottenham", Herald (28/05/1887).
93   "The Tottenham Deaconess Institution and Hospital", Daily News (08/101894). Fisk (1923), p. 189.
94   Baggs et al. (1976), pp. 345–348.
95   HAS: PW 6/6, p. 1. The Franco-Prussian War was fought in 1870–1871. The Turco-Servian War was fought between the Ottoman Empire and the Principality of Serbia in 1876–1877.
96   Fisk (1923), p. 193.
97   Morris (1990), pp. 412–413.
98   HAS: PW 6/9, undated typescript, "Information from Royal College of Nursing Records". I was unable to find the source of these notes in the *Royal College of Nursing*.
99   Watkin (1967), p. 14.

was not considered adequate by the *Medical Council*. By the 1890s, systematic training, examinations and nursing certificates were the norm in major London hospitals. A report on nursing at the hospital from the *Medical Council*, dated 1896, suggested a restructure which prioritised professionalising the nursing staff and required a Superintendent of Nurses with 'full hospital training'.[100] Once implemented, this effectively removed the nursing staff out of Dundas's control.

Michael Laseron managed this hospital as Director, but Deaconess Dundas had a noteworthy amount of input as Laseron's "co-labourer, a sister in Christ". These were words he used in describing the kind of partnership he was looking for in the 1860s.[101] In 1869, one press article declared that "the director and lady superintendent are to be regarded as the legitimate heads of the establishment".[102] Deaconess Dundas was considered a woman of great piety, but also one with great administrative ability and a 'forceful personality'.[103] Annual reports included a list of trustees as well as a *Medical Council* but one wonders how much decision-making responsibility they had; it appears the hospital was managed by Laseron as Director and Dundas as Lady Superintendent.

With the death of Laseron, Dundas's management role became redundant. The *Medical Council* restructured the management of the hospital, with guidance from the *Charity Commission*, into a management committee of 21 members which included subscribers, donors and representatives of the medical committee.[104] Notably, there was no hospital management role for the Lady Superintendent of the Hospital, Deaconess Mary A. Apted, or Deaconess Dundas as Superintendent of the Institute.[105] The new position created by the restructure was more narrowly defined as the 'Superintendent of Nurses', whose responsibilities only pertained to the nursing staff. The joint management of the hospital intended by Laseron was a thing of the past. The Superintendent of Nurses was selected by the newly constituted *Hospital Council* and *Medical Committee*. She reported to the *Medical Council* and *Medical Committee* rather than to the Director. Many of her decisions regarding nursing, including the hiring of ward nurses and courses of lectures, were confirmed or determined by the *Medical Committee*.[106] Dundas was retained, as Lady Superintendent of Deaconesses, but in a reduced capacity and with little influence over

100 HAS: PW8/3 "Report of the Medical Council (as revised by the sub-committee) on the Nursing Department", 28/01/1896, p. 1. "Full hospital training" is nowhere described in the report, but it was three years of training.

101 HAS: Laseron, A Narrative, p. 16.

102 "Community of Deaconesses", Liverpool Mercury (04/05/1869).

103 HAS: PW6/3 "An Outline of the History of the Prince of Wales General Hospital", undated typescript, p. 1. She had a separate income and census records indicate that she came from a well-to-do family in Edinburgh with servants.

104 Watkin (1967), p. 24.

105 Mary Apted was listed as Superintendent of the Hospital in the 1891 census.

106 HAS: PW8/3 "Report of the Medical Council (as revised by the sub-committee) on the Nursing Department", 28/01/1896, p. 2.

the nurses or the running of the hospital. This new structure gave much more decision-making power to the *Medical Council*, and particularly the *Medical Committee*, and met with the Charity Commissioner's approval. In 1899 the evangelical deaconesses "surrendered control to a committee" and the institution was renamed *Tottenham Hospital*.[107] This restructure was not welcomed by all; resident historian of Tottenham, Fred Fisk, notes that the new scheme "estranged many ardent workers of the original institution". He then commented that the new structure was "managed by a committee appointed by the subscribers, thus taking the control from the 'sisters'".[108]

Deaconess Dundas, in her description of these events, intimated that the *Medical Council* did not understand the religious ethos of the work. Though the new hospital was "conducted on Christian lines", she observed "it has lost the special aroma of a voluntary Christian work."[109] The religious ethos remained to some extent; members of the nursing staff were required to be "in sympathy with the religious principles of the Institution, as incorporated in the 'Deed of Trust' and if possible, should be willing to become a deaconess.[110] Dundas opined that the new nursing was

> to have paid certificated nurses like other hospitals, – and to give no promise of mainte-
> nance in illness or old age. The management therefore fell out of the hands of the Dea-
> conesses, who had to scatter and find their way elsewhere.[111]

Dundas and some of the more senior deaconesses left the hospital entirely in 1897.[112] Many of the Sunderland deaconesses and those in some of the other outstations became paid nurses and severed their relationship with the deaconess institution.[113] Deaconess Stella Arthur left for the *York Union*, Daisy Button and Maud Chambers went to the *Dublin Union*.[114] Some deaconesses remained at *Tottenham Hospital*, though several left after a few years. Deaconesses Nellie Cleary and Lily Kean felt the call of the missions and left for South Africa in 1902. Others like deaconess Frances eventually left, being "unable to agree with [the] Head Sister".[115] The elderly deaconesses were maintained by the hospital. One anonymously written typescript recorded that

> Their presence lent something of an old world atmosphere to the hospital, serving to
> remind the twentieth century student nurse, coping with the General Nursing Council
> curriculum [sic] and preparing for State Examinations, of the pioneer work of two genera-
> tions ago.[116]

107 Baggs et al. (1976), pp. 345–348.
108 Fisk (1923), p. 192.
109 Fisk (1923), p. 190.
110 HAS: PW8/3 "Report of the Medical Council (as revised by the sub-committee) on the
     Nursing Department", 28/01/1896, p. 1.
111 Fisk (1923), p. 190.
112 HAS: PW8/52 Nursing staff records.
113 HAS: PW8/52 Nursing staff records. Fisk (1923), p. 190.
114 HAS: PW8/52 Nursing staff records.
115 HAS: PW1/1–95 Photographs.
116 HAS: PW6/8, typescript account of the history of the Tottenham Hospital, p. 2.

The deaconess tradition did not disappear entirely. Deaconess E. Margaret Fox, who nursed at the *Evangelical Protestant Deaconesses' Institute and Training Hospital* from 1889–1893, left to train at *Guy's Hospital* in 1893. She returned to *Tottenham Hospital* as the Superintendent of Nurses in 1899, a post she held until 1915.[117] She was replaced by Theodora Bickerton, who was also a deaconess and was matron from 1915–1934.[118]

The conclusions derived from this case study reflect the primacy of the model of the voluntary hospital. Maintaining the funding of a growing hospital became difficult at a time of increasing technological developments, as costs rose and individual funders of such institutions disappeared. As the *Evangelical Protestant Deaconess Institute and Training Hospital* transitioned to the more secular model of the medical marketplace, the management and medical committee, gendered male, gained more power and authority as the role of the Superintendent of Nurses was made redundant and the deaconess nurses were marginalised. The professionalisation of nursing, with a more rigorous nurse training regime that led to 'certificated' nurses, became an important marker of the professional and secular space of the hospital. The religious ethos of the hospital was also diminished by the effective removal of the deaconess nurses as well as the name change to *Tottenham Hospital.*

Conclusion

By the end of the nineteenth century, nursing by religious communities of women, including deaconess institutions, was regarded with a degree of reservation.[119] The assumption that religious nurses prioritised care for the soul over care for the body was embedded in cultural understanding. The adequacy of the medical training of such religious nurses was being questioned. Both case studies reflect a tension between the religious underpinnings of the role of the deaconess and the professionalisation of nursing. In the Anglican example, the London deaconesses refocused on their ministerial role as deaconesses once they left institutional nursing. As parish deaconesses or even as nurses in convalescent homes in the nineteenth century, they could use their practical knowledge of nursing as a means of healing the body while ministering to the soul. In the second case study, the evangelical Protestant deaconesses were edged out of their nursing roles in *Tottenham Hospital* when the charitable model of medical care was replaced by the secular model of the voluntary hospital that expected a professional nursing body. The growing complexities of the medical marketplace were significant to both case studies. The voluntary hospital was becoming a more secularised place where medical science and professionalised 'charity' reigned.

---

117 "Appointments", The British Journal of Nursing (13/05/1916), p. 422.
118 Watkin (1967), pp. 34–35; HAS: PW1/1–95 Photographs.
119 Bashford (1998), pp. 48–53.

Bibliography

Allchin, A. M.: The silent rebellion. Anglican religious communities 1845–1900. London 1958.
Baggs, A. P.; Bolton, Diane K.; Scarff, Eileen; Tyack, G. C.: Tottenham. Public services. In: Baker, T. F. T.; Pugh, R. B. (ed.): A history of the county of Middlesex, Volume 5: Hendon, Kingsbury, Great Stanmore, Little Stanmore, Edmonton Enfield, Monken Hadley, South Mimms, Tottenham. London 1976, pp. 345–348. British history online. Web. 4/3/2015. http://www.british-history.ac.uk/vch/middx/vol5/pp345-348
Baggs, A. P.; Bolton, Diane K.; Hicks, M. A.; Pugh, R. B. (ed.): Hornsey, including Highgate: Churches. In: Baker, T. F. T.; Erlington, C. R. (ed.): A history of the county of Middlesex, Volume 6: Friern Barnet, Finchley, Hornsey with Highgate. London 1980, pp. 172–182. British history online. Web. 5/3/2015. http://www.british-history.ac.uk/report.aspx?compid =22527
Bancroft, Jane E.: Deaconesses in Europe and their lessons for America. New York 1889.
Bashford, Alison: Purity and pollution. Gender, embodiment and Victorian medicine. Houndsmills; Basingstoke 1998.
Bebbington, David: Evangelicalism in modern Britain. London 1989.
Blackmore, Henrietta (ed.): The beginning of women's ministry. The revival of the deaconesses in the 19th-century church of England. Woodbridge 2007.
Blackmore, Henrietta: Autonomous mission and ecclesiastical authority. The revival of the deaconess order in the church of England, 1850–1900. Diss University of Oxford, 2004.
Brown, Callum G.: The death of Christian Britain. Understanding secularisation, 1800–2000. London; New York 2001.
Clarke, W. Fairlie: The medical charities of London. In: Golden hours. A monthly magazine for family and general reading (January 1872), pp. 51–57.
Clavin, Patricia: Defining transnationalism. In: Contemporary European History 14 (2005), pp. 421–439.
Daggers, Jenny: The Victorian female civilising mission and women's aspirations towards priesthood in the Church of England. In: Women's History Review 10 (2001), pp. 651–670.
Day, Elsie: The London diocesan deaconesses. In: The Times (21 February 1873), p. 12.
Ducrocq, Francoise: The London biblewomen and nurses mission, 1857–1880. Class relations / women's relations. In: Harris, Barbara J.; McNamara, Jo Ann K. (ed.): Women and the structure of society. Selected research from the fifth Berkshire conference on the history of women. Durham; N. C. 1984, pp. 98–107.
Fisk, Fred: The history of the ancient parish of Tottenham. Tottenham 1923.
Flew, Sarah: Money Matters. The neglect of finance in the historiography of modern Christianity. In: Clarke, Peter D.; Methuen, Charlotte (ed.): The church on its past. Woodbridge 2013, pp. 430–446.
Flew, Sarah: Financial crisis. A case study of the Laity's declining financial support of Anglican home-missionary organisations, 1856 to 1914. http://www.academia.edu/8315968 accessed 30 October 2014.
Gill, Sean: Women and the Church of England from the eighteenth century to the present. London 1994.
Granshaw, Lindsay: The rise of the modern hospital in Britain. In: Wear, Andrew (ed.): Medicine in society. Historical essays. Cambridge 1992, pp. 197–218.
Grierson, Janet: The deaconess. London 1981.
Hawkins, Sue: Nursing and women's labour in the nineteenth century. The quest for independence. London; New York 2010.
Heeney, Brian: The women's movement in the Church of England 1850–1930. Oxford 1988.

Huntsman, R. G.; Bruin, Mary; Holttum, Deborah: Twixt candle and lamp. The contribution of Elizabeth Fry and the institution of nursing sisters to nursing reform. In: Medical History 46 (2002), pp. 351–380.

Helmstadter, Carol; Godden, Judith: Nursing before Nightingale, 1815–1899. Farnham; Surrey 2012.

Iriye, Akira: Transnational history. In: Contemporary European History 13 (2004), pp. 211–222.

Ludlow, J. M.: Deaconesses, or Protestant sisterhoods. In: Edinburgh Review 87 CLXXVI, pp. 438–448.

Ludlow, John Malcolm Forbes: Woman's work in the church. London 1865.

Mangion, Carmen M.: Women, religious ministry and female institution-building. In: DeVries, Jacqueline; Morgan, Sue (ed.): Women, gender and religious cultures in Britain, 1800–1940. Abingdon 2010, pp. 72–93.

Mangion, Carmen M.: Voluntary hospitals and sectarianism in nineteenth-century England. Forthcoming 2016.

Lees, Florence S.: Handbook for hospital sisters. London 1874.

Morris, R. J.: Clubs, societies and associations. In: Thompson, F. M. L. (ed.): The Cambridge social history of Britain, Volume 3: social agencies and institutions. Cambridge 1990, pp. 395–444.

Mumm, Susan: Stolen daughters, virgin mothers. Anglican sisterhoods in Victorian Britain. London 1998.

Prelinger, Catherine M.: The female diaconate in the Anglican Church. What kind of ministry for women? In: Malmgreen, Gail (ed.): Religion in the lives of English women, 1760–1930. London 1986, pp. 161–192.

Prochaska, F. K.: Bible nurses and the poor in Victorian London. In: Historical Research 60 (1987), pp. 336–348.

Sewell, Elizabeth M.: Anglican deaconesses. In: MacMillan's Magazine 28 (1873), 167 (September), pp. 463–467.

Sister Joanna: The deaconess community of St Andrew. In: Journal of Ecclesiastical History 12 (1961), pp. 215–230.

Summers, Anne: The mysterious demise of Sarah Gamp. The domiciliary nurse and her detractors, C. 1830–1860. In: Victorian Studies 32 (1989), 3, pp. 365–386.

Vicinus, Martha: Independent women. Work and community for single women, 1850–1920. London 1985.

Waddington, Keir: Charity and the London hospitals, 1850–1898. Woodbridge 2000.

Watkin, Brian: The Prince of Wales's General Hospital. Tottenham; London 1967.

White, Teresa Joan: The (deaconess) community of St Andrew 1861–2011. London 2011.

Williamson, Lori: Soul sisters. The St John and Ranyard nurses in nineteenth century London, In: International History of Nursing Journal 2 (1996), pp. 33–49.

Archives

Deaconess Community of St Andrew, Lambeth Palace Archives
[These uncatalogued materials were viewed in the Community's archives which have now been relocated to the Lambeth Palace Archives.]
Annual Reports
Ancilla Domini
'Directions for Sisters Nursing in Hospitals', autograph undated thought to be written by Elizabeth Ferard
Finance Committee Notes 1881–1942
Inner Council minutes (1868–1888)
S. Michael's Home for Men and Women Annual Reports (1855–1971)

Tottenham Hospital, Haringey Archives Service
923.3 Newspaper Clippings
PW 1/1–95 Photographs
PW 6/2 Michael Laseron, A Narrative of the Origin and Progress of the Girls' Industrial Or-
    phan Home, and the Evangelical Protestant Deaconesses' Institution and Training Hospi-
    tal (1875)
PW 6/3 'An Outline of the History of the Prince of Wales General Hospital', undated, anony-
    mous typescript
PW 6/6 history of Tottenham Hospital, undated, anonymous typescript
PW 6/8, Account of the history of the Tottenham Hospital, undated, anonymous typescript
PW 6/9, 'Information from Royal College of Nursing Records', undated, anonymous type-
    script
PW 8/3 'Report of the Medical Council (as revised by the sub-committee) on the Nursing
    Department', 28 January 1896
PW 8/52 Nursing staff records

Great Northern Hospital, London Metropolitan Archives
Great Northern Annual Reports
H33/RN/A2/1 Great Northen [sic] Hospital Minute Book Medical Committee
H33/RN/Y11/1 Cuttings Book, 1860–1872

St Andrew's House, Portsmouth History Centre
CHU 1/90/3/1/4 Winchester Diocesan Deaconess Home, Portsmouth Annual Report

'How to meet the needs of the Church'. On the history of deaconesses in the Lutheran motherhouse in Baltimore, Maryland, USA, in the twentieth century

Doris Riemann

In 1885, representatives of the *General Synod*, one of the associations of the Lutheran Churches in America at the time, informed the members of the Church public:

> After four years of preparation and six years of work as a Board, we are permitted to place [...] the practical accomplishment of the task we were appointed to. We have secured and trained an adequate number of sisters for the establishment of a Deaconess Mother-house and Training School, and now offer to the Church an institution prepared to undertake the duty of training its daughters in appropriate spheres of Christian ministry.[1]

These sentences announced the foundation of the *Baltimore Motherhouse of Deaconesses (BMD)* in the US state of Maryland.[2] This was an ambitious project that was under a lot of pressure to be successful because of the Church leadership's conviction that a *formal women's ministry* was not only a necessity but a crucial part of the Church if it was to be whole and institutionally complete, existing alongside the *ministry of the Word*. The *BMD* was therefore the only motherhouse to emerge directly from a project initiated by the Church leadership. In this it differed significantly from the German prototypes on which it was modelled. However, it also differed from the other motherhouses that had been established in various countries, including the US, from the 1840s onwards. It was at the centre of the formation of the Lutheran Church at the beginning of the twentieth century. For this reason, the *General Synod* did not just perceive it as a local institution but as a "vital part of the church intended finally to benefit every congregation throughout the General Synod of the United States",[3] or, as one pastor put it, with an obvious reference to the effective Gettysburg Address given by US president Abraham Lincoln in 1863: "The deaconess role proposed was organized '*in* a Church, *by* a Church and [created] *for* the Church."[4]

---

1   Extracts from the Report of the Deaconess Board to the General Synod at Hagerstown, June 1895. In: Hand-Book of the Deaconess Board of the General Synod of the Evangelical Lutheran Church in the United States of America, Philadelphia, 1895, Evangelical Lutheran Church in America (ELCA) Archives, ULCA 61/8/1, Box 2, p. 13.
2   The article is based on a research project entitled "Rationalization of Nursing in Western Germany and the United States. A Comparative History of the Exchanges of Ideas and Practices, 1945 to 1975", directed by Susanne Kreutzer and sponsored by the *German Research Foundation*. I would like to thank Susanne Kreutzer and Karen Nolte for their helpful comments.
3   Baltimore Deaconess Motherhouse and School, Scrapbook, cited after Zerull (2011), p. 306.
4   At the inauguration of a graveyard for soldiers during the American Civil War, the 16th president of the United States, Abraham Lincoln, sketched out his idea of a democratic

In 1895, six trained women moved into the new motherhouse and began very successfully to work in the communities and in families as nurses, teachers and parish sisters.[5] At the end of the century, so many families and communities were asking for help that they had to reject applicants and rent an additional building. Here they organised a day-care centre for children and a "colored night school", and they offered women the opportunity to learn how to sew at an "industrial school".[6] They had a broad network of contacts beyond the realm of the Church and their advice was respected in many places. Their work was based on the idea that nursing the body and nursing the soul were inextricably linked. For this reason, the sisters also understood providing for patients and religious training as an *Inner Mission*, i. e. as religious nursing of the soul.

However, the situation changed radically after World War I, when the *General Synod* merged with other Lutheran Churches to form the *United Lutheran Church in America* (*ULCA*). The numbers of deaconesses stagnated, pastors increasingly preferred to use secular nurses and there were frequent discussions about the future of deaconesses. In this article I pursue the question of how the *BMD* and the Church leaders succeeded in securing the institutional survival of the deaconesses. In hindsight we can see that they believed the only option was to abandon the sisters' traditional area of expertise and skills. The history reveals a departure from genuinely feminine knowledge gained through experience and the advent of a process of scientification and occupationalisation of their work. This paved the way for the transformation of the Lutheran Church into an institution that provided social services, and established the principle of competition as the basis for action.

To back up this argument, I start by outlining the foundation years of the *BMD* within the context of American society, before following the efforts of the Church leaders during the twentieth century to establish deaconess work as an "office of the church".[7] There is little existing work for me to draw on. Lisa Zerull delineated the history of the foundation of the *BMD*, pointing out that the motherhouse corresponded to the ideal of 'separate spheres' for men and women – with men in the public and women in the domestic domain – that had developed in the nineteenth century.[8] In contrast, Susanne Kreutzer compares the history of Lutheran deaconess houses in West Germany and the US and shows that the imported German model of community nursing care failed as early as the 1930s in the United States.[9] Yet the further history of the *BMD* within the Lutheran Church-related structure and the larger social

---

state as a "government of the people, by the people, for the people." Lincoln, Abraham, cited after Boyer (2012), p. 60.
5   A Hand-Book issued by the Deaconess Motherhouse of the General Synod of the Evangelical Lutheran Church in the United States, Philadelphia, 1903, p. 25, ELCA Archives, ULCA 61/8/1, Box 2.
6   Zerull (2011), p. 240.
7   Minutes of the Board of Deaconess Work (BDW), cited after: Zerull (2011), p. 144.
8   Cf. Zerull (2011).
9   Cf. Kreutzer (2010), pp. 134–150.

framework of the US have not been investigated at all. For this reason my work is not only a contribution to the history of denominationally attached, pious women and their spheres of activity within the Lutheran Church, but it also adds to the history of female employment in the United States far into the second half of the twentieth century.

My work is based on archival material of the *ULCA* and the *Evangelical Lutheran Church in America* (*ELCA*) that has not been analysed before. These sources primarily enable a reconstruction of the organisational and conceptual history of the motherhouse. However, they do not provide a picture of the sisters' daily lives in their community, their personal experiences and conflicts. The personal files mainly contain application documents or obituaries and, only in a few rare cases, letters. An exception are the memoirs of Sister Mildred Winter who, in 1989, wrote a retrospective of the Sisterhood in Baltimore from her point of view as a senior sister during the 1940s and 1950s. Yet it is possible to depict the organisation of the motherhouse, changes in training and working conditions, and the position of the institutionalised sphere of female activity and its significance for the Church using the minutes of the Church boards, publications of the motherhouse and personal letters.

"The Board may not have known exactly what those young deaconesses were to do, but they knew"[10]: The founding years

The *General Synod* had been considering the idea of building a deaconess motherhouse from as far back as 1883. In the context of a general lack of pastors,[11] severe social hardship due to industrialisation and, finally, the high number of immigrants, a group of theologians had suggested to the synod that they form a *female ministry*. The idea was that unmarried women or widows would take care of the sick, bring up children in the Christian faith, and support pastors in their work. After long and intensive discussions, the members of the synod welcomed the suggestion and put the newly established *Board of Deaconess Work* (*BDW*) in charge of implementing the project.[12] This decision by the Church leadership found further support at the end of the nineteenth century in the growth of the *Social Gospel Movement*, whose members believed that the Church had a responsibility to address people's hardship. This simultaneously helped the movement become one of the driving forces of American Protestantism at the start of the twentieth century.[13] The welfare state did not exist and was only slowly coming into existence,[14] plans to establish a

---

10 Winter, Mildred, I remember…, Recollections I of Sister Mildred Winter, December 1988, pp. 12–13, ELCA Archives, ELCA 127/6/1, Box 32.
11 Cf. Meuser (1980), p. 359.
12 Cf. Lundeen, Catherine, Administrative History of the Board of Deaconess Work in the United Lutheran Church in America, ELCA Archives, ULCA 22.
13 Cf. Zerull (2011), pp. 57–59; Meuser (1980), pp. 385–387.
14 Cf. Gräser (2009).

motherhouse were in limbo, both from the point of view of the Church and of society.

The members of the *BDW* based their work on the concept of the first deaconess motherhouse in Germany. Pastor Theodor Fliedner had founded it in 1836 in the context of the revival movement in a town near Düsseldorf called Kaiserswerth. Fliedner's goal had been to provide an opportunity for unmarried women to live in a community and to pursue tasks defined by their 'nature' and by 'creation', i. e. to engage in the nursing care of people who were unwell and/or old. This idea rested on the conviction that care of the body and care of the soul formed an inextricable union and that the *Inner Mission* could serve as a starting point for the renewal of personal faith.[15] The *BDW* found here a theological and organisational concept that it could use to justify the establishment of a completely new field of work within the Church and to promote its practical realisation. Nonetheless, the American project differed dramatically from the German template, since – as a project of the Church leadership – it played a central role in setting up and establishing the Lutheran Church organisation.

The people in charge began eagerly with the implementation, searching for women who were willing to be trained as deaconesses, to live in a motherhouse, and to wear a uniform that was intended to make them recognisable in the public sphere and protect their status as unmarried women. After their training and consecration they were to be granted the right to call themselves 'deaconess' and to become a member of the Community of Sisters. They were not supposed to receive a salary but the Church leadership promised to finance their training and to provide lifelong security in all matters. The *BDW* was under enormous pressure to achieve success: after rejecting ten applicants, they eventually found six women they trusted to set up a motherhouse and perform the work. While two of them were trained in American motherhouses, the other four were sent to Kaiserswerth and were subsequently consecrated as deaconesses in Baltimore in 1895. They moved into a house that the Lutheran Church parishes had provided for them. Faced with a growing number of Catholics and Catholic sisterhoods that were heavily involved in social issues, they hoped that the foundation of the motherhouse would enable them to strengthen the position of Lutheran Protestantism within society and enlarge its area of influence.

The motherhouse served both as a place to live and as the training school for the deaconesses. At this time it was organised according to the contemporary ideal of a family: at the top of the sisterhood there was a pastor as the house-father and a 'head sister' as the house-mother. The *BDW* appointed both of them after an election process. It also set up committees to carry out management tasks so that the pastor of the motherhouse and the head sister were free to focus on internal issues. The sisterhood formed a "council"[16] that

15 Cf. Köser (2006).
16 Organization and Government of the Motherhouse. In: Hand-Book, Philadelphia, 1895, p. 11.

organised matters relating to everyday communal life. The model, the contemporary image of the family, was regarded as an expression of a Christian lifestyle for both men and women and was based on the conviction – promoted and justified by practical theology – that the order of marriage and family as well as that of the Church reflected God's relationship with the people. This idea guided the Church's policies and influenced the communal life of the sisters, the organisation of the motherhouse, and the understanding of their office, on which their work was based. The female office, the *ministry of helpfulness and mercy*, was simultaneously coequal and subordinate to the *ministry of the Word* and thus constituted a complementary relationship between men and women. The deaconesses gained a status "beside and under the direction of the ministry of the Word".[17]

The sources barely describe, or even mention, the conditions and situation of the people in need. In a noteworthy contrast to the expansive explanations of the organisation of the motherhouse and its integration within the Church, those in need are referred to in formulaic terms as those people who constituted the target of the sisters' work: "These may be the sick, the poor, the unchurched, the indifferent, the orphan, the widow, the child, the aged, the tempted, the erring, and those in need of teaching or of succour".[18] The idea that personal hardship should be seen as an expression of poverty of faith becomes apparent here – a notion that had also guided Theodor Fliedner's work. In the US this idea joined the conviction that poverty was a matter of individual character and a proof of personal failure. The American political scientist Nancy Fraser and the historian Linda Gordon emphasise the pioneering role of the US in promoting this form of personal independence, which was explained in moral and psychological terms and linked the notion of 'being dependent' to a personal stigmatisation. The term 'dependence' had lost all connotations of an economic, political, or social status other than one that had been caused by a person's own actions. In the US, these broader connotations had been very weak to begin with and the term developed into a key concept in welfare state building in America.[19] Poverty and other social hardships had a strong negative connotation. In other words, social ascent and economic independence were regarded as proof of a person's capability, his positive character, and also his strong faith. As Marcus Gräser points out in his investigation of the formation of the welfare state in the US, the demarcation of socially disadvantaged people could thus become a constitutive part of the middle class,[20] but also, in a special way, of the Lutheran Church. Without doubt, this development strengthened the significance of the *BMD* for the Church because its development could be regarded as essential to the establishment and self-image of the Church institution as a whole.

---

17   The Female Diaconate. In: A Hand-Book, Philadelphia, 1903, pp. 11–12.
18   Rev. Manhart, F. P., When can every Lutheran Church in the Land be supplied with a Deaconess and a Kindergartner?, p. 2, ELCA Archives, ULCA 61/1/1, Folder 7.
19   Cf. Fraser/Gordon (1997), pp. 131–132.
20   Cf. Gräser (2009), p. 65.

Considering this scope, it seems a natural decision that, in contrast to other motherhouses, the *BMD* focused very quickly on training the deaconesses for work in parishes. The guiding principle of the family, justified from a theological point of view, proved to be the perfect match for the concept of order in this large clerical project: it provided women with a professional sphere of action within the Church, where they could contribute their experience and skills. The deaconesses administered an area that resembled a household and was incredibly large and non-specific. Their actions derived from their respective situations in families or parishes and guaranteed them a high level of independence from institutional guidelines. Their work could not be accounted for in financial terms or in terms of time because they were an inseparable presence in the families and parishes they served. They constituted a "ministry of presence"[21] on the basis of the motherhouse as "an ever present community".[22] In terms of status, they were subordinate to the male figure of authority but they were allowed to act autonomously and independently within their area of expertise. While the Church leadership monitored them closely – the leaders had to produce daily or at times weekly reports[23] and the sisters' performance was reviewed annually[24] – the sisters' testaments document their enthusiasm and high level of contentment during these years. Mildred Winter described the founding years as a time when "the Board may not have known exactly what those young deaconesses were to do, but they knew and they lost no time in doing it".[25] Thus, the establishment of the *BMD* was a success story. At the end of the nineteenth century, the first six deaconesses started looking after patients, taking care of children, helping youngsters and women who had got into trouble, and supporting pastors with their parish work.

Without a doubt, this project was an expression of clerical, conservative ideas of femininity (up)held by the Church leaders. They regarded "gentleness, patience [and] fidelity" as "women virtue[s]" through "the Saviour [was] still ministering to the needs of a sinning and sorrowing world".[26] The leadership understood the concept of living the life of a deaconess as a vital model for all women, so that it seemed logical to offer training for Church work not only to future deaconesses but also to married women. As early as 1901, when the sisters moved into a bigger house, women who did not want to become deaconesses could attend courses at their own expense. In this way they contributed to the financial upkeep of the *BMD*. Just ten years later, this training service was established as an independent department within the training

---

21 Zerull (2011), p. 259.
22 Zerull (2011), p. 321.
23 Cf. Organization and Government of the Motherhouse. In: Hand-Book, Philadelphia, 1895, p. 11.
24 Cf. Zerull (2011), p. 172.
25 Winter, Mildred, I remember …, Recollections I of Sister Mildred Winter, December 1988, pp. 12–13, ELCA Archives, ELCA 127/6/1, Box 32.
26 An Attractive Calling. In: A Hand-Book. Philadelphia, 1909, p. 25.

school and the *BMD* emphasised its focus on parish work, thus differentiating itself from other motherhouses.[27]

As well as having to provide various certificates and references when applying to become a parish sister, the women also had to justify their motivation for wanting to live as a deaconess. As the *BDW* specified: "The chief requisite in an applicant is the right spirit". This included

> a strong desire to serve Christ in labors of service and mercy, and a willingness to meet the necessary requirements of associated life in a motherhouse and training in an institution, and to work under its direction and that of Christian pastors and churches.[28]

In response, some women generically expressed their "strong desire to become a Deaconess",[29] but others passionately emphasised "that there has come to me a definite call to enter the diaconate".[30] This sample sentence reveals that the term 'profession' (in German *Beruf*) was still understood as a 'calling' (*Berufung*) or as a 'call' *(Ruf)* from God[31] that the women followed when they applied to be enrolled in the motherhouse. They used this term to describe a personal experience of faith that demanded their obedience to God. While the Church leadership could demand or at least desire such faith, it resisted a hierarchical disciplinary enforcement and could not be artificially created. Rather, those appointed to the *ministry of the Word* and the women appointed to the *ministry of mercy* were all placed equally 'beneath the Word'. The *General Synod* subjected the female sphere of work to a process of professionalisation, without, however, establishing a profession in the modern sense of the word – one marked by vocational training, a salary, and limited working hours. This is where discrepancies emerge within the institutional conquest of female nursing care: neither the physical care nor the care for the soul that the women performed in response to a 'calling' was accounted for in terms of time or money. This work was merely regarded as a function or requirement that the women had to fulfil as efficiently as possible, since this was their contribution to successfully building and growing the Church.

The policies of the *General Synod* and the *BDW* attest from the very beginning to their efforts to establish the motherhouse in its clerical function as efficiently as possible. In defining the work of the motherhouse as 'clerical needs', the leadership was able to justify the experience-based work of the sisters as institutional interests, rather than explaining it as a response, borne out of faith, to the hardships of the people. The term 'need' is gender-neutral, ab-

---

27 Cf. Lundeen, Catherine, United Lutheran Church in America, Lutheran Deaconess Motherhouse and Training School, Baltimore, Maryland, Administrative History, ELCA Archives, ULCA 61.

28 Requirements for Admission. In: A Hand-Book, Philadelphia, 1903, pp. 26–29, here: p. 29.

29 Bingaman, Mildred K., Sketch of my Life – Requirements for Admission, n. d. [1906], ELCA Archives, ELCA 127/6/1, Box 27.

30 Shirey, Miriam Kathleen, Sketch of My Life, n. d., ELCA Archives, ELCA 127/6/1, Box 26.

31 Cf. Rendtorff (1971), Vol. 1, Col. 833.

stract, meaningless, and functional.[32] Using this term allows one to deviate from concrete conditions or real-life situations and to link vastly different spheres with a unifying logic. 'Needs' can be ascribed to people and groups, but also to institutions, and they reveal a possessive relationship. People or organisations have 'needs' that they can claim themselves and that others can ascribe to them. This concept of needs developed its impact in the history of modern Western organisations because it allows one to merge personal motivations and institutional interests. It became a central term in the twentieth century. The 'fulfilment' of needs could be claimed as a right and investigated as an 'issue' by researchers. It also helped to justify institutional interests.[33] In terms of the history of the deaconesses in Baltimore, this meant that their personal experience of the 'call' and their actions were not regarded as clerical tasks. Instead, the *BDW* could ask the following question to guide its actions: "How to meet the needs of the Church?"[34]

It was a perspective used by the *BDW* to justify the establishment of the motherhouse, to emphasise its significance for society, and to explain all the measures designed to secure and expand the scope of the women's work. Understanding clerical activity not as a task but as an institutional function by using the phrase 'clerical needs' made it possible to link them to contemporary methods that had been used by the social sciences and humanities to promote the professionalisation of helping since the end of the nineteenth century.[35] Simultaneously, it relieved the leaders of the necessity of putting matters of substance at the centre of the discussion. It was more important to win the pastors' support because they were expected to find trainees for the motherhouse and deploy deaconesses as members of staff. The *BDW* faced the task of creating a 'demand' for the new deaconess 'offer': it stated in its constitution that it had to evoke a "general interest in our churches".[36] For this reason, the *BDW* initiated advertising campaigns, developed the institution according to the 'needs' of the parishes, and disciplined the sisters' lives in order to establish the *BMD* as a new leadership 'product' of the Church on the religious market. For the deaconesses this meant that their care work did not derive from the specific hardship of individuals and families. Instead, it had to be brought in line with the 'needs' of the Church for institutional growth and significance in society. They themselves were to be the representatives fulfilling this institutional 'need'. In other words, the inextricable care of body and soul, which they understood as a response to a call from God, did not align with the 'needs' of the Church and had thus become ideologically dysfunctional.

---

32 Cf. Kim-Warrzinek/Müller (1972), p. 441.
33 Cf. Illich (1993), pp. 47–70; Gronemeyer (2002).
34 For instance in: Letter from Rev. Foster to Rev. Lang 26/02/1930, ELCA Archives, ULCA 22/7, Box 1, Folder 1.
35 Cf. Gräser (2009), pp. 208–248.
36 Constitution of the Deaconess Board of the General Synod of the Evangelical Lutheran Church in the United States of America. In: Hand-Book, Philadelphia, 1895, p. 6.

Nursing course a "debatable equipment"[37]: The crisis of the 1920s and 1930s

After only a few years, the sisters' work came under pressure. On the one hand, the consensus in society about women's status in the family and in society began to fall apart. In particular, women of the white upper and middle classes began to fight for the right to vote and began to question their position in the family and in the working world.[38] They were not prohibited by law from working outside the home after they married and, increasingly, more women decided to earn their own money independently of their husbands. For unmarried women, taking on an unpaid job as an alternative to getting married made less and less sense.[39] In addition, the service sector exploded, offering women improved means of earning a living.[40] These included working as secular nurses, whose influence grew because they had completed an academic, science-based training course and offered patients care at home through the framework of local organisations, such as the *Visiting Nurse Associations* (*VNAs*). Their work was based on the conviction that training according to scientific nursing care standards would ensure the best care – in contrast to the deaconesses, whose work was merely based on the women's experience.[41]

Within the Church itself, the situation was also becoming more difficult for the deaconesses. There had been numerous attempts to unite the various Lutheran denominations in the US into one Lutheran Church. However, the parishes insisted on their autonomy, so these endeavours often failed due to theological and practical differences. The immigrant Lutherans, typically from Germany or Scandinavia, celebrated the religious traditions of their countries of origin and thus emphasised their distinctiveness within American society, even if they were united in their aversion to the Churches with links to the state in their home countries. World War I changed the situation dramatically because the parishes that were dominated by Germans faced a difficult situation, both politically and within society. While the Lutherans had largely welcomed the outbreak of war on the European continent, they faced considerable accusations after the US joined the war. In everyday life this became obvious in the problems they faced when speaking German. The Church leaderships reacted with a change of policy, assuring the US of their support and their commitment "to adjust church and individual life quickly to American ways".[42] Simultaneously, the 400th anniversary of the Reformation in 1917 offered an opportunity to remember their commonalities. The *General Synod* took charge of preparing

---

37 Letter from Rev. Frederick B. Clausen, St. John's Evangelical Lutheran Church, to Rev. Foster U. Gift, Lutheran Deaconess Motherhouse 26/02/1930, ELCA Archives, ULCA 61/6/1, Box 1, Folder 1.
38 Cf. Heinemann (2011).
39 Cf. Kreutzer (2010), p. 143.
40 Cf. Heinemann (2011), p. 3.
41 Cf. Kreutzer (2010), p. 145.
42 Meuser (1980), p. 399.

these festivities and was instrumental in paving the way for the amalgamation of the Lutheran denominations into the *United Lutheran Church in America* (*ULCA*) in 1918.[43] The *BDW* became part of the new *Lutheran Church*[44] and again had to justify the work of the deaconesses in this significantly larger organisation. After the war, this task was doomed.

The numbers speak for themselves: by 1926, only 79 deaconesses had been consecrated in Baltimore and during this period the numbers of those joining was much smaller than the number of those leaving the *BMD*.[45] Other motherhouses in the US struggled with similar challenges. In 1930 a member of the church reported that "of the seven deaconess motherhouses not connected with the ULCA [...] only two made any gain at all in the decade of 1918 to 1928, and they increased their number one each, and the other five actually registered a loss of 47 deaconesses. The whole number of deaconesses connected with these seven motherhouses dwindled from 227 to 182 deaconesses during the ten years referred to".[46] A study of the personal files reveals that, especially during the 1920s and 1930s, the sisters often decided after only a brief period of time to leave the motherhouse again. In the few written explanations that have survived, it is striking that the sisters talk about the problem of 'dependence'. The women felt restricted by their life in the sisterhood and the lack of payment, complained in the parishes about their dependence on the pastors, and their poor image, which they blamed not least on their working conditions. Ethel Mosteller, for instance, did not even wait for her consecration in 1924, but left the motherhouse during her training period: "At the close of the scholastic year I desire to be released from the diaconate, as I feel that I can do more efficient work by working independently rather than under supervision".[47] A year later, Estella Hansen asked for her release because "it seems best that I should take a position with a salary. You may not know, but some of the Sisters know that I am very independent, and one of the most difficult things for me to do is to ask favors of anyone". Furthermore, she added: "I want to tell you that if any of the other Parish Sisters have experiences like I have had, many embarrassing situations arise, in working only for our support, and many times we feel like we are being treated like objects of charity."[48]

43 Cf. Meuser (1980), p. 392.
44 Cf. Lundeen, Catherine, United Lutheran Church in America, ELCA Archives, ULCA 61.
45 Cf. Report of the Committee on Survey to the Board of Deaconess Work of the United Lutheran Church in America, dated 24/04/1930, ELCA Archives, ULCA 22/7, Box 1, Folder 1.
46 Report of the Committee on Survey to the Board of Deaconess Work of the United Lutheran Church in America, dated 24/04/1930, ELCA Archives, ULCA 22/7, Box 1, Folder 1.
47 Letter from Ethel Mosteller to the BDW 08/04/1924, ELCA Archives, ELCA 127/6/2, Box 13, Ethel Mosteller.
48 Letter from Estella Hansen to Dr Hay 10/10/1920, ELCA Archives, ELCA 127/6/2, Box 7, Estella Hansen.

While the sources vividly show that this form of female ministry was already starting to lose its credibility after the first generation of deaconesses, the letters also reveal the women's serious interest in working within the Church without becoming deaconesses. From the beginning, a large number of women received training at the training school in various subjects so as to work within the Church. In 1922, an additional two-year programme was set up.[49] From 1927, Mildred Winter also attended as a 'special student' and reported that there was a high demand for these courses: "I remember in 1927 when I enrolled in the Motherhouse School as a special student it was filled to capacity." However, of the 40 students "possibly twelve [...] were preparing for the diaconate; the rest of us were classified as 'special students'". She concluded that "women were seeking to serve the Church"[50] – yet obviously not primarily as deaconesses.

The search for the reasons and for possible strategies to resolve the issue began. The *BDW* founded committees and commissions that were given the task of analysing the situation, outlining the problems and searching for solutions. Following the ideals of contemporary social science research methods, they conducted surveys, carried out interviews, analysed organisational structures, created opinion pieces based on questionnaires and figured out 'needs'. The *BDW* records provide vivid evidence that the goal of this project was "to meet the needs of the Church".[51] Theological concepts and considerations relating to the social situation of the women or those they visited in families and communities are mentioned very rarely.

The results of the surveys were devastating and revealed that the work of the deaconesses as parish sisters had failed. Even though many parish pastors could imagine having a deaconess as a member of staff, the majority of them wanted a secretary or other members of staff but not necessarily a deaconess. Nursing care played hardly any role in the survey responses. Instead, it was regarded as a "debatable equipment" because "most large cities have visiting nurses associations". Instead, the deaconesses were to receive "some training in office efficiency"[52] or, as someone else suggested, specialise in "parish education" so that they could work as "primarily directors of religious education".[53] More critical voices did not discuss areas of the deaconesses' work that had a future but regarded the concept of the deaconess itself as outdated. One pastor joined the discussion claiming that the uniform "raises a barrier between the deaconess and the people whom she meets" and another held the opinion that "the day of the deaconess in modern Twentieth Century con-

49   Cf. Lundeen, Catherine, United Lutheran Church in America, ELCA Archives, ULCA 61.

50   Winter, Mildred, Recollections II, p. 4, ELCA Archives, ELCA 127/6/1, Box 32.

51   E. g. Letter from Rev. Foster to Rev. Lang 26/02/1930, ELCA Archives, ULCA 22/7, Box 1, Folder 1.

52   Letter from Rev. Frederic B. Clausen to Rev. Foster U. Gift 26/02/1930, ELCA Archives, ULCA 61/6/1, Box 1, Folder 1.

53   Letter from Rev. Frederick R. Knubel to Rev. Foster U. Gift 04/03/1930, ELCA Archives, ULCA 61/6/1, Box 1, Folder 1.

gregation is done".[54] The reviewers summarised the opinions of the critical pastors stating that other female members of staff were "better fitted naturally, by family inheritance and social background".[55]

The *Committee on Survey of the Field* recommended to the *BDW* to open a course in 'office training' and to convince more women to live the life of a deaconess through a campaign within the Church.[56] When the members of the committee stated that "there is no doubt that the Church needs more trained, full-time women workers"[57] they mainly thought of the women working in sisterhoods. At the time, the deaconesses were still the only representatives of a female ministry who were expected to complete their tasks on the basis of an "impulse of an inner call to a work [...] that is not to be regarded professionally or as a mere career". The reviewers considered it would be dangerous to expand the number of courses for women who did not want to become deaconesses and they asked "whether the constant intermingling in the classroom and otherwise of the candidates for the diaconate and those with less serious intentions is altogether favorable to the earnestness of spirit". Because, they thought, "when a deaconess drops out of the ranks a few weeks or months after her consecration, there must be a defect somewhere".[58]

For the committee it seemed a natural step to ask the parish pastors in circular letters or standardised questionnaires which opportunities for employment they saw within their parish for a deaconess and which requirements she would have to fulfil. In doing so, they were employing investigational methods that had been developed during the first decade of the twentieth century in the US in the context of the *Social Survey Movement*. Since 1914, particularly in the north-eastern states, these methods had become established as a common means of collecting comparable and measurable data on the social situation of the people.[59] While the investigations of the *BDW* did not correspond to the scientific standards of the time, this form of internal Church communication involving people who were not board members made it possible to engage parishes as decision-makers in the development of necessary solutions without infringing on their autonomy. Furthermore, the surveys facilitated, and maybe even established, the perception within the Church that the

54 Report of Committee on Survey of the Field, n.d. [1929], ELCA Archives, ULCA 22/7, Box 1, Folder 1.
55 Report of the Committee on Survey to the Board of Deaconess Work of the United Lutheran Church in America dated 24/04/1930, ELCA Archives, ULCA 22/7, Box 1, Folder 1.
56 Cf. Report of the Committee on Survey to the Board of Deaconess Work of the United Lutheran Church in America dated 24/04/1930, ELCA Archives, ULCA 22/7, Box 1, Folder 1.
57 Report of the Committee on Survey to the Board of Deaconess Work of the United Lutheran Church in America dated 24/04/1930, ELCA Archives, ULCA 22/7, Box 1, Folder 1.
58 Report of Committee on Survey of the Field, n.d. [1929], ELCA Archives, ULCA 22/7, Box 1, Folder 1.
59 Cf. Bulmer (1991), pp. 291–315; Desrosière (1991), pp. 217–244; Converse (1987), pp. 11–53.

ULCA was a homogeneous space. As a result, both the parishes and the deaconesses faced a public opinion within the Church that had been created by the leadership and that was based on standardised questions.[60] While the surveys formally preserved the parishes' autonomy, they also forced the pastors into a situation where they had to deal with questions that had previously had little or no relevance to their work.[61] By implying a specific point of view on a problem within the survey, those asking the questions delineated the framework within which the pastors were to base their thoughts and decisions.

At the end of the 1920s, this resulted in unintended consequences for the deaconesses. On the one hand, the surveys revealed the scope and variety of their areas of work, but on the other, this vastness emerged as the key problem. Until then, the deaconesses' strength had been precisely that they knew what had to be done, whereas now the pastors were being asked to put into words what they thought the deaconesses should do. The deaconesses' strength – their incomparable work that escaped standardisation – was juxtaposed with the pastors' answers, who called for the deaconesses' work to be systematised and split into professional categories linked to concrete actions, in accordance with institutional demands. According to this logic, a decision to cut back whole areas of tasks, for example, or to change the training, did not require any further debate. These measures were justified by the 'needs of the Church' that had been identified by those asking the questions and which needed to be fulfilled. Neither the deaconesses, the special students nor the people they took care of could contribute their views to the discussion because of the logic that guided the process.

"The new area"[62]: The long 1940s

At the end of the 1930s, criticism of the training and work of the deaconesses and the *BDW* became increasingly forceful and opinions gained influence according to which "our parish deaconesses are not meeting the needs of our United Luthcran Church" and "the BDW and the Administration of the Motherhouses seem not to be sufficiently aware of the situation".[63] However, the critics did not aim to abolish the female diaconate. Their goal was a fundamental modernisation: improving the search for suitable women through better advertising campaigns, toughening the requirements for enrolment, and implementing insights from social sciences and the humanities, not only in the training of the deaconesses but also in the organisation of the diaconate as a whole. They hoped that this would result in more efficient work that

---

60   Cf. Osborne/Rose (September 1999), pp. 365–396.
61   Cf. Bourdieu (1993), pp. 60–71.
62   Report by the President Rev. Harvey Hoover. In: Minutes of the Meeting of the BDW on 27/06/1940, p. 9, ELCA Archives, ULCA 22/3, Box 2.
63   Statement as attachment to a letter from Rev. Teichmann to Rev. Simon 23/07/1935, ELCA Archives, ULCA 61/6/1, Box 1.

would improve the poor image of the diaconate within the Church and outside it. Their pleas were the expression of a "new climate"[64] within Lutheran
Protestantism. As it was slowly recovering from the Great Depression and
enjoying increasing financial means, World War II began to cast its shadow.
The *ULCA* played a significant role in this new beginning because it was regarded as liberal within the ensemble of the various conservative orthodox
Lutheran Churches.[65] The requests for another reorientation of deaconess
work during the 1940s were able to take hold because of the President of the
BDW at the time, Rev. Harvey Hoover. Mildred Winter wrote about him, in
hindsight, that he "had vision and a deep feeling for women's work and place
in the life of the Church".[66] It was thanks to his efforts that the cornerstones
were laid for a fundamental transformation of the female diaconate into a
modern profession for women, without which the modernisation of the *ULCA*
into a social service organisation would have been unthinkable. For Hoover,
the central issue was to develop a self-image of the diaconate "in a broader
way", i. e. as a "fellowship of those that serve". Within this framework women
merely had a "special status".[67]

Hoover built on the modernisation policies of the *BDW* that had been
started at the end of the 1930s. They had tightened up the high-school requirements for enrolment in the sisterhood, extended the training by a year
(from two to three years), firmly integrated sociology, psychology, and education into the curriculum and provided significantly more space for matters of
Church organisation and administration.[68] He strongly supported the idea
that more women should have the opportunity to work in a paid position
within the *Lutheran Church*. In his justifications he linked the lack of workers
within the Church – because of the "call of men into military training and
service" – to an overall positive view of women working outside the home. He
emphasised "the appeal of financial returns, personal independence, individual initiative and professional advancement". He believed there was no question that "the general church work demands the services of trained women".[69]

In 1943 his efforts started to be successful. The *BDW* managed, together
with the leading deaconesses, to firmly anchor their interests as 'needs of the
Church' within the institution. For seven years they put women in charge of
both motherhouses. The family ideal can no longer be found here as a guiding principle for the organisation and the direction of deaconess work. Rather,
the *BDW* completely reorganised the work: three deaconesses formed the

---

64 Meuser (1980), p. 465.
65 Cf. Meuser (1980).
66 Winter, Mildred, Recollections II, p. 6.
67 Memorandum on the Organizational Structure of the BDW of the ULCA dated
    13/07/1953, p. 1, ELCA Archives, ULCA 22/7, Box 1, Folder 21.
68 Cf. Catalogue issued by the Lutheran Deaconess Motherhouse and Training School,
    Baltimore 1942–1943, 1943–1944, p. 8.
69 Rev. Hoover, Report by the President. In: Minutes of the Meeting of the BDW of
    01/03/1940, ELCA Archives, ULCA 22/3, Box 2.

Cabinet of Secretaries.[70] They were responsible, alongside those women who had been in charge of executive tasks for the *BMD* and the second mother-house of the *ULCA* in Philadelphia (*PMD*) up to that point, and who now constituted the *Board of Management*,[71] for the fate of deaconess work. Sister Anna Ebert was appointed to the post of executive secretary, Sister Martha Hansen became the director of the motherhouse and the training school, and Sister Mildred Winter was the new field secretary. The pastor retained his status as spiritual advisor.[72]

The *Cabinet of Secretaries* was well aware of how it had to act in terms of Church policy to draw attention to its own concerns.

> We learned early that one could not go to the Church convention with a drastically new idea and expect approval upon first presentation. [...] Usually it was wise first to seek authorization for a study to be made with the promise of reporting to the next convention. Also [...] it was necessary to ask permission to involve representatives of other boards and agencies [...] [and] this procedure usually was advisable.[73]

As early as 1942, the *BDW*, in collaboration with the *Board of Education*, managed to secure a commission from the Convention to investigate the situation of the motherhouses within the framework of a "total responsibility of the Diaconate to the work of the church at large".[74] This meant that deaconess work could be re-examined and the situation of women within the Church could be brought directly to the Church leaders' attention. Soon afterwards, in 1943, the *BDW* issued an invitation to the First Council of Women in Full-Time Service in the Church, held at the *PMD*, and simultaneously began to investigate the deaconesses' situation. In the following years, women working within the Church teamed up and met at the Councils, which now took place annually. At the same time, numerous surveys were conducted. During this time, Hoover and the *Cabinet of Secretaries* managed to portray the work of the deaconesses as an issue linked to the Church's establishment, and an institution in which women were transformed into a "great resource of the Church" whose 'better use' would allow the Church "to fulfil its function more effectively".[75]

The surveys of these years illustrate that a "modern idea of the profession" based on professional training, fair wages and limited working hours had without doubt gained acceptance. In this context the survey responses from the people in charge caused distress: in addition to criticising means of payment, the uniform, and the communal life together, the women's work was

---

70 Cf. Winter, Mildred, Recollections II, pp. 6–7.
71 Cf. Lundeen, Catherine, United Lutheran Church in America, Administrative History of the Lutheran Deaconess Home and Training School, Baltimore, ELCA Archives, ULCA 61/6/1.
72 Cf. Minutes of Minneapolis Convention 11–17/10/1944, p. 401, ELCA Archives, ULCA 2/1, Box 1.
73 Winter, Mildred, Recollections II, p. 11.
74 Minutes of the Louisville Convention 14–21/10/1942, p. 473, ELCA Archives, ULCA 2/1, Box 1.
75 Cf. Rev. Hoover, Report of the BDW, Minutes of the Minneapolis Convention 11–17/10/1944, p. 402, ELCA Archives, ULCA 2/1, Box 1.

seen as unprofessional and it was lamented that "neither in secretarial work, nor in religious education, nor in social work [...] [did] the church establish any standards". Following the failure of parish nursing in the 1930s, it was now the turn of parish work to come under attack because, in the opinion of those asking the questions, it was still a "very vague and undefined type of work".[76] Similarly, the responses provided by full-time women workers "were shocking to most who read them"[77] because they revealed that the women did not have appropriate training, did not earn enough money, and did not have limited working hours.[78]

The Convention rapidly responded and commissioned the *BDW* to develop personnel standards for all women and to search for ways to open up equal access to training opportunities within the Church and thus, subsequently, to the labour market within the Church, to both women and men. In addition, the *BDW* was charged with developing ideas for areas of work: they wanted to give new clerical tasks to women with appropriate qualifications who worked in the Church, and not only consecrate deaconesses and send them to their posts.[79] In this way, against the backdrop of World War II, Hoover and the *Cabinet of Secretaries* managed to position themselves as a *Church resource* and to place themselves at the forefront of what one could call a clerical women's movement. Fighting for improved and equal opportunities for work outside the home, they contributed significantly to the development of a sizeable labour market within the Church. At the same time, they helped describe and delineate the entire realm of women's labour within the Church in a completely new fashion, adopting a perspective of qualification and professionalism.

The *Cabinet* enthusiastically fulfilled these tasks and designed a "comprehensive program for the expansion of the diaconate".[80] It proposed two major reforms in this programme: on the one hand, the theological training institutions would be opened up more widely to laypeople, including women,[81] and a new status was to be established within the Church, in addition to the *ministry of the Word* and the *female ministry*: that of "full-time commissioned Church worker".[82] Furthermore, the programme's authors developed personnel standards, differentiating between professionals and non-professionals, which they hoped would become mandatory throughout the *ULCA*. Here

---

76 Report on "The training program for deaconesses and the deaconess Motherhouses at Philadelphia and Baltimore", n. d. [1943], pp. 3 and 8, ELCA Archives, ULCA 22/7, Box 1, Folder 4.

77 Winter, Mildred, Recollections II, p. 10.

78 Cf. Rev. Hoover, Report of the BDW, Minutes of the Minneapolis Convention 11–17/10/1944, p. 402, ELCA Archives, ULCA 2/1, Box 1.

79 Cf. Cf. Rev. Hoover, Report of the BDW, Minutes of the Minneapolis Convention 11–17/10/1944, p. 402, ELCA Archives, ULCA 2/1, Box 1., p. 412, ELCA Archives, ULCA 2/1, Box 1.

80 Minutes of the Des Moines Convention 4–12/10/1950, p. 691, ELCA Archives, ULCA 2/1, Box 1.

81 Cf. Report by Anna Ebert during the meeting of the BDW 19/06/1946, pp. 15–18.

82 Report by Anna Ebert during the meeting of the BDW 19/06/1946, p. 19.

they showed their conviction that deaconesses should take on tasks in the fields of education and social work, while regarding domestic tasks as possibly even harmful. Hoover expressed this unambiguously:

> We belittled our cause and our Church by calling women to be deaconesses, consecrating them, garbing them in the uniform of the glorious Church of Lord Jesus Christ, and assigning them to positions where they were required to be scrub women, workers at laundry tubs or doing unskilled labor of the lowest order.[83]

The devaluation of domestic work illustrates how thoroughly the idea of complementary areas of activity had lost its legitimacy. This link had been the basis for the female diaconate as a *ministry of presence* as opposed to the *ministry of the Word*. The previously female ministry was increasingly divested of its gender-specific character so that even here a professional education and a salary of one's own could become guarantees of personal independence. This was the logic behind the discrediting of domestic work. Hoover could be sure that everyone involved would agree with him when he rhetorically asked whether an appropriate wage and social security were not better than "our parental oversight and control?"[84]

Now the path was clear to proceed with the fundamental modernisation of deaconess work and to discuss the issue of wages and whether or not the uniform was outdated. The *Cabinet of Secretaries* suggested establishing various groups of women and having them decide for themselves whether they wanted to belong to the "traditionally garbed sisters", the "non-garbed deaconess[es]", or the *Deaconess Extension Corps*. These groups were supposed to differ not only in terms of uniform but also payment. The idea was that deaconesses would have the opportunity to decide for themselves whether they wanted to receive financial remuneration in the form of a "salaried plan"[85] or whether they wanted to continue to receive their security in the way it had been granted before. By providing a choice, the head sisters hoped to alleviate the lingering conflict between the younger and older deaconesses that had emerged during the debate about appropriate changes. By leaving the decision to the sisters, they could push ahead with the modernisation process without having to completely discredit former beliefs. The deaconesses themselves had thus permanently given up their status of significance.

Even though the *BDW* and the *Cabinet of Secretaries* failed with their proposals for personnel standards and the introduction of the status of 'commissioned Church worker' throughout the Church at the Convention of 1950,[86] all the necessary measures were nonetheless put in place over the following

---

83 Rev. Hoover, Report by the President. In: Minutes of the Meeting of the BDW 17/01/1946, p. 4, ELCA Archives, ULCA 22/3, Box 2.

84 Rev. Hoover, Report by the President. In: Minutes of the Meeting of the BDW 17/1/1946, p. 4, ELCA Archives, ULCA 22/3, Box 2, p. 6.

85 Report of the Cabinet of Secretaries during the meeting of the BDW 07/09/1945, ELCA Archives, ULCA 22/7, Box 1, Folder 8.

86 Cf. Minutes of the Des Moines Convention 04–12/10/1950, p. 1057, ELCA Archives, ULCA 2/1.

years to transform the former female diaconate into a modern profession for women. Collaboration between the training schools of *BMD* and *PMD* and cooperation with other colleges was intensified and a period of clinical experience was also integrated into the training programmes.[87] As early as 1952 the Convention decided to introduce a salary plan, which coincided with the end of the placement principle for deciding where the deaconesses should work, and the establishment of a social security concession that was similar to an insurance plan.[88] The deaconesses were now allowed (and supposed) to decide on the status and location of their work for themselves. The *BDW* was supposed to serve as a "placement agency"[89] that served to advise both the deaconesses and the parishes. Whereas, during the 1940s, the *BDW* and the *Cabinet of Secretaries* succeeded in becoming the mouthpiece of the women demanding improved access to the labour market within the Church, during the 1950 and 1960s, as we will see in the final analysis, the deaconesses lost their significant status in institutional growth as the *ULCA* merged with other Lutheran churches through the foundation of the *Lutheran Church in America* (*LCA*). They became one possible choice among many of being gainfully employed within the realm of the enlarged Church.

"What is a deaconess?"[90] – The mergers of the 1950s and 1960s

Neither the deaconesses nor the *BDW* could have anticipated the far-reaching consequences of a policy that asked women to declare their interests regarding access to a professional labour market within the Church. Their motivation had not been the question of a female ministry. Rather they wanted to utilise their institutional significance to provide women with more importance within the Church and they wanted to secure their status and improve the deaconesses' image, which was regarded as old-fashioned and outdated. As they increasingly began to understand the diaconate 'in a broader way', as a ministry that was supposed to be open to both men and women, thereby divesting it of its gender-specific character, they challenged its very existence: they found themselves in competition with the spheres of work of other boards that also depended on and tried to attract laypeople to work within the Church. The argument that they were the only board that dealt with women's labour increasingly lost its power of persuasion.

Advice by Sister Anna Ebert to two missionaries who wanted to open a motherhouse in India reveals how fragile their position and self-image had become. She wrote to them that they should not make "the same mistake" in

---

87 Cf. Catalogue issued by the Lutheran Deaconess Motherhouse and Training School, Issued 1946–47, Calendar 1947–48, p. 7.

88 Cf. Minutes of the Seattle Convention 08–15/10/1952, p. 910, ELCA Archives, ULCA 2/1.

89 Minutes of the Seattle Convention 08–15/10/1952, p. 910, ELCA Archives, ULCA 2/1, p. 883.

90 Minutes of the meeting of the BDW 28/10/1953, ELCA Archives, ULCA 22/3, Box 3.

India that "has been made in the United States", and she asked: "Do you not fear that the introduction of a diaconate as we know it in Europe and the United States will cause unhealthy competition between it and existing personnel?" She urged them to consider what the motherhouse was to be called because they knew "how unpopular the name 'Motherhouse' has been in the United States". She wondered whether *ashram*[91] might be a possibility. The *BDW* dealt with similar questions but found in 1950 no reason for "dropping the term Motherhouse in promotional work and replacing it with some new term, such as Deaconess Fellowship Center and School".[92] Nonetheless, only half a year later it asked women who were interested in becoming deaconesses whether "the name 'deaconess' appeal[s] to you as equally appropriate for all women engaged in full time service in the church?"[93]

In the following years it emerged that the *BDW*'s efforts to make the training more professional, to increase advertising and to implement the salary plan had not had the desired success. Despite the fact that wartime had resulted in a "huge expansion"[94] of the Churches and a strong interest in deaconesses within the motherhouses,[95] the number of applicants was stagnant. The motherhouses did not get the opportunity to benefit from the expansion of clerical work. At the same time, their agenda became enmeshed in the bureaucracy of the Church leadership, whose president, Rev. Franklin Fry, wanted to unify and modernise the organisation of the Church. This goal marked the beginning of the end of the *Cabinet of Secretaries* and initiated a struggle between the individual boards for maximum areas of competency and interpretational sovereignty. The *BDW* and the leading sisters found themselves in a situation in which they had to defend their previous competencies and areas of responsibility while simultaneously working on the modernisation of deaconess work.

Sister Mildred Winter, who was to become the Executive Secretary of the *BDW*, warned as early as 1950 of "things to come". She reported on a conversation with Fry about the job description for this position and felt that the previous orientation of her work was threatened: "the authority with which he would invest the Office, I fear, far exceeds anything either of the motherhouses has in its thinking".[96] Nonetheless, Mildred Winter took up the post and faced a president of the Church who regarded the autonomous work and position of the motherhouses as a thorn in his side. He wrote in another letter:

91 Letter from Anna Ebert to Sr. Margret Fry and Sr. Edna Hill 15/04/1949, pp. 2–3, ELCA Archives, ULCA 61/5/2/1, Box 1, Folder 4.

92 Minutes of the Committees on the Preparation and the Projection of a Comprehensive Program for the Expansion of the Diaconate 28/06/1950, ELCA Archives, ULCA 22/7, Box 1, Folder 12.

93 Minutes of the meeting of the BDW 24/01/1951, ELCA Archives, ULCA 22/3, Box 3.

94 Nelson (1980), p. 482.

95 Cf. Minutes of the Des Moines Convention 04–12/10/1950, p. 772, ELCA Archives, ULCA 2/1.

96 Letter from Sr. Mildred Winter to Dr Baughman 22/12/1949, ELCA Archives, ELCA 127/6/1, Box 32.

"I hope for the day that deaconesses will wear the cross of the United Lutheran Church in America, with their loyalty and identification there, rather than the cross of their Deaconess House".[97]

In 1953, a *Commission on Organizational Structure* (*COS*) began its work and the situation of the motherhouses became even more precarious. Its task was to investigate the organisation of the *ULCA* "in view of the continuous growth of The *United Lutheran Church* in America and of its expanding program".[98] The *COS* had hired a management consulting firm, *George Fry & Associates*, to analyse the organisational structure of the work. This consulting firm presented various proposals that would have restricted the previous competencies of the leading sisters in the motherhouses, and furthermore rejected the request by the *BDW* to be in charge of training laypeople. Accordingly, the deaconesses were no longer represented in the *BDW*, were to hand over the task of organising work placement and mentorship to the *BDW* and shorten the training in line with courses provided by other training institutions. The concepts of 'consecration' and 'commissioning' were to be abandoned completely and to be replaced with the phrase 'setting apart'.[99] Faced with these recommendations, the *BDW* asked the question "What is a deaconess?" and put it as its "key question" at the core of its response. It lamented that "many in the church interpret the deaconess merely in terms of their own experience – the visible graduates of Philadelphia and Baltimore. If this be all, the function of the BDW is simply to administer two motherhouses and their graduates".[100] For this reason, it suggested replacing the *BDW* with a *Board of Women's Work* or establishing a *Board of Christian Service*. This was an attempt to address the by now 'familiar question'[101] of their right to exist and, simultaneously, to emphasise the *BDW*'s opinion "that there be a board whose sole responsibility be recruitment, education, setting apart, and placement of all full-time workers except the clergy".[102] However, this suggestion was rejected and in the following years the directors of the motherhouses had to curtail their training courses for laypeople[103] and align the programmes of the *BMD* and *PMD* into a "unified program of education for deaconesses and other lay workers".[104]

---

97 Letter from Rev. Franklin Fry to Sr. Mildred Winter 13/06/1952, p. 3, ELCA Archives, ULCA 22/7, Box 1, Folder 18.

98 Report of the Commission on Organizational Structure to the 1954 Convention of The United Lutheran Church in America, p. 1, ELCA Archives, ULCA 22/7, Box 2, Folder 1.

99 Cf. Report of the Commission on Organizational Structure to the 1954 Convention of The United Lutheran Church in America, p. 1, ELCA Archives, ULCA 22/7, Box 2, Folder 1, pp. 26–28.

100 Minutes of the meeting of the BDW 28/10/1953, ELCA Archives, ULCA 22/3, Box 3.

101 Cf. Appendix to the Memorandum on the Organizational Structure of the Board of Deaconess Work of The United Lutheran Church in America, pp. 3–5.

102 Winter, Mildred, Recollections II, p. 21.

103 Cf. Minutes of the Harrisburg Convention 10–17/10/1956, p. 888, ELCA Archives, ULCA 2/1.

104 Cf. Minutes of the Toronto Convention 06–13/10/1954, p. 762, ELCA Archives, ULCA 2/1.

At the end of the 1950s, projects were on the horizon for another unification of Lutheran Churches in America and instigated the merging of the training schools of the *BMD* and *PMD* to form the *Professional Schools for Church Workers of the United Lutheran Church in America.*[105] Thus, in the context of the newly founded *LCA*, they were well prepared when, in 1962, the training schools merged to form the *Lutheran Deaconess House and School (LDHS)*[106] and, only a few years later, the *Lutheran Deaconess Community (LDC)* emerged as a result of combining all the sisterhoods of the *LCA*,[107] now however under the *Board of College Education and Church Vocation (BCECV)* that had been appointed against the express desire of the *BDW*.[108] While the deaconesses had survived the complete reorganisation of the Lutheran Church landscape, they had lost their central status within the institutional structure of the Church. They had become one of many social institutions and had the role of providing social services and education within the service sector of the Church. Their previous vast sphere of activity, which only they as women could 'manage' had fallen prey to the power of definition by contemporary experts and had been newly mapped into gender-neutral 'occupations' and 'jobs'. Caring activities, such as nursing care and domestic and family work, had been largely erased. As a side effect of this reorientation of deaconess work, a self-image emerged that did not prescribe how the women should live and that promised them the opportunity to make educated choices for themselves from the available options. However, this obscured the fact that it was the Church leaders and not the women who decided on the available options and guided the women in making their decision. In this way, the ideology of "How to meet the needs of the Church" once again incorporated the women's desires as a "way of thinking of being at [someone's] disposal"[109] so that these would match the Church's interests as 'needs'.

The American sociologist of religion Peter L. Berger coined the term "heretic imperative"[110] for the in-between options – a term which is useful for describing the self-image of Lutheran women in the twentieth century. Recalling the meaning of the Greek term *hairesis* as selection or choice, he describes how the American Church landscape clearly distinguishes itself in that both the believers and potential members of the congregation face the necessity of choosing from the various options of parishes. This phenomenon is deeply linked to the foundation of the United States and without it the right to a free and personal practice of religion would be unthinkable. Whereas, until the beginning of the twentieth century, the Lutherans had based their Church

---

105 Professional Schools for Church Workers of The United Lutheran Church in America, Catalogue 1960–62, ELCA Archives, ULCA 61/6/1, Box 1, Folder 16.
106 Lutheran School For Church Workers, Lutheran Deaconess House and School Baltimore, Maryland, ELCA Archives, ULCA 22/8/1, Box 1, Folder 10.
107 Cf. Lundeen, Catherine, Lutheran Church in America, Deaconess Community of the Lutheran Church in America, Administrative History, ELCA Archives, LCA 108.
108 Cf. Winter, Mildred, Recollection II, p. 21.
109 Duden (2010), p. 451.
110 Cf. Wenzel (2007).

membership on their place of origin, this approach was seriously shaken up by World War I. Yet the history of the deaconess in the twentieth century reveals how the "remnants of the past [...] were adapted to the prevalent moral code"[111] by elevating the "value of success gained through competition",[112] which was regarded as an ultimate and original American value, to an orientation guide within the Church, so that advertisement, scientification, and the principle of selecting between options could presumably fill the gap previously filled by people's place of origin. The history of the motherhouse in Baltimore vividly illustrates the failure of these efforts. It neither managed to increase the number of deaconesses nor to bestow a clerical significance on its actions and its organisation. Instead, the financial and organisational reforms led by experts can be seen as rationalisation measures used by the people in charge to address the merciless competition that resulted from the clerical mergers. Women proved to be an institutional resource whose demands for improved working conditions and equal access to the Church labour market attracted particular attention at a time when there was a conspicuous shortage of labour. The experience and skills in (nursing) care that had given these women status and respect became invisible and even discredited in the wake of the substantial reorganisation. Their professional actions became the subject of interpretation by researchers in the humanities. The new orientation of clerical work doubtlessly secured women improved access to the clerical service sector. Yet because of the guiding ideology of 'How to meet the needs of the Church', the time women spent with families in need and the care they provided based on experience became a delimited professional asset in the competition for clerical and social significance within the Lutheran institution.

Conclusion in the context of the history of the deaconess motherhouses in West Germany

In hindsight we can see the enormous difficulties that the Lutheran deaconesses in Baltimore had been facing since the foundation of the motherhouse in 1885. In the nineteenth century in Germany, a model of Protestant parish care had been established that was based on the conviction that body and soul form a unit. Simultaneously, it opened up a field of work within the Church as an institution that incorporated a large area of tasks. Deaconess work was practised until the 1960s in West Germany. In contrast, the history of the *BMD* in the United States illustrates that the deaconesses could barely survive as an institution and had to sacrifice parish nursing care as an area of activity in the early decades of the twentieth century. At the same time, their work in households and similar locations was discredited or dismissed and thus made invisible. Yet the flipside of the coin was that the deaconesses' activities were increasingly supported by and based on scientific methods and

---

111 Berger (1962), p. 89.
112 Berger (1962), p. 47.

subsequently regarded more as a profession. The reasons for the German success and the American failure to import the German model of the mother-house stem from the interrelationships and differences in the modernisation processes in the clerical and social systems of both countries during the twentieth century. Professionalism, efficiency and standardisation were set as the goals during these developments. The result was contradictory for those women who, on both sides of the Atlantic, were at the centre of the transformation of the Lutheran Churches into religious social service centres within the market of professional care services in the twentieth century.

The conditions for establishing deaconess motherhouses in the nineteenth century in Germany and the US were fundamentally different. Germany was marked by a generally homogeneous religious landscape and the formation and shape of the nation state was closely linked to the existence of the two large Christian Churches.[113] This close connection provided the fertile ground for establishing numerous Protestant motherhouses that successfully represented a concept of nursing that combined care for both the patient's body and soul – a notion of nursing that had an impact on German care practices until the second half of the 1950s.[114] The key founding father was the Protestant pastor Theodor Fliedner who, in 1836 in Kaiserswerth, gave unmarried women the opportunity to receive training in nursing care and to be subsequently sent out into communities, to hospitals, or to private posts. He supplied the training and lifelong provision for the deaconesses while they, in return, had to commit their lives to the service of the motherhouse and its mission.

By contrast, American society was characterised by a vast religious diversity and variety. With the end of the *frontier*, around 1890, the different Christian congregations faced a situation in which they had to stand up to each other and hold their own within a limited space.[115] Within the Protestant denominations, in addition to the issue of the confession of faith, it was a person's origin that decided the parish to which he belonged. The parishes were united in rejecting the bureaucratic Church structures in their original countries of origin and Church life was characterised by an emphasis on independence. Nonetheless, the founding of the *BMD* illustrates that at the end of the nineteenth century Church leaders looked to Western Europe for their innovations within the Church organisation. However, in the US, the work of the deaconess as a parish sister was only successful in the first few years. During this time, the scope of deaconess work was assessable and was most often located in close proximity to the motherhouse, enabling the motherhouse to establish itself as an exemplary institution in Baltimore. It was structured like a family and provided a space for the sisters in which they could use their own experience and skills as women to respond to specific difficulties in the fami-

---

113 Cf. Lässig/Prätorius (2008), pp. 65–96.
114 Cf. Kreutzer (2014).
115 Cf. Lässig/Prätorius (2008).

lies and households that they served. They carried out a large number of tasks autonomously, and were apparently very happy doing so.

At the beginning of the twentieth century, this situation changed significantly. Since this female way of life was not very attractive to American women, there was a lack of suitable applicants for the formal women's ministry. Women who were interested in the Church preferred the training that was on offer to qualify for paid or voluntary positions within the Church, but they did not necessarily want to become deaconesses. Furthermore, in these years nursing care in the US was increasingly becoming established as a paid profession for women based on a secular and scientific view of disease, rather than on training founded on experience. Whereas in West Germany up until the 1960s there were still enough women who were willing to live their lives in a motherhouse and stick to training based on knowledge gained from experience, as early as the start of the twentieth century, the deaconesses of the *BMD* were faced with an approach to nursing care based on theoretical and scientific standards.[116] Ultimately, World War I marked the end of the successful period for deaconesses because when the US entered the war, the German immigrants were brought into disrepute and their Protestant parishes lost their integrational power. Furthermore, the *General Synod* united with several other Lutheran Churches.

In this context it is not surprising that the leadership based their actions on the question of 'How to meet the needs of the Church' so that they could tap into the established methodological skillsets provided by the sciences and humanities. Thus, psychological tests seemed to promise more suitable candidates, advertising ensured a higher number of candidates, academisation offered a higher training status and the secular scientific notion of disease provided better nursing care. Finally, a crucial method employed by the Church leadership during decision-making processes was to use surveys to analyse the 'needs within the Church' to gain a better understanding of the modernisation that was deemed necessary for the *BMD*. In this context, parish nursing had served its time because the parishes signalled no 'need', since they had enough secular nurses to take care of any patients. Religious education and administrative work became the professional focus, but there was still a lack of individuals seeking deaconess training.

During World War II and the first years after the war the deaconesses managed to define the interests of all women who worked within the Church as 'needs of the Church' and subsequently advanced the modernisation of the *BMD*. By banking on the professionalism of their work and by understanding the diaconate 'in a broader way' as a ministry for both women and men, the women themselves, along with the new merger of Lutheran Churches into the *LCA*, contributed significantly to a situation in which the very identity of the deaconess was called into question: "What is a deaconess?" The German model of a female diaconate had at last become obsolete.

---

116 Cf. Kreutzer (2012), pp. 221–243.

By contrast, in Germany, parish nursing care established itself as the central area of work for the motherhouses. It was based on a "broad understanding of need",[117] just as it had been for the American sisters during the early years. Due to a lack of men, there was no problem with recruitment until the 1950s, and in parishes, where deaconesses were often the only other full-time working female staff next to the male pastors, they were treated with the utmost respect and appreciation. They did not have to fear secular competitors and were able to stay largely unaffected by scientific and technological findings. Only during the 1960s did their 'labour of love' develop into a modern profession for women,[118] so that training based on experience lost its legitimacy and the lifelong security that the motherhouse granted the sisters was replaced by regular wages and fixed working hours: from that time life as a deaconess was regarded as outdated in West Germany. In contrast to the US, it was not the deaconesses who were the pioneers of what we might call a 'women's movement' within the Church, nor did they raise the issue of the status of women within the Church. In Germany, this question emanated from female theologians, who demanded access to the ministry.[119] However, the history of motherhouses in Germany and the US reveals unambiguously that while professionalisation and professionalism were the gates for women to enter employment in the Protestant Church, this only occurred at the cost of discrediting and renouncing both the status that had earned them appreciation and respect, and their broad, subordinate yet autonomous sphere of work.

Bibliography

Berger, Peter Ludwig: Kirche ohne Auftrag. Am Beispiel Amerikas. Stuttgart 1962.

Bourdieu, Pierre: What talking means. In: Sociology in question, translated by R. Nice. London 1993, pp. 60–71.

Boyer, Paul S.: American history. A very short introduction. Oxford 2012.

Bulmer, Martin: The decline of the social survey movement and the rise of American empirical sociology. In: Bales, Kevin; Bulmer, Martin; Kish Sklar, Kathryn (ed.): The social survey in historical perspective 1880–1940. Cambridge 1991, pp. 291–315.

Converse, Jean M: Survey research in the United States. Roots and Emergence 1890–1960. Berkeley; Los Angeles; London 1987, pp. 11–53.

Desrosière, Alain: The part in relation to the whole. How to generalise? The prehistory of representative sampling. In: Bales, Kevin; Bulmer, Martin; Kish Sklar, Kathryn (ed.): The social survey in historical perspective 1880–1940. Cambridge 1991, pp. 217–244.

Duden, Barbara: Von den liebsten Leichnamen. In: Tag, Brigitte; Groß, Dominique (ed.): Der Umgang mit der Leiche. Sektion und toter Körper in internationaler und interdisziplinärer Perspektive. Frankfurt/Main; New York 2010, pp. 447–461.

Fraser, Nancy; Gordon, Linda: A genealogy of 'dependency'. Tracing a keyword of the U.S. welfare state. In: Fraser, Nancy (ed.): Justice interruptus. Critical reflections on the 'postsocialist' condition. New York; London 1997, pp. 121–149.

---

117 Kreutzer (2010), p. 140.
118 Cf. Kreutzer (2005).
119 Cf. Riemann (2015).

Gräser, Marcus: Wohlfahrtsgesellschaft und Wohlfahrtsstaat. Bürgerliche Sozialreform und Welfare State Building in den USA und in Deutschland 1880–1940. Göttingen 2009.

Gronemeyer, Marianne: Die Macht der Bedürfnisse. Überfluss und Knappheit. Darmstadt 2002.

Heinemann, Isabel: "Concepts of motherhood". Öffentliche Debatten, Expertendiskurse und die Veränderung von Familienwerten in den USA (1890–1970). In: Zeithistorische Forschungen / Studies in Contemporary History, online edition, 8 (2011), 1, p. 3, <http://www.zeithistorische-forschungen.de/16126041-Heinemann-1-2011> accessed 28/07/2014.

Illich, Ivan: Bedürfnisse. In: Sachs, Wolfgang (ed.): Wie im Westen so auf Erden. Ein polemisches Handbuch zur Entwicklungspolitik. Hamburg 1993, pp. 47–70.

Kim-Warrzinek, Utta; Müller, Johann-Baptist: Bedürfnis. In: Brunner, Otto; Conze, Werner; Koselleck, Reinhart (ed.): Geschichtliche Grundbegriffe. Historisches Lexikon zur politisch-sozialen Sprache in Deutschland. Vol. 1, Stuttgart 1972, pp. 440–489.

Köser, Silke: Eine Diakonisse darf kein Alltagsmensch sein. Kollektive Identitäten Kaiserswerther Diakonissen 1836–1914. Leipzig 2006.

Kreutzer, Susanne: Vom "Liebesdienst" zum modernen Frauenberuf. Die Reform der Krankenpflege nach 1945. Frankfurt/Main; New York 2005.

Kreutzer, Susanne: Nursing body and soul in the parish. Lutheran deaconess motherhouses in Germany and the United States. In: Nursing History Review 18 (2010), pp. 134–150.

Kreutzer, Susanne: Rationalisierung evangelischer Krankenpflege. Westdeutsche und US-amerikanische Diakonissenmutterhäuser im Vergleich, 1945–1970. In: Medizinhistorisches Journal 47 (2012), pp. 221–243.

Kreutzer, Susanne: Arbeits- und Lebensalltag evangelischer Krankenpflege. Organisation, soziale Praxis und biographische Erfahrungen, 1945–1980. Göttingen 2014.

Lässig, Simone; Prätorius, Rainer: Religion, Glaube und Kirche. In: Mauch, Christof / Patel, Kiran Klaus (ed.): Der Wettlauf um die Moderne. Die USA und Deutschland 1890 bis heute. Munich 2008, pp. 65–96.

Meuser, Fred W.: Facing the twentieth century. In: Nelson, E. Clifford (ed.): The Lutherans in America. Philadelphia 1980, pp. 359–541.

Nelson, E. Clifford: The church in war and in peace. In: Nelson, E. Clifford (ed.): The Lutherans in America. Philadelphia 1980, pp. 472–494.

Osborne, Thomas; Rose, Nikolas: Do the social sciences create phenomena? The example of public opinion research. In: British Journal of Sociology 50 (1999), 3, pp. 365–396.

Rendtorff, Trutz: Beruf. In: Ritter, Joachim (ed.): Historisches Wörterbuch der Philosophie, Vol. 1. Freiburg; Stuttgart 1971, Col. 833–835.

Riemann, Doris: Protestantische Geschlechtergeschichte und sozialtechnische Modernisierung. Zur Geschichte der Pfarrfrauen. Leipzig 2015.

Wenzel, Uwe Justus: "Wir sind alle Häretiker. Eine Erörterung der Frage: Was ist eine gute Religion?" In: Neue Züricher Zeitung 26/05/2007.

Zerull, Lisa [Martha]: Nursing out of the parish. A history of the Baltimore lutheran deaconesses 1893–1911. Michigan 2011.

Archives

Evangelical Lutheran Church in America (ELCA) Archives
ULCA 61 United Lutheran Church in America
ULCA 22 Board of Deaconess Work
ULCA 2/1 United Lutheran Church in America Convention Minutes
ELCA 127 Deaconess Community of the ELCA

Deaconess nurses in Germany, Sweden, and the United States. Transformations of a female model of life and work in the twentieth century

Susanne Kreutzer

The deaconess motherhouses – as they were founded in Germany in the nineteenth century – saw themselves as communities of faith and service. Their members were unmarried women who regarded their work as a 'labour of love' rooted in Christian faith, rather than as a means of earning a livelihood. To be a sister encompassed their entire life, which also meant sharing the values and behavioural code of the community. The deaconess motherhouses represented a specific understanding of nursing that was based on caring for the body and the soul as one entity. In addition to the nursing activities in the stricter sense, the sisters also performed pastoral tasks. Thus, the deaconesses' work was situated between the tasks of physicians and pastors.

The training of the deaconesses also had a dual objective: as well as teaching the sisters nursing techniques and medical knowledge, an important goal was to form the 'personality of the nurse'. A 'good' nurse had to be a nurse 'at heart' and this – according to the concept of the training – could not be developed through theoretical instruction but only through practical hands-on work and the life within the community of sisters.

This model could not be transferred in its entirety to other countries and during the twentieth century it came increasingly under pressure. The following depiction[1] investigates the transformation of the work and life model of a deaconess in Germany, Sweden, and the US during the twentieth century when the framework of Protestant nursing care underwent fundamental, albeit different, changes in all three countries. The key changes were: the establishment of a scientific understanding of disease, a forced professionalisation, specialisation and increased use of technology in nursing care, changes in gender relations, and finally the expansion of the welfare state. Due to these societal changes, the motherhouses in all three countries faced new challenges that varied according to the national context. This article pursues the question of how the deaconess motherhouses dealt with these challenges in Germany, Sweden and the US. To what extent did they develop different concepts of nursing care and how can we explain these differences? The organisation of nursing training is of particular interest.

By focusing on Germany, Sweden and the US we are able to investigate three different paths of development of the motherhouse diaconia. In Germany the motherhouse system of the nineteenth century succeeded as the dominant organisational form of nursing, and the Christian model of uniting

1   This article is based on a project funded by the *German Research Foundation* on the topic: Rationalisation of nursing care in West Germany and the United States: A comparative history of the exchanges of ideas and practices, 1945 to 1975.

care of body and soul shaped the history of nursing in West Germany until the second half of the 1950s. By contrast, in the US nursing became a gainful occupation for (unmarried) women as early as the nineteenth century and the idea of basing healthcare on scientific standards fell on fertile ground. The deaconess motherhouses were merely a footnote. Finally, in Sweden in the nineteenth century the deaconesses played a central role in establishing both a healthcare system and systematic training in nursing care. Yet, at the end of the nineteenth century, the life and work model of the deaconesses came under noticeable pressure and became gradually less important.

One Lutheran motherhouse shall serve as an example for each country: firstly, I look at the *Henriettenstiftung* in Hanover, Germany, which was founded in 1859/60 and transformed into the largest deaconess motherhouse in the region of Lower Saxony. The deaconesses worked in numerous hospitals and parish nurse stations all over Lower Saxony and Schleswig Holstein. Secondly, I analyse the American deaconess motherhouse in Philadelphia that was founded in 1884 and followed the German tradition. The motherhouse in Philadelphia developed into the largest institution for deaconesses in the US, focussing its central area of work on hospital nursing care. Thirdly, I introduce the *Ersta* deaconess motherhouse in Stockholm, Sweden, that began its work as early as 1851 – that is only 15 years after the motherhouse in Kaiserswerth had been established. It provided nurses for hospitals, parish nurse stations and other social institutions all over Sweden.

At this point it should be noted that this article is based on varying degrees of knowledge of the individual motherhouses. I conducted a systematic transfer-history research project on the German and American motherhouses, analysing the extensive archives of the motherhouses, including personal records, documents written by the nurses, and files on the structure of the motherhouses, the training and the sisters' areas of work. By contrast, the remarks on the Swedish deaconess motherhouse are mainly based on my analysis of the scattered corpus of research on the history of nursing and deaconesses in Sweden. Until now I have been able to conduct only initial research at the *Ersta* deaconess institution in Stockholm, focussing on the training the nurses received.

Deaconesses in Germany: A success story lasting into the second half of the twentieth century

In Germany, the life and work model of the deaconesses shaped the history of nursing until well into the second half of the twentieth century. There had been new formations of so-called 'free' communities of nurses founded at the end of the nineteenth century, which offered their members more independence. Nonetheless, the position of the motherhouses was untouched for a long period of time. Not even the anti-church politics of the National Socialists had been able to change this. National Socialism made it difficult for Protestant – as well as Catholic – motherhouse organisations to recruit new members, in particular because the denominational institutions were suspected of promoting an 'unworthy' life due to their belief in Christian love. Yet, as an organisation, the motherhouses remained intact. Immediately after the war, the deaconess motherhouses experienced a real boom of new recruits. During the hard times of the post-war years they offered women an attractive training and benefits package. This applied particularly to many young female refugees who came to the Western occupation zones from the former Eastern territories of the German Reich. The motherhouses offered them not only financial stability but also a new social home.[2]

The high regard for denominational nursing increased during the post-war period because, in contrast to 'free', independent nurses, the Christian nurses were not suspected of having been actively involved in the National Socialist politics of genocide.[3] A Christian ethos was therefore regarded as a guarantee of a 'good', caring type of nursing. Even public hospitals were very interested in delegating nursing care to Christian nurses because such a move had a positive effect on the reputation of the hospital.

Furthermore, the West German welfare state granted denominational institutions a privileged position. Independent welfare organisations received public funds and support from the state after World War I.[4] The *subsidiarity principle* – the policy of giving preference to independent welfare organisations over public welfare bodies – had its roots in the Weimar welfare state (1918–1933) and was finally and fully recognised in the Federal Republic of Germany. It rewarded hospitals that had a specifically charitable approach to welfare.[5]

In this context, the deaconesses succeeded in preserving their tradition from the nineteenth century until well into the post-war period. This became particularly apparent in the training of the next generation. From the beginning of the twentieth century, and initially in Prussia, training in the area of nursing was subject to some initial regulations.[6] Yet the motherhouses managed to restrict that influence to a large extent. Until the middle of the 1960s,

2   Kreutzer (2014), pp 60–66.
3   The largest 'free' community of nurses, the professional organisation of nurses in Germany, had been dissolved in 1938. Its successor was the *Association of Free Nurses and Carers of the German Reich* (*Reichsbund freier Schwestern und Pflegerinnen*) that had a National Socialist leadership. Because of the colour of their uniform, the nurses of the *Reichsbund* were called Blue Nurses. In 1942, the distinction between Blue and Brown Nurses became obsolete when both groups united into the *NS Reich Association of German Nurses* (*NS-Reichsbund deutscher Schwestern*). For this reason, at the end of World War II, it was no longer possible to distinguish between former members of the professional organisation and Brown Nurses. Cf. Steppe (2001), pp. 65–66. The fact that deaconess motherhouses were regarded as politically unsuspicious after World War II does not mean, however, that the deaconesses had not been involved in implementing National Socialist health and population policies. For instance, enforced sterilisations were also conducted in deaconess hospitals. On the history of deaconess motherhouses during National Socialism, cf. Kaminsky (1995) and Lauterer (1994).
4   Cf. Kaiser (2008), p. 60.
5   Cf. Schmuhl (2010), p. 162.
6   Cf. Schweikardt (2008).

the legal guidelines provided only a rough framework, such as prerequisites, duration of the training, and the number of hours of theoretical instruction. The *Nursing Act* of 1938, which regulated the training requirements, required only 200 hours of theory, spread out over one and a half years. By 1957 the training time had increased to three years but the proportion of theory was still quite small – now 450 hours.[7]

Students spent the majority of their training doing practical work on the wards. They learned the necessary skills from the older nurses and simultaneously absorbed their work ethic.[8] The nurse trainer at the *Henriettenstiftung* who was in charge of the deaconess students explained in 1954 that the proper pastoral attitude was "not only taught through services and sermons or in the courses and other classes […] but from the first day onwards through the entire atmosphere of the house, the exchanges between the sisters and the role model the older sisters represent".[9]

The high value placed on practical training is apparent even in the structure of the curriculum. The students were sent to the wards from their very first day at the school. They had some individual lessons with physicians ("doctor hours") that took place preferably during the lunch break or in the evening when everybody involved was tired. The main part of the theoretical training took place as one block towards the end of the programme. There were no legal regulations for the practical training, i. e. the main portion of the programme, and the *Henriettenstiftung* was able to design the curriculum for nursing training largely as it saw fit. All roles that were crucial for the training of the next generation, i. e. teaching staff and especially the ward nurses who supervised the practical training, were filled by deaconesses. Students who completed their training at the beginning of the 1950s at the *Henriettenstiftung* were firmly integrated into the community of deaconesses on site. This applied even to students who did not want to become deaconesses, but only chose to complete their nursing training in a Protestant institution.[10]

The erosion of the life and work model of the deaconess in West Germany during the 'long 1960s'[11]

Only from the end of the 1950s did the Christian understanding of nursing start to come under pressure in West Germany, when West German society as a whole underwent fundamental changes.[12] The original and guiding princi-

7   Cf. Kreutzer (2005), pp. 231, 246.
8   Cf. Kreutzer (2014), pp. 157–165.
9   Sister Martha Koch, On the basic principles. Presentation given at the general meeting of the sisters on 28/06/1954, Archive of the Henriettenstiftung, S - 4.
10 Cf. Kreutzer (2006), pp. 161–168.
11 For a while, the year 1968 was regarded as a deep rupture in the history of West Germany. Newer time-historical accounts embed 1968 into a longer transformational period: the so-called 'long 1960s' spanning the period from 1958/59 to 1973/74.
12 Cf. among others Frese/Paulus (2003), Herbert (2007), and Schildt (2007), pp. 30–53.

ple of the celibate 'labour of love' rapidly lost its support. The ideal of self-sacrifice was increasingly at odds with the emerging consumer society. Hardly
any woman was willing to dedicate her entire life to altruistically serving her
neighbour, and the influx of new applicants dried up almost completely. As a
result of the growing wealth of West German society, it was possible to expand
the healthcare sector significantly.[13] Yet there was a serious threat that the new
hospitals could be jeopardised by the increasing shortage of nurses. If the
hospitals wanted to attract new nurses and keep them in the profession, they
had to adapt the working conditions to the life plans of the new generation of
women. This changed the essence of the traditional Christian understanding
of nursing.

During the 1960s, nursing was changed into a female profession regulated
by labour laws and wage contracts with fixed working hours and wage categories.[14] Even Christian hospitals had to follow the new zeitgeist if they wanted
to attract and retain nursing staff. Particularly significant were the reductions
in weekly working hours that had been implemented in 1956/57. These reductions were the starting point for comprehensive rationalisation measures
in nursing because working time developed into a precious possession that
had to be treated efficiently. The manager of the *Annastift Hospital* in Hanover,
where deaconesses from the *Henriettenstiftung* worked, explained in 1957 in
the journal *Die evangelische Krankenpflege* (*Protestant Nursing*) that the introduction of shorter working hours was a clear sign "that the internal production
reserves of the people working at the hospital had to be fully exhausted".[15]
This fundamentally changed the understanding of nursing care. The nurse
was transformed from a servant of God into an economic factor of production. By extracting nursing from its religious interpretation and moving it into
the context of industrial production, the profession was opened up to the logic
of economic cost-benefit calculations.

Furthermore, a biomedical understanding of medicine based on scientific
concepts also found its way into the Christian hospitals of West Germany in
the 1960s.[16] The new physicians were not really interested in working with
religious deaconesses and demanded to work with nurses who matched the
professional standards of the modern hospitals equipped with new technology.

The *Nursing Act* of 1965 reflected this development. The theoretical part of
the training was increased significantly to 1,200 hours in total. In addition, the
Henriettenstiftung now organised the theoretical training in parallel with the
practical work. Thus, learning the theory became a regular component of the
curriculum. The practical training was also more strictly regulated. A card
system was introduced to structure the order of learning: each card stated

---

13   The number of hospital beds increased from 575,300 in 1956 to 665,500 in 1968, cf.
      Krukemeyer (1988), pp. 85, 98–99.
14   Cf. Kreutzer (2005), pp. 164–229.
15   Arnstorf (1957), p. 53.
16   Cf. Kreutzer (2014), pp. 93–101.

what tasks the students had to learn in which semester.[17] The new control measures document the increasing mistrust of the traditional practices, which were based on the experiences the nurses had gained in their everyday work on the wards. In addition, they illustrate the fact that the *Henriettenstiftung* was slowly departing from its traditional understanding of education and training, which had centred around establishing ethical conduct in the everyday work and life practices of the nurses, rather than on learning standardised skills that could be tested.

When a more scientific understanding of disease took hold, the nursing staff began to focus more on caring for the body. The tasks that fell under care of the soul were transferred entirely to the pastors' area of competence and it was the pastors who now provided spiritual care in the hospitals. This meant a separation of physical and spiritual care – two areas that had been inextricably linked until then. In contrast to deaconesses, the hospital chaplains had not been integrated into the everyday practice on the ward. In addition, hospital chaplains looked after numerous patients. During the 1970s in the deaconess motherhouse of the *Henriettenstiftung* they had to care for more than 120 patients, while also performing other tasks such as holding services and fulfilling roles in the training and further education facilities.[18] As a general rule, there will not have been much time for the individual patient. Furthermore, as Dreßke and Göckenjan have shown in a study, if the help of hospital chaplains was called for, they were regarded not as part of a religious service but as a psychosocial service.[19] The care for the soul that had previously been practised by the deaconesses had now lost its established position within patient care – both in the daily care of the patients and also in the self-understanding and the organisational logic of the scientifically oriented hospitals.

Deaconesses in the US: How the model failed

Whereas in Germany the motherhouse principle of the nineteenth century became the dominant organisational form of nursing, institutions for deaconesses in the US were rather unsuccessful.[20] The first attempt at establishing a Protestant motherhouse in Pittsburgh towards the end of the 1840s failed due to a lack of apprentices.[21] Only at the end of the 1880s was there a successful,

---

17 Cf. Kreutzer (2006), pp. 176–177.
18 Principal Pastor Helbig, Report on the work of the Henriettenstiftung, presented at the committee meeting on 04/12/1974, Archive of the Henriettenstiftung, S-9-3-2; Work report Pastor Schomerus, n. d. [1977/78], Archive of the Henriettenstiftung, S-9-3-2.
19 Cf. Göckenjan/Dreßke (2005), p. 246.
20 Cf. Nelson (2003), pp. 134–142. Compare also the article by Doris Riemann in this volume.
21 Cf. Köser (2006), p. 118, and Doyle (1929).

yet modest wave of new institutions for deaconesses.[22] One of them was the *Philadelphia Motherhouse of Deaconesses*, which, despite being the largest deaconess motherhouse in the US, had only 109 nurses in 1946 – approximately one fifth of the membership of the *Henriettenstiftung*.[23] The US American deaconesses thus always formed a minority.

Initially, the *Philadelphia Motherhouse of Deaconesses* followed the German model and was set up as a motherhouse system by seven deaconesses who had been specifically recruited from Germany.[24] The main area of work for the sisters was the *Lankenau Hospital* (until 1917: *German Hospital*) which had originally been set up to provide for the German immigrants in the area. It also served as a training hospital for the deaconesses. In terms of institutional ownership, the sisters of the *Philadelphia Motherhouse of Deaconesses* were in a weaker position locally than those at the *Henriettenstiftung*.

At the *Henriettenstiftung* in Hanover, the hospital and nursing school belonged to the sisters as a matter of course. In Philadelphia, the motherhouse was closely connected to the *Lankenau Hospital*[25] but the sisters did not own it. Rather, the motherhouse agreed in a contract to provide the hospital with nurses. Thus in Philadelphia – unlike Hanover – the deaconesses were not the owners of the institution but only contractual partners. The hospital itself belonged to a public body.

The position of the American deaconesses was further weakened by the fact that the *Lankenau Hospital* saw itself explicitly as a non-denominational institution. Since it had originally been founded as a *German Hospital*, it had been conceptualised as a place the entire German community in Philadelphia could use. In contrast to the *Henriettenstiftung*, a distinctly Protestant orientation of the nursing students would have been less welcome here. This became evident when the nursing school of the *Lankenau Hospital* hired Ida F. Giles, a leading representative of the professionalisation movement in Pennsylvania, as the full-time teaching nurse in 1909.[26] As a result, even future deaconesses received their training from a secular nurse – a situation that would have been unthinkable at the *Henriettenstiftung* even in the 1950s.

22 These were in particular the motherhouses in Philadelphia, Brooklyn, Omaha, Minneapolis, Milwaukee, Baltimore, Chicago, St. Paul, Brush, and Axtell, cf. Weiser (1960), p. 168. On the foundation of the motherhouse in Baltimore cf. Zerull (2010).

23 In 1946 the total number of deaconesses in the US was 450. Minutes of the Fifteenth Biennial Convention of the United Lutheran Church in America, Cleveland, Ohio, 5–12.10.1946, p. 545, Archive of the Evangelical Lutheran Church of America (ELCA-Archives), ULCA 2/1, Box 5. In 1949 the *Henriettenstiftung* alone had 650 sisters. Retrospective on the year 1949, Archive of the Henriettenstiftung, S-8-8.

24 Cf. Schweikardt (2010).

25 Cf. Schweikardt (2010).

26 Sister Louise Burroughs, A Short History of the Lankenau Hospital School of Nursing, 22.4.1974, Barbara Bates Center for the Study of the History of Nursing, School of Nursing, University of Pennsylvania (Bates Center archives), MC 98, Series I, Box 1, Folder 2.

The transformation of Protestant nursing care in the US during the twentieth century

As the recruitment of Ida F. Giles in 1909 shows, the deaconesses in the US came under the pressure of professionalisation much sooner than the *Henriettenstiftung*. The fact that, in the US, the development of the health insurance system did not start until the 1940s had far-reaching consequences for the history of Protestant nursing.[27] Only hospitals that offered the best possible patient care were able to survive the competition when it came to attracting the few affluent, paying patients. The so-called standardisation movement that went beyond the healthcare profession, was promoted in the healthcare system mainly by secular organisations and here foremost by the *American College of Surgeons*. At the beginning of the twentieth century it made sure that the standards of 'good' nursing care were based on a biomedical understanding of nursing.[28] American hospitals at that time were therefore mostly interested in professionally qualified nurses.

Because they were so few in number, the American deaconess motherhouses were not in a position to counter this development. Even the Catholic sisterhoods, which were much bigger than the deaconess institutions, followed the general trend for standardisation at the beginning of the twentieth century.[29] If the deaconess motherhouses wanted to train a workforce that was in demand and if they wanted to offer an appealing training programme to the young women, they had to adapt to these new requirements. While the costs of the standardisation process were a subject of controversy at the beginning of the twentieth century, during the 1920s the criticism gave way to broad approval. For instance, the head nurse of the *Lankenau Hospital*, deaconess Marie Koeneke, followed the contemporary trend and published 'Nursing Procedures' in 1927 that established standardised working processes for nursing such as bathing, bedding and catheterising of patients, measuring pulse and temperature and distributing drugs.[30]

In contrast to the *Henriettenstiftung*, the school of the *Lankenau Hospital* already regarded a professional qualification very highly at the beginning of the twentieth century. This perspective determined the further development of the school. The first curriculum from Philadelphia that has been preserved is from 1925/26 and it already contains a preparatory course with 300 hours of theory to prepare the students for their practical work. This curriculum also included an introduction to psychology.[31] Thus there were obviously early efforts to make personal dealings with the patients more scientific.[32] At the

---

27   Cf. Stevens (1999), p. 259.
28   Cf. Mann Wall (2005), pp. 167–171.
29   Cf. Mann Wall (2005), pp. 175–185 and Kaufmann (1995), pp. 168–192.
30   Cf. Koeneke (1927).
31   Lankenau Hospital Training School for Nurses, Curriculum, 1925–1926, Bates Center archives, MC 98, Series III, Box 20, Folder 152.
32   In West Germany only the training and examination regulations of 1966 required an introduction into psychology, pedagogy and sociology. Cf. Ausbildungs- und Prüfungsord-

beginning of the 1950s the theoretical part of the training comprised a total of 900 hours.[33] In 1962, the school had 13 teaching nurses who all held an academic degree. Five of them were deaconesses. The school also employed its own librarian.[34]

The willingness of the *Lankenau Hospital* to align its nursing training with the scientific standards of the time was further supported by the accreditation process of the nursing schools. As in Germany at the beginning of the twentieth century, nursing training in the US became subject to federal regulation, which however was much stricter than in Germany. From the beginning of the twentieth century, the *State Board of Examiners for Registration of Nurses* set the requirements for the training curricula and the general training and working conditions for nursing students. In the 1920s in Pennsylvania, the *State Board* consisted of leading proponents of the concept of nursing as a profession based on science, rather than as a skill acquired by experience.[35] The *State Board* not only gradually increased requirements for the theoretical and practical training; it also began to regulate the living conditions in the dormitories of the nurses, e. g. the minimum size of the accommodation.[36] Those schools that did not pass the check-ups by the *State Board* lost their federal approval, after which they found it very difficult to attract further trainees.

Particularly effective for the implementation of new training standards were comparisons between the nursing schools, i. e. the rankings the schools received from the *State Board* to ensure greater transparency of the performance of the various institutions. The ranking system did much to promote competition between the schools.[37]

After 1945 the accreditation process of the *National League for Nursing* – the association of leading teachers in nursing schools and colleges – was added, which, from the 1950s onwards, became *the* quality label. The fact that

---

nung für Krankenschwestern, Krankenpfleger und Kinderkrankenschwestern [Training and Examination Regulations for Nurses and Paediatric Nurses] (1966), Section 1, Paragraph 2, p. 462.

33 Lankenau Hospital Training School for Nurses, Curriculum, 1950–51, Bates Center archives, MC 98, Series III, Box 20, Folder 152.

34 The leading teaching nurse, Ada Mutch, had a master's degree in nursing didactics from the *Teachers College of Columbia University* in New York – the 'motherhouse of college education' in the US. Her deputy, the deaconess Sister Amalie Schaeffer, held a bachelor's degree in nursing didactics from *Temple University* in Philadelphia. State Board of Nursing Education and Licensure, Department of Public Instruction, Annual Report of School of Nursing for the Year Ending May 31, 1962, Bates Center archives, MC 98, Series III, Box 14, Folder 61.

35 Cf. West (1939), p. 120–141.

36 Pennsylvania State Board of Nurse Examiners, Handbook for Schools of Nursing in the Commonwealth of Pennsylvania, 1952, Bates Center archives, MC 98, Series III, Box 22, Folder 190; Commonwealth of Pennsylvania, Department of Public Instruction, Mary A. Rothrock and Mr Hosford, Administrator of Lankenau Hospital, 05/07/1955, Bates Center archives, MC 98, Series III, Box 15, Folder 66.

37 Minutes of the Nursing Committee of the Board of Trustees, 11/06/1951, Lankenau Hospital archives.

the *Lankenau Hospital* participated in the very first accreditation process of the *National League* in 1951/52 illustrates that the hospital did not wait for external pressure before it decided to take part. Rather it wanted to be one of the first institutions to differentiate itself from its competitors with the new quality seal of the *National League*.[38]

The *National League for Nursing* consistently increased the requirements for the theoretical training of both the students and the teachers and thus massively interfered with the training practice of the nursing schools. While the *State Board* followed the logic of minimum standards and mainly controlled the standardised framework, such as the number of working hours, the breakdown of the lessons within the curriculum, and the size of the rooms for students, the *National League* targeted a meticulous regulation of the nursing training and organisational structure of the nursing schools to promote 'excellence' in nursing training.[39] For this reason the nursing schools suspected that the policies of the *National League* were designed to force nursing training out of the hospitals and into the realm of higher education. Indeed, small nursing schools in particular struggled to survive from the middle of the 1950s onwards due to the – in their opinion – excessive demands of the *National League*.[40]

Under the pressure of the accreditation process, the nursing school of the *Lankenau Hospital* became an increasingly bureaucratic organisation that tried to fulfil the requirements of the *National League* with a new committee structure. A significant part of the work of the numerous school committees seems to have been to keep defining new working goals and to check whether targets were reached. To this end, they used an ongoing evaluation and self-evaluation process that included the teachers, the students and the committees themselves.[41] These optimisation practices resulted in an incredibly large portfolio of files has been preserved from the nursing school in Philadelphia. By contrast, the *Henriettenstiftung* left hardly any documents, since its teaching nurses could teach as they saw fit until the 1960s, based on their own experience.

In addition to representatives of professional organisations in the US becoming active in the *State Board* and the *National League for Nursing*, the state itself became increasingly active in the professionalisation and academisation process. The US economy was strengthened after World War II. In this time of new affluence the university system and the entire healthcare system was

---

38 Minutes of the Nursing Committee of the Board of Trustees, 09/07/1951, Lankenau Hospital archives; National League for Nursing, Division of Nursing Education, Accrediting Your School of Nursing, 1956, Bates Center archives, MC 98, Series III, Box 10, Folder 7.

39 National League for Nursing, Department of Diploma and Associate Degree Programs, Towards Excellence in Nursing Education. A Guide for Diploma School Improvement, 1964, Bates Center archives, MC 98, Series III, Box 10, Folder 7.

40 Minutes of the Nursing Committee of the Board of Trustees, 17/03/1958, Lankenau Hospital archives.

41 Protocols of the curriculum committee, Bates Center archives, MC 98, Series IV, Box 36, Folder 46 to 51.

expanded. The proportion of people with health insurance increased from approximately a quarter of the population in 1945 to about 70 per cent in 1960.[42] Socially disadvantaged groups had better access to healthcare when, in 1965, the social security programmes *Medicare* and *Medicaid* were introduced. Along with this development the demand for nursing staff increased and at the same time there was a demand to improve the quality of nursing care. From 1964 onwards, there were federal funds specifically for the establishment of nursing care programmes and students in nursing could also receive student loans.[43] For colleges and universities it thus paid well to set up degrees in nursing care.

At the same time, many hospitals began to recalculate the costs of their nursing schools. Under the pressure of the accreditation process many schools had become expensive affairs that were no longer sustainable in the eyes of the healthcare providers. During the 1960s, many hospitals closed their schools. This development further supported the trend towards a more academic approach.[44] At the *Lankenau Hospital*, that continuance of the nursing school was not seriously put up for renegotiation during the time period under investigation – possibly due to the lasting tradition of the deaconesses.

In the context of the general trend towards academisation, from the middle of the 1960s onwards the school found it increasingly difficult to attract new students. As a result, it began to conduct some of its training in cooperation with nearby colleges, to increase the attractiveness of the training programme.[45] It was not until 1992 that the *Lankenau Hospital* closed down the school completely – at a time when less than ten per cent of future nurses opted to attend a nursing school linked to the hospital.[46]

Deaconesses in Sweden: A success story in the nineteenth century

In contrast to the US, the deaconess motherhouses in the Lutheran Scandinavian countries were very successful during the nineteenth century. The first Swedish deaconess motherhouse was established in 1851 in Stockholm – only 15 years after the foundation of the motherhouse in Kaiserswerth. The *Society for the Preparation of a Deaconess Institution in Stockholm* drew heavily on the German programme of the *Inner Mission* and considered nursing care as an essential vehicle for converting the population. For this reason, the nurses were to be trained mainly in physical and spiritual care.[47]

---

42   Cf. Stevens (1999), p. 259.
43   Cf. Lynaugh (2008), pp. 13–28.
44   Cf. Mann Wall (2011), pp. 13–15.
45   Minutes of the Nursing Committee of the Board of Trustees, 8.9.1969, Bates Center archives, MC 98, Series IV, Box 42, Folder 97.
46   "Lankenau Nursing School Closes When Freshman Class Graduates", Main Line Times, 01/02/1990, Bates Center archives, MC 98, Series III, Box 11, Folder 18.
47   Cf. Green (2011), pp. 38–39.

The motherhouse developed into a significant agent for expanding the healthcare system and professionalising nursing care in Sweden. After modest beginnings, Stockholm saw the development of a large deaconess hospital that received financial support for its new construction in 1907 from the city council. In return, the hospital provided beds to take care of the city's impoverished citizens.[48] In addition, the hospital served as a training hospital for the deaconesses.

The deaconess institution was the first institution in Sweden that offered any kind of systematic training in nursing, even though it was conceptualised more as an all-round programme for all tasks linked to nursing and social work. Such a broad, non-specialised qualification was important for enabling the sisters to work as flexibly as possible after their graduation, in any area of the larger institution for deaconesses. Some deaconesses worked locally in Stockholm. Most sisters, however, were sent to hospitals, parishes, orphanages or other social institutions all over Sweden. Usually they took on a leading role there and thus were highly influential in the everyday life of these houses. As Todd Green has shown, in the nineteenth century, deaconesses were regarded as highly qualified and sought-after workers. Only rarely do we find complaints about eager missionary efforts by the sisters. Overall, the motherhouse struggled to even barely meet the demand for deaconesses.[49]

The transformation of Protestant nursing care in Sweden during the twentieth century

In the middle of the nineteenth century, the institution for deaconesses in Stockholm occupied a pioneering position in the training of nurses in Sweden. However, it subsequently lost this significant function. From approximately 1870 onwards, the institution faced competition. New training facilities emerged that drew on English nursing traditions and Florence Nightingale. One of these was the nursing school of the *Red Cross* in Uppsala and another the *Sophia Home* (*Sophiahemmet*) in Stockholm. Both institutions adopted some elements of the motherhouse: for example, the *Sophia Home* was also structured as a surrogate family, the sisters lived in celibacy and wore the same uniform, and the *Sophia Home* sent them to their ultimate work destinations.[50] To that extent, the deaconess tradition lived on. In contrast to the institution for deaconesses, however, the young women received a more secular and more specialised training, and those who started their education here could be certain of working as nurses after their graduation. Finally, the *Sophia Home* offered noticeably better pay than the deaconess motherhouse and began to expand the theoretical part of the training at a very early stage. With these changes, the *Sophia Home* succeeded in establishing itself as the leading train-

48   Cf. Green (2011), pp. 128–33.
49   Cf. Green (2011), pp. 139–141.
50   Cf. Bohm (1972), pp. 153–154.

ing institution for nursing. It successfully drew in daughters of the upper class who were purposefully trained to take on leading roles in nursing.[51] While the deaconess motherhouse still offered thorough training, it slowly lost its importance.

As Andersson shows in her analysis of the concept of a female calling in the Swedish history of nursing, another factor was that, at the beginning of the twentieth century, a more secular understanding of a calling took hold, and nursing increasingly gained the qualities of a secular profession, which nonetheless still posed special requirements on its members. These included first and foremost the capacity for self-sacrifice.[52] In Sweden – as in Germany – there was still the unchanged expectation at the beginning of the twentieth century that nurses had to adapt their lives to the needs of their patients. Naturally the women were unmarried, lived in the flats provided by the hospitals, and effectively worked around the clock.[53]

When, in 1910, the *Swedish Society of Nursing* (*Svensk Sjuksköterskeförening*) was founded as a professional organisation of caregivers, it initially promoted a non-occupational concept of nursing. Even at the beginning of the 1920s, the *Swedish Society of Nursing* still strongly opposed shorter working hours in nursing because, it argued, on the one hand patient care would suffer and, on the other hand, the profession of nursing would lose its special characteristic that had differentiated it from other occupations. The *Swedish Society of Nursing* saw its main task not in shaping the working conditions but in working for longer training with a better theoretical basis.[54]

The argument of the nurses' special position in society lost its persuasive power, however, as early as the 1930s. The image of female nurses as a special and unique group of professionals was increasingly at odds with the concept of the developing Swedish welfare state, which emphasised equality and aimed at a standardisation of living conditions.[55]

Another complicating factor for the deaconesses was that the Swedish social-democratic welfare state was by default sceptical about any Christian charity endeavour, regarding it as unprofessional.[56] Social tasks were supposed to be handled by the state and the idea was to restrict denominational charity, if possible, exclusively to the realm of the Church. The conflicts between Protestant nursing traditions and governmental social policy that drew on scientific ideas emerged most obviously in the domain of parish nursing. Since the 1920s the Swedish councils had been employing more and more public health nurses, who threatened to supersede the deaconesses. At the end of the 1930s, the whole country was divided into districts. Each district had to hire a public health nurse who had undergone special training. Deaconesses without ap-

---

51   Cf. Andersson (2002), pp. 92–102.
52   Cf. Andersson (2002), pp. 63–70.
53   Cf. Emanuelsson (1990), p. 62.
54   Cf. Bohm (1972), p. 213, Nicklasson (1995), pp. 284–285 and Emanuelsson (1990), p. 98.
55   Cf. Kolbe (2002), pp. 35–40.
56   Cf. Christiansson (2006), pp. 141–143.

propriate training were no longer employed. This regulation put the deaconesses under immense pressure to professionalise and many sisters were sent for further training. This is just one example of how the Swedish welfare state began to influence the training and nursing practice of deaconesses.[57]

Pressure to professionalise also increased for the schools providing training in nursing care. As early as the 1930s, the Swedish nursing schools were offering training that lasted three years.[58] In 1952, the Swedish deaconess motherhouse split its training programme into two separate tracks: one for nursing and one for social work.[59] This specialisation of the educational programme marked a clear break from the German training tradition that had been based on an all-encompassing schooling of the nurses. The detailed training regulations in which the Swedish health administration laid down the structure for nursing care training at the beginning of the 1950s speak of the comparatively high level of professionalisation. 800 hours of theory were intended, including psychology.[60] In Sweden, the denominational institutions in particular emphasised the high significance of practical training because experience had shown "that the personal encounter with the patients has a high educational value."[61] Nonetheless, they were forced to adapt their training practices to the government guidelines.

Finally, during the 1950s, the work and life model of the deaconess completely lost its justification in Sweden. After fierce internal debates within the association, the *Swedish Society of Nursing* had been expanded during the 1930s into a union that was in favour of organising the profession in accordance with labour and wage laws.[62] The fact that in 1945 a total of 94 percent of nursing staff were organised in a union is evidence of the high acceptance of professionalised nursing care in Sweden.[63] In 1957, a third of all nurses were married. The Swedish institution for deaconesses responded by substantially reforming its structures in the 1960s. Celibacy was abolished. From now on, the sisters could choose their area of work for themselves and enter their own employment agreements.[64] The institution for deaconesses in Sweden said a final farewell to the motherhouse system it had adopted from Germany – a path the motherhouse in Philadelphia had already taken in the 1950s.[65]

---

57 Cf. Markkola (2000), pp. 113–114.
58 Cf. Holmdahl (1994), p. 193.
59 Cf. Iversson (1988), p. 155.
60 Kungl. Medicinalstylrelsens cirkulär med föreskrifter och anvisningar rörande undervisningen vid godkände sjuksköterskeskolor, 11/11/1952, Ersta archives, F 8/11.
61 Bethanienstiftelsens styrelse till kungliga Medicinalstyrelsen, 30/07/1948, Ersta archives, F 8/19.
62 The communal employers recognised the *Swedish Society of Nursing* as social partners in 1940, cf. Bohm (1972), p. 198.
63 Cf. Bohm (1972), p. 213.
64 Cf. Green (2011), pp. 75, 170.
65 Compare the article by Doris Riemann in this volume.

Conclusion

The history of the deaconesses serves as a perfect lens for the transnational history of nursing, medicine, the Church, gender, and the welfare state. Deaconesses worked in many countries, albeit with varying degrees of success. While the Swedish deaconesses played a significant role in the nineteenth century in setting up qualified training and expanding social institutions throughout the country, the life and work model of the deaconess found little support in the US and the deaconess motherhouses remained in a minority.

In both countries, the deaconesses referred to the German tradition. However, they had to adapt it to the specific local context. This history of nursing training illustrates that the US American deaconesses came under intense pressure to professionalise comparatively early on. If they wanted to stand a chance in the US they had to be open to a more scientifically oriented understanding of nursing. Theoretical training was already quite important in the American motherhouse at the beginning of the twentieth century. Overall, we can note that the deaconesses from the American motherhouse were willing to follow the new scientific trends. The Swedish deaconesses followed this course a little later and more noticeably during the 1930s. In contrast, German deaconesses were opposed to a scientific approach in nursing for a long time – not because the nurses were 'backward' but because they prioritised a different type of knowledge based on learning from experience and providing an ethical education. This comparison shows that the idea of 'good' nursing and its implementation in reality varies significantly, both historically and culturally.

The comparison of the motherhouses furthermore reveals that professionalisation did not automatically lead to an increased autonomy of the members of groups that became more professional. The policy-motivated accreditation process in the US significantly restricted freedom in training practice. In Sweden it was mainly the state that increased the pressure to professionalise during the 1930s and interfered with training practice. In contrast, the deaconesses of the *Henriettenstiftung* were able to maintain a much greater degree of independence and insisted on keeping their own tradition for a much longer period of time. Until the 1960s, the deaconesses in West Germany were largely able to train their students as they saw fit. This meant they felt the changes of the 1960s even more drastically when the deaconesses slowly became a minority within their own organisation.

Bibliography

Literature

Andersson, Åsa: Ett högt och ädelt kall. Kalltankens betydelse för sjuksköterskeyrkets formering 1850–1930. Umeå 2002.

Arnstorf, Verwaltungsleiter des Annastifts: Bericht über die Durchführung der Arbeitszeitverkürzung im Annastift [Report on implementing a shortening of the working hours at the Annastift]. In: Die evangelische Krankenpflege 7 (1957), pp. 52–55.

Ausbildungs- und Prüfungsordnung für Krankenschwestern, Krankenpfleger und Kinderkrankenschwestern 02/08/1966 [Training and examination regulations for male and female nurses and paediatric nurses]. In: Bundesministerium für Justiz (ed.): Bundesgesetzblatt (1966), Part I, Bonn, pp. 362–365.

Bohm, Eva: Okänd, godkänd, legitimerad. Svensk Sjuksköterskeföreningens fösta 50 År. Stockholm 1972.

Christiansson, Elisabeth: Kyrklig och social reform. Motiveringar till diakoni 1845–1965. Skellefteå 2006.

Doyle, Ann: Nursing by religious orders in the United States. Part IV: Lutheran deaconesses, 1849–1928. In: American Journal of Nursing 29 (1929), pp. 1197–1207.

Emanuelsson, Agneta: Pionjärer i vitt. Professionella och fackliga strategier bland svenska sjuksköterskor och sjukvårdsbiträden, 1851–1939. Huddinge 1990.

Frese, Matthias; Paulus, Julia; Teppe, Karl (ed.): Demokratisierung und gesellschaftlicher Aufbruch. Die sechziger Jahre als Wendezeit der Bundesrepublik. Paderborn u. a. 2003.

Göckenjan, Gerd; Dreßke, Stefan: Seelsorge im Krankenhaus. Zeit haben von Berufs wegen. In: Bollinger, Heinrich; Gerlach, Anke; Pfadenhauer, Michaela (ed.): Gesundheitsberufe im Wandel. Soziologische Beobachtungen und Interpretationen. Frankfurt/Main 2005, pp. 239–262.

Green, Todd H.: Responding to secularization. The deaconess movement in nineteenth-century Sweden. Leiden; Boston 2011.

Herbert, Ulrich (ed.): Wandlungsprozesse in Westdeutschland. Belastung, Integration, Liberalisierung, 1945–1980. Göttingen 2007.

Holmdahl, Barbro: Sjuksköterskans historia. Från siukwakterska till omvårdnadsdoktor. Stockholm 1994.

Iverson, Yngve: Tro verksamhet i kärlek. En bok om Ersta. Stockholm 1988.

Kaiser, Jochen-Christoph: Evangelische Kirche und sozialer Staat. Diakonie im 19. und 20. Jahrhundert. Stuttgart 2008.

Kaminsky, Uwe: Zwangssterilisation und "Euthanasie" im Rheinland. Evangelische Erziehungsanstalten sowie Heil- und Pflegeanstalten 1933 bis 1945. Köln 1995.

Kaufmann, Christopher: Ministry and meaning. A religious history of Catholic health care in the United States. New York 1995.

Koeneke, Sister Marie (ed.): The Lankenau Hospital. Nursing procedures. Philadelphia 1927.

Köser, Silke: Denn eine Diakonisse darf kein Alltagsmensch sein. Kollektive Identitäten Kaiserswerther Diakonissen 1836–1914. Leipzig 2006.

Koivunen Bylund, Tuulikki: Frukta icke, allenast tro. Ebba Boström och Samariterhemmet 1882–1902. Stockholm 1994.

Kolbe, Wiebke: Elternschaft im Wohlfahrtsstaat. Schweden und die Bundesrepublik im Vergleich 1945–2000. Frankfurt/Main; New York 2002.

Kreutzer, Susanne: Vom "Liebesdienst" zum modernen Frauenberuf. Die Reform der Krankenpflege nach 1945. Frankfurt/Main; New York 2005.

Kreutzer, Susanne: Aus der Praxis lernen? Umbruch in den pflegerischen Ausbildungskonzepten nach 1945. In: Medizin, Gesellschaft und Geschichte. Jahrbuch des Instituts für Geschichte der Medizin der Robert Bosch Stiftung 25 (2006), pp. 155–180.

Kreutzer, Susanne: Arbeits- und Lebensalltag evangelischer Krankenpflege. Organisation, soziale Praxis und biographische Erfahrungen. Göttingen 2014.

Krukemeyer, Hartmut: Entwicklung des Krankenhauswesens und seiner Strukturen in der Bundesrepublik Deutschland. Analyse und Bewertung unter Berücksichtigung der gesamtwirtschaftlichen Rahmenbedingungen und der gesundheitlichen Interventionen. Bremen 1988.

Lauterer, Heide-Marie: Liebestätigkeit für die Volksgemeinschaft. Der Kaiserswerther Verband deutscher Diakonissenmutterhäuser in den ersten Jahren des NS-Regimes. Göttingen 1994.

Lynaugh, Joan: Nursing the great society. The impact of the Nurse Training Act of 1964. In: Nursing History Review 16 (2008), pp. 13–28.

Mann Wall, Barbra: Unlikely entrepreneurs. Catholic sisters and the hospital marketplace, 1865–1925. Columbus 2005.

Mann Wall, Barbra: American Catholic hospitals. A century of changing markets and missions. New Brunswick; New Jersey; London 2011.

Markkola, Pirjo: Promoting faith and welfare. The deaconess movement in Finland and Sweden, 1850–1930. In: Scandinavian Journal of History 25 (2000), pp. 101–118.

Markkola, Pirjo: Women's spirituality, lived religion, and social reform in Finland, 1860–1920. In: Perichoresis 9 (2011), pp. 143–182.

Nelson, Sioban: Say little, do much. Nursing, nuns, and hospitals in the nineteenth Century. Philadelphia 2003.

Nicklasson, Stina: Sophiasystern som blev politiker: Bertha Wellin. Pionjär för moderat politik. Stockholm 1995.

Schildt, Axel: Die Sozialgeschichte der Bundesrepublik Deutschland bis 1989/90. München 2007.

Schmuhl, Hans-Walter: Der Neubeginn sozialer Staatlichkeit nach 1945. In: Kaiser, Jochen-Christoph; Scheepers, Rajah (ed.): Dienerinnen des Herrn. Beiträge zur weiblichen Diakonie im 19. und 20. Jahrhundert. Leipzig 2010, pp. 148–163.

Schweikardt, Christoph: Die Entwicklung der Krankenpflege zur staatlich anerkannten Tätigkeit im 19. und frühen 20. Jahrhundert. Das Zusammenwirken von Modernisierungsbestrebungen, ärztlicher Dominanz, konfessioneller Selbstbehauptung und Vorgaben preußischer Regierungspolitik. München 2008.

Schweikardt, Christoph: The introduction of deaconess nurses at the German Hospital of the City of Philadelphia in the 1880s. In: Nursing History Review 18 (2010), pp. 29–50.

Steppe, Hilde (ed.): Krankenpflege im Nationalsozialismus. Frankfurt/Main 2001.

Stevens, Rosemary: In sickness and in wealth. American hospitals in the twentieth century. Baltimore; London 1999.

Weiser, Frederik: Serving love. Chapters in the early history of the diaconate in American Lutheranism. Pennsylvania 1960.

West, Roberta: History of nursing in Pennsylvania. Pennsylvania 1939.

Zerull, Lisa: Nursing out of the parish. A history of the Baltimore Lutheran Deaconesses 1893–1911. Virginia 2010.

Archives

Archive of the Barbara Bates Center for the Study of the History of Nursing, School of Nursing, University of Pennsylvania (Bates Center Archives)

MC 98 Lankenau Hospital School of Nursing Records, 1871–1992
- Series I: Lankenau Hospital, 1895–1992
- Series III: School of Nursing, 1901–1992
- Series IV: Commitee records, 1955–1992

Archive of the Ersta deaconess institution (Ersta archives)

F 8/11 Education/School of Nursing

Archive of the Evangelical Lutheran Church in America (ELCA-Archives)
ULCA 2/1 United Lutheran Church in America Convention Minutes
Archive of the Henriettenstiftung
– S-4 Kaiserswerth Association
– S-8 Motherhouse
– S-9 Foundation
Lankenau Hospital archives
Minutes of the Nursing Committee of the Board of Trustees

List of Authors

Annett Büttner, Dr.
Archiv der Fliedner Kulturstiftung Kaiserswerth (Archives of the
Fliedner Cultural Foundation Kaiserswerth), Zeppenheimer Weg 20,
D-40489 Düsseldorf
buettner@fliedner-kulturstiftung.de

Susanne Malchau Dietz, PhD, MSc (Nursing), RN
Nurse Historian, Nordre Fasanvej 78, 4.th, DK-2000 Frederiksberg, Denmark
s-malchau@mail.tele.dk

Matthias Honold, M. A.
Zentralarchiv der Diakonie Neuendettelsau, Wilhelm-Löhe-Straße 23,
D-91564 Neuendettelsau
Matthias.Honold@diakonieneuendettelsau.de

Uwe Kaminsky, Dr.
Evangelisch-theologische Fakultät, Christliche Gesellschaftslehre,
Ruhr-Universität Bochum, Universitätsstr. 150, D-44801 Bochum
dr.uk@web.de

Susanne Kreutzer, Prof. Dr.
Muenster University of Applied Sciences, Muenster School of Health,
Leonardo-Campus 8, D-48149 Münster
kreutzer@fh-muenster.de

Carmen M. Mangion, Dr.
Department of History, Classics and Archaeology, Birkbeck,
University of London, Malet Street, London WC1E 7HX
c.mangion@bbk.ac.uk

Pirjo Markkola, Prof. Dr.
School of Social Sciences and Humanities, University of Tampere,
FI-33014 Tampereen yliopisto
pirjo.markkola@uta.fi

Karen Nolte, PD Dr.
Institut für Geschichte der Medizin (Institute for the History of Medicine),
University of Wuerzburg, Oberer Neubergweg 10a, D-97074 Wuerzburg
Karen.nolte@uni-wuerzburg.de

Doris Riemann, Dr.
Kirchstraße 12, D-29308 Winsen (Aller)
Doris.Riemann@gmx.de

Ruth Wexler
12, Halamedhei St., Jerusalem 9366112
ruth.wexler@gmail.com

MEDIZIN, GESELLSCHAFT UND GESCHICHTE — BEIHEFTE

Herausgegeben von Robert Jütte.

Franz Steiner Verlag   ISSN 0941–5033